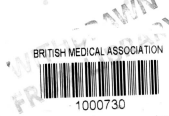

Frontiers of Hormone Research

Vol. 45

Series Editor

Ezio Ghigo Turin

Co-Editors

Federica Guaraldi Turin
Andrea Benso Turin

Imaging in Endocrine Disorders

Volume Editors

Michael Buchfelder Erlangen
Federica Guaraldi Turin

141 figures, 33 in color, and 9 tables, 2016

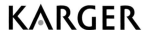

Basel · Freiburg · Paris · London · New York · Chennai · New Delhi ·
Bangkok · Beijing · Shanghai · Tokyo · Kuala Lumpur · Singapore · Sydney

Frontiers of Hormone Research

Founded 1972 by Tj.B. van Wimersma Greidanus, Utrecht
Continued by Ashley B. Grossman, Oxford (1996–2013)

Michael Buchfelder, MD, PhD
Department of Neurosurgery
University of Erlangen-Nürnberg
Erlangen, Germany

Federica Guaraldi, MD, PhD
Division of Endocrinology, Diabetes and Metabolism
Department of Medical Sciences
University of Turin
Turin, Italy

Library of Congress Cataloging-in-Publication Data

Names: Buchfelder, Michael, editor. | Guaraldi, Federica, editor.
Title: Imaging in endocrine disorders / volume editors, Michael Buchfelder,
  Federica Guaraldi.
Other titles: Frontiers of hormone research ; v. 45. 0301-3073
Description: Basel ; New York : Karger, 2016. | Series: Frontiers of hormone
  research, ISSN 0301-3073 ; vol. 45 | Includes bibliographical references
  and index.
Identifiers: LCCN 2016004459| ISBN 9783318027372 (hard cover : alk. paper) |
  ISBN 9783318027389 (electronic version)
Subjects: | MESH: Endocrine System Diseases--diagnosis | Diagnostic
  Imaging--methods
Classification: LCC RC649 | NLM WK 140 | DDC 616.4/075--dc23 LC record available at http://lccn.loc.gov/2016004459

Bibliographic Indices. This publication is listed in bibliographic services, including Current Contents® and PubMed/MEDLINE.

© Copyright 2016 by S. Karger AG, P.O. Box, CH-4009 Basel (Switzerland)
www.karger.com
Printed in Germany on acid-free and non-aging paper (ISO 9706) by Kraft Druck GmbH, Ettlingen
ISSN 0301–3073
e-ISSN 1662–3762
ISBN 978–3–318–02737–2
e-ISBN 978–3–318–02738–9

Contents

Online supplementary material: www.karger.com/book/toc/271322

Preface

The suspicion of an endocrine disorder is based on the patient's history, clinical signs and the phenotypic appearance. However, the exact scientific diagnosis is then usually confirmed by laboratory hormonal measurements or imaging, and sometimes by both modalities. Both of these technologies have undergone revolutionary changes during the last decades. Direct depiction of anatomical and pathological structures has been possible since the introduction of computed tomography (CT) and magnetic resonance imaging (MRI) scanning.

'Imaging' is considered to be the depiction of structures or functions without the particular use of visible light. Metabolic imaging using radionucleotides, CT and MRI are in this context the main investigational tools used today.

In this multiauthor book, distinguished experts, who have published extensively in their fields, have contributed concise and well-illustrated chapters that cover imaging of all the organs that are involved in endocrine disorders. Metabolic and structured imaging of the thyroid and parathyroid glands, the pancreas, the adrenals, the gonads, the pituitary and sellar region, and neuroendocrine tumors and involved tissues are thoroughly covered. Both benign and malignant diseases are covered in detail. A specific asset of this book is the provision of readers with online-accessible videos of some dynamic diagnostic and therapeutic procedures.

This volume has been conceived to primarily address endocrinologists, who have to interpret the results of the examinations obtained by the various imaging techniques, radiologists and nuclear physicians, who should correlate images to the respective endocrinological background information. At the same time, it represents a valuable reference for internists and general practitioners to appropriately manage the essential diagnostic workup in patients with suspected endocrine disorders, before referring them to the specialist.

We are very grateful to the authors for their dedication, and to Professor Carlo Monti, Director of the Service of Radiology, Casa di Cura Madre Fortunata Toniolo, Bologna, Italy, for his precious support in the selection and labeling of radiological images and for expert manuscript revision. Our special thanks go to Miriam Schulz, Rebecca Ganz and Thomas Nold at Karger Publishers in Basel, Switzerland, for their generous support through all stages of the production of this book.

Michael Buchfelder, Erlangen
Federica Guaraldi, Turin
Ezio Ghigo, Turin

Buchfelder M, Guaraldi F (eds): Imaging in Endocrine Disorders.
Front Horm Res. Basel, Karger, 2016, vol 45, pp 1–15 (DOI: 10.1159/000442273)

Sonography of Normal and Abnormal Thyroid and Parathyroid Glands

Massimiliano Andrioli[a] · Roberto Valcavi[b]

[a]EndocrinologiaOggi, Centro Medico, Rome, and [b]Poliambulatorio Privato, Centro Palmer, Reggio Emilia, Italy

Abstract

Ultrasonography (US) represents the most sensitive and efficient method for the evaluation of the thyroid and parathyroid glands. Infectious and autoimmune thyroiditis are common diseases, usually diagnosed and followed up by clinical examination and laboratory analyses. Nevertheless, US plays an important role in confirming diagnoses, predicting outcomes and, in autoimmune hyperthyroidism, in titrating therapy. Conversely, in nodular thyroid disease US is the imaging method of choice for the characterization and surveillance of lesions. It provides consistent clues in predicting the risk of malignancy, thus directing patient referral for fine-needle aspiration (FNA) biopsy. Suspicious US features generally include marked hypoechogenicity, a shape taller than it is wide, ill-defined or irregular borders, microcalcifications and hardness at elastographic evaluation. Finally, the role of US in thyroid cancer is to evaluate extension beyond the thyroid capsule and to assess nodal metastases or tumor recurrence. The main application of US in parathyroid diseases is represented by primary hyperparathyroidism. In this condition, US plays a role after biochemical diagnosis, and it should always be strictly performed for localization purposes. In both thyroidal and parathyroid diseases, US is recommended as a guide in FNA biopsies.

© 2016 S. Karger AG, Basel

The thyroid and parathyroid are endocrine glands located in the neck. For their superficial position, ultrasonography (US) represents the most sensitive and cost-efficient method for their evaluation, providing accurate information about size, shape and texture. Besides these glands, an accurate ultrasonographic examination of the neck should always include the salivary glands, lymph nodes and any possible abnormal neck mass. For an optimal US evaluation, the patient should be scanned in the supine position with the neck mildly hyperextended, using a 10–14 MHz linear probe. US equipment may need to be adjusted to operate at the optimal frequency, balancing resolution and beam penetration. Deep targets should be evaluated with lower frequencies (5.0–7.5 MHz) or using convex transducers. However, the lower portions of thyroid lobes in the case of large mediastinal goiters or ectopic parathyroids may be hidden to US assessment. Despite these limits, US remains the first-line technique for the evaluation of normal and abnormal thyroid and parathyroid glands.

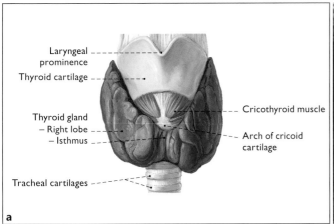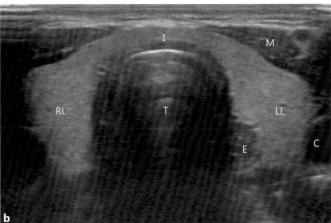

Fig. 1. Anatomic illustration (**a**) and ultrasonographic appearance (transverse scan, **b**) of the normal thyroid gland. At US evaluation (**b**), thyroid parenchyma is homogeneous, bright and slightly hyperechoic with respect to the surrounding muscles. C = Common carotid artery; E = esophagus; I = isthmus; LL = left lobe; M = muscles; RL = right lobe; T = trachea. **a** Reproduced with permission from Köpf-Maier [37].

Thyroid Ultrasonography

Normal Anatomy

The thyroid resides in the midline of the lower neck. The gland is composed of a right and a left lobe, typically interconnected by an isthmus, lying anterolateral to the larynx and trachea at approximately the level of the second and third tracheal rings. The gland is bordered laterally by the common carotid arteries and sternocleidomastoid muscles, anterolaterally by the jugular veins, anteriorly by strap muscles and posteriorly by the longus colli muscles. The recurrent laryngeal nerve runs along the inferior thyroid artery, but it is not usually visible at US. The thyroid is attached to the larynx and trachea and, therefore, moves with the larynx during swallowing (fig. 1a).

The ultrasound appearance of a healthy thyroid parenchyma is usually homogeneous, bright and slightly hyperechoic with respect to the surrounding muscles (fig. 1b). Thyroid US also provides adjunctive information about the thyroid size, shape and texture.

Thyroid Anomalies

US is useful in detecting thyroid anomalies due to embryologic disorders, such as hemiagenesis or presence of aberrant thyroid tissue along the midline. In thyroid hemiagenesis the left lobe is the most commonly absent, with the right lobe and isthmus in the right place. The isthmus, instead, is lacking more frequently in the rarer cases of right lobe hemiagenesis. Ectopic thyroid tissue can be found anywhere along the normal path of thyroid descent, but is most commonly found at the base of the tongue (lingual thyroid). Aberrant thymic and parathyroid tissues within the thyroid gland, although extremely rare, can also be detected by US. The latter are usually hypoechoic, without significant internal vascularity on US and can easily be mistaken for thyroid nodules. Finally, US is helpful in evaluating thyroglossal duct cysts, which are usually medial, from brachial cysts, mostly placed more laterally in the neck.

Thyroiditis

The inflammation of the thyroid, i.e. thyroiditis, causes follicular changes in its parenchyma, resulting in the gland losing its uniform and bright ultrasonographic appearance. The various types of thyroiditis usually present specific ultrasonographic features.

Acute Thyroiditis

The thyroid gland is generally resistant to acute infection due to its high blood flow, iodine content, excellent lymphatic drainage and protective capsule. Therefore, acute suppurative thyroiditis, predominantly caused by Gram-positive aerobes, is rare. There is no gender predisposition and the majority of patients have an underlying thyroid disorder, such as goiter, chronic thyroiditis or a history of di-

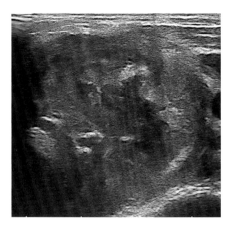

Fig. 2. Ill-defined, hyperechoic, heterogeneous abscess in the left thyroid lobe in the context of thyroiditis. Transverse scan.

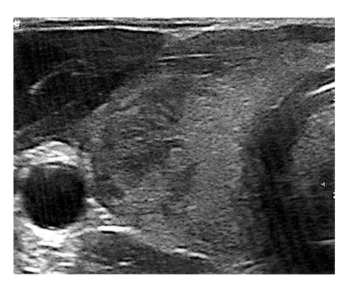

Fig. 3. Ultrasonographic appearance of subacute thyroiditis. Focal hypoechoic areas with ill-defined margins in the right lobe can be identified. This feature may change during follow-up. Transverse scan.

rect thyroid trauma. The clinical presentation varies depending on the route of spread, type of organism and the immunocompetence of the host, but there is typically a warm, firm mass in the anterior neck that is mobile with swallowing and painful to palpation. There may be fever, dysphagia, dysphonia, hoarseness and palpable cervical adenopathy. On US imaging, the thyroid gland may be regionally or diffusely edematous. US usually demonstrates a gland with diffusely decreased echogenicity, sometimes bearing a focal abscess [1]. Abscesses are ill-defined hypoechoic, heterogeneous masses with internal debris and bright echoes from gas (fig. 2). In this context, US may also be useful in providing guidance for diagnostic or therapeutic aspiration.

Subacute Thyroiditis
Subacute granulomatous de Quervain thyroiditis is a transient, self-limited, inflammatory disorder of the thyroid gland of viral origin, representing the most common cause of a painful thyroid mass. It presents with rapid onset of thyroid tenderness, neck pain, generalized malaise, low-grade fever and occasional dysphagia, often with a history of preceding viral upper respiratory tract infection. One or both thyroid lobes may be involved and the gland may be enlarged [2]. The typical sonographic findings are focal patchy areas of marked hypoecogenicity, which may elongate along the long-axis of the gland. They may be unilateral, bilateral or migrate over time. The involved parenchyma may appear

quite hypoechoic on US, with ill-defined margins, sometimes mimicking carcinoma (fig. 3). Ultrasonographic follow-up and possibly fine-needle aspiration (FNA) biopsy may be necessary to achieve the proper diagnosis.

Tuberculous Thyroiditis
Tuberculosis involving the thyroid gland is extremely rare in developed countries. Although different ultrasonographic patterns have been described, the most common clinical presentation is a solitary thyroid mass that may be visible on US as a round heterogeneously hypoechoic nodule or as an anechoic lesion (abscess) with internal echoes and ill-defined irregular borders [3]. Inflammatory changes usually produce obscuration of the surrounding tissues and fat planes.

Hashimoto's Thyroiditis
Hashimoto's lymphocytic thyroiditis (HT) is the most common cause of hypothyroidism in developed countries (prevalence 1–1.5 cases/1,000 people). It occurs predominantly in women (F:M = 20:1) and in patients with other autoimmune disorders. It is characterized by autoimmunity to thyroid antigens causing lymphocytic infiltration and fibrosis, sometimes resulting in glandular enlargement. In the early stages of the disease, the patient may be euthyroid, but as thyroid parenchyma becomes increasingly replaced by fibrous tissue, hypothyroidism ensues. Both benign and malignant nodules, including lymphoma, may be present in this setting.

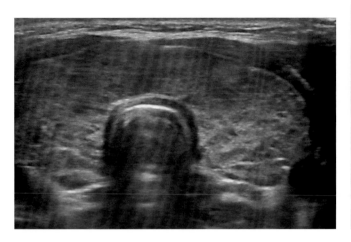

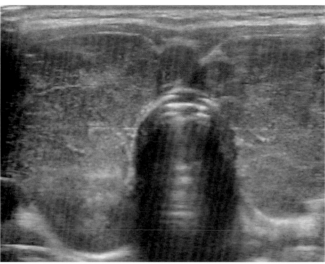

Fig. 4. Ultrasonographic appearance of autoimmune thyroiditis. The thyroid gland appears enlarged, predominantly hyperechoic and diffusely heterogeneous. The parenchyma presents an irregular echotexture, with poorly defined hyperechoic regions separated by fibrous strands ('Swiss cheese' or 'honeycomb' pattern). Transverse scan.

Fig. 5. Ultrasonographic appearance of GD. The thyroid gland is typically enlarged, diffusely heterogeneous and hyperechoic. Transverse scan.

The sonographic appearance of HT varies depending on the length and severity of the disease. Generally, thyroid echogenicity decreases as lymphocyte infiltration progresses, approaching and sometimes exceeding that of the surrounding strap muscles. With mild disease the gland may appear normal or slightly decreased in size, irregular and only mildly hypoechoic. With more advanced disease the gland may be enlarged and diffusely heterogeneous, but predominantly hypoechoic (online suppl. video 1; for all online suppl. material, see www.karger.com/doi/10.1159/000442273). The parenchyma may have an irregular echotexture, with poorly defined hypoechoic regions separated by fibrous strands simulating a multinodular goiter (fig. 4). When treated with levothyroxine, in the late stages, the gland may be very small, heterogeneous and hypoechoic.

In summary, reflecting the histopathologic features and the dynamic nature of chronic inflammatory disease, a variety of ultrasonographic patterns can be observed in HT: (a) hypoechoic and heterogeneous, in cases of mild and diffuse lymphocytic infiltration; (b) pseudomicronodular, in cases of more discrete areas of lymphocytic infiltration, forming localized hypoechoic pseudonodules (usually subcentimetric) and with the same appearance, which may vary over time – this pattern is also called 'Swiss cheese' or 'honeycomb' if very little fibrotic parenchyma separates the hy-

poechoic pseudonodules; (c) pseudomacronodular, when the pesudonodules are larger; (d) markedly hypoechoic when the ultrasonographic thyroid appearance is homogeneous and profoundly hypoechoic (usually in cases of the parenchyma completely replaced by lymphocytes); (e) fibrous when the fibrosis development generates hyperechoic bands separating the typical hypoechoic tissue; (f) hyperechoic and heterogeneous when, in the late stage of the disease, the fibrosis is diffuse and the thyroid may appear hyperechoic, and (g) speckled (very rare) with numerous punctate densities scattered throughout the parenchyma, often challenging the differential diagnosis with diffuse sclerosing papillary carcinoma [4, 5].

The vascularity of HT is variable, ranging from avascular to hypervascular. The possibility of malignancy in thyroiditis should be considered in case of atypical large pseudonodules, especially if calcifications, infiltrative margins or cervical lymphadenopathy are present.

Enlarged lymph nodes with reactivity features are almost invariably present in HT. The prominent nodes are in the paratracheal and pretracheal space (level VI), and near the isthmus. Lymph nodes in level VI tend to appear rounded, with a variable presence of a hilum.

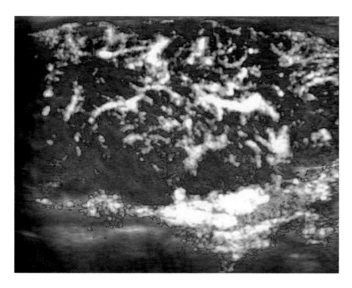

Fig. 6. Power Doppler evaluation of GD. The enlarged thyroid gland typically presents a markedly increased vascularity appearing as increased color flow throughout the thyroid parenchyma ('thyroid inferno'). Longitudinal scan.

Graves' Disease

Graves' disease (GD) is a common cause of hyperthyroidism, with a higher prevalence in women (F:M = 5:1). It is characterized by thyromegaly, hyperthyroidism and, in some patients, orbitopathy. Autoantibodies stimulating the TSH receptor cause the thyroid gland to grow, become more vascular and increase its hormone production. GD and HT probably represent the same autoimmune disease at different ends of the spectrum. In fact transition between the two forms may occur, complicating their ultrasonographic differential diagnosis. Their ultrasonographic appearances are also often similar, with both potentially presenting with a hypoechoic and heterogeneous echotexture. On grayscale examination, the thyroid gland in GD is typically enlarged and diffusely hypoechoic [6] (fig. 5). The initial hypoechogenicity of the gland is associated with TSH receptor positivity and patients with hypoechoic glands at presentation are more likely to relapse after medical therapy [6]. The echotexture is usually inhomogeneous and may demonstrate numerous small hypoechoic foci (2–3 mm in size), but its heterogeneity is usually less than that seen in HT. Moreover, the hypoechogenicity is not as pronounced and in some cases the thyroid gland may tend to be hyperechoic.

In GD, the thyroid gland typically shows marked hypervascularity. On US, this is seen qualitatively as an increase in color flow throughout the thyroid parenchyma, referred to as a 'thyroid inferno' (fig. 6). Nevertheless, there can be some crossover between the vascular appearances of GD and HT, since both entities may sometimes present clearly increased parenchymal blood flow [7, 8]. A more quantitative assessment of thyroid blood flow, such as the peak systolic velocity obtained in the infrathyroidal artery, usually markedly increased in GD, may be helpful in making a differential diagnosis [7, 8]. Nevertheless, findings on both grayscale and color-Doppler US may vary considerably depending on the course of the disease: patients who are acutely hyperthyroidal have larger glands and more prominent vascularity than those observed in remising patients.

Painless Thyroiditis

Painless thyroiditis includes both silent and postpartum thyroiditis. Silent thyroiditis is considered an autoimmune process, with autoantibody titers lower than in HT. When it presents within 1 year after delivery it is termed postpartum thyroiditis. Ultrasound evaluation shows hypoechogenicity similar to other forms of autoimmune thyroid diseases, but with less fibrosis and hypoechogenicity.

Riedel's Thyroiditis

Riedel's ligneous thyroiditis is an extremely rare chronic inflammatory thyroid disease. It is believed to be a primary autoimmune disease and it can occur as an isolated disorder or as part of a multifocal fibrosclerosis syndrome. It is characterized by the replacement of normal parenchyma by dense fibrosis, extension beyond the thyroid capsule and, sometimes, invasion of adjacent structures of the neck. The gland is enlarged, firm and attached to contiguous structures. Riedel thyroiditis is usually associated with hypothyroidism, hypoparathyroidism, compression of adjacent structures and invasion of bordering muscles and mediastinum. The limited data available from the literature on the ultrasonographic appearance of this disease report an enlarged diffusely hypoechoic gland with fibrous septations and hypovascularity. In contrast to HT, there may be carotid artery encasement.

Granulomatous Thyroiditis

Although granulomatous lesions can be detected in subacute thyroiditis, and more rarely in HT, the main granulomatous thyroiditis are sarcoidosis, Wegener's granulomatosis and Langerhans cell histiocytosis. In these very rare conditions, the thyroid usually appears hypoechoic and inhomogeneous on US and, sometimes, especially in cases of Langerhans cell histiocytosis, may be enlarged.

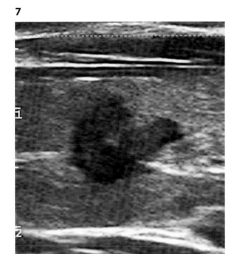
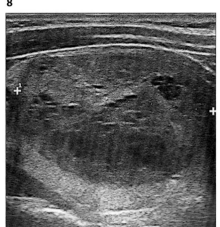

Fig. 7. Ultrasonographic appearance of a papillary thyroid carcinoma presenting an irregular shape and irregular speculated margins. Longitudinal scan.

Fig. 8. Ultrasonographic appearance of a thyroid nodule presenting as an oval hypoechoic lesion almost entirely occupying the thyroid lobe, finely heterogeneous for some spongiform features, presenting well-defined and regular margins. Longitudinal scan.

Nodular Diseases

A thyroid nodule is defined as a discrete lesion within the thyroid gland that is ultrasonographically distinct from the surrounding thyroid parenchyma. It can be unique or associated with other lesions. Nodular thyroid disease is a common finding, especially in females and in the elderly population. Thyroid nodules are found in 5% of the general population with the use of palpation, but high-resolution US allows their detections in up to 67% of subjects [9]. Malignancy comprises approximately 5% of all thyroid nodules [10] but its incidence has been increasing around the world in recent years.

According to the AACE/AME/ETA (American Association of Clinical Endocrinologists/Associazione Medici Endocrinologi/European Thyroid Association) and ATA (American Thyroid Association) guidelines, it is suggested to perform US in any palpable nodule with the aim of sonographically confirming a nodule corresponding to the palpable abnormality, detecting additional nonpalpable lesions, identifying the sonographic characteristics of the lesions and guiding FNA. When a physical examination is conducted instead, US should be performed only in case of a prior history of head/neck irradiation or familiar history of thyroid cancer.

It is the general opinion that US is the imaging method of choice for the characterization of thyroid nodules and surveillance of multinodular goiter [11]. US evaluation of nodular features may provide consistent clues for predicting the probability of malignancy, thus directing patient referral for FNA biopsy. Therefore, an adequate US examination should always document the position, extracapsular relationships, number of lesions and the following characteristics: shape, internal content, echogenicity, echotexture, presence of calcifications, margins, vascularity and size [12].

Any thyroid lesion can be described as approximately located in either the superior third, the medium third, the inferior third or in the isthmus. Thyroid nodules are seldom located in the pyramidal lobe, and very rarely they can be ectopic.

US may evaluate extracapsular relationships, detecting possible deformation or infiltration of the hyperechoic thyroid capsule and the invasion of adjacent structures. Based on their ultrasonographic shape, nodules can be classified as: ovoid (anteroposterior diameter less than transverse diameter), round (anteroposterior diameter equal to transverse diameter), taller-than-wide (anteroposterior diameter longer than transverse diameter) or irregular (neither ovoid/round nor taller-than-wide). A taller-than-wide shape is reported to be more frequently associated with thyroid malignancy [13, 14]. Malignant lesions often present an irregular shape (fig. 7), but this can also be noticed in some benign lesions [15].

On the basis of internal content, thyroid nodules can be: solid (liquid portion ≤10% of the nodule volume), mixed predominantly solid (liquid portion >10% but ≤50% of the nodule volume), mixed predominantly cystic (liquid portion >50% but ≤90% of the nodule volume), cystic (liquid portion >90% of the nodule volume) and spongiform (>50% of the nodule volume characterized by aggregation of multiple microcystic areas separated by thin septations that are interspersed within solid tissue; fig. 8). Cystic nodules can

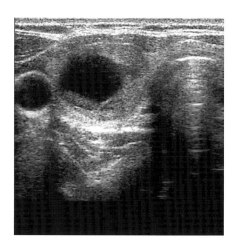

Fig. 9. Ultrasonographic appearance of a papillary thyroid carcinoma presenting as a cystic lesion with a thick parenchymal wall in the right lobe. Transverse scan.

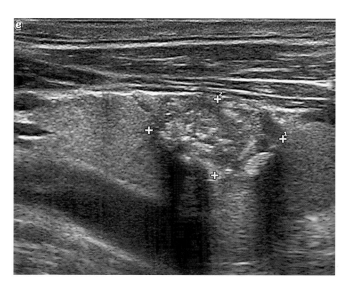

Fig. 10. Inhomogeneous benign thyroid nodule with coarse calcifications. Longitudinal scan.

be pure cysts (without internal septa) that are almost always benign, or polyconcamerated cysts (one or more internal septae) or cysts with thick walls that, instead, may harbor a risk of malignancy (fig. 9) [16].

Based on US echogenicity, a thyroid lesion can be markedly hypoechoic (nodule hypoechoic relative to the adjacent strap muscles), hypoechoic (nodule hypoechoic relative to the thyroid parenchyma), isoechoic (nodule with the same echogenicity of the thyroid parenchyma), hyperechoic (nodule more echoic than thyroid parenchyma) or anechoic (in cystic lesions with fluid content with through transmission of sound waves). Marked hypoechogenicity seems to be highly specific for malignant nodules [17].

Based on their echotexture, nodules can be homogeneous, finely inhomogeneous or markedly inhomogeneous. Nevertheless, the nodule echotexture plays a marginal role in a differential diagnosis between benignant and malignant lesions.

Calcifications are features detectable by US in up to a third of both benign and malignant thyroid nodules. They are defined as prominent echogenic foci, with or without posterior shadowing, and can be microcalcifications (<1 mm, intranodular punctate hyperechoic spots without posterior acoustic shadowing), macrocalcifications (coarse and large calcifications >1 mm causing posterior acoustic shadowing; fig. 10) or peripheral rim/eggshell calcifications (peripheral eggshell calcifications surrounding the nodule).

Microcalcifications are thought to represent the calcified psammoma bodies of papillary thyroid cancer (PTC) and are highly specific for thyroid cancer. Eggshell calcifications should be evaluated for interruption as calcification breaches may be suspicious for malignancy. Macrocalcifications, instead, may also occur in 'old' degenerating benign nodules.

The margins of thyroid nodules may be well defined (clear demarcation with normal thyroid tissue) or ill defined (lack of clear demarcation with normal thyroid parenchyma), regular (without irregularities and imperfections) or irregular (with edges and irregularities). The latter can be further divided into spiculated (one or more spiculations on the surface; fig. 7) and microlobulated (one or more smooth lobules on the surface; fig. 11). Poorly defined and irregular, both spiculated and microlobulated margins are usually reported to be suggestive of malignancy [15, 17, 18]. US can also evaluate the presence of the halo sign, a hypoanechoic ring that may, completely or incompletely, surround a nodule. Unlike an irregular thick halo (fig. 12), a thin regular halo, especially if accompanied by peripheral vascularity on power Doppler, is a finding usually suggestive of a benign lesion.

The vascularity of thyroid lesions, evaluated with Doppler imaging, may be absent (no or scarce blood flow), perinodular (vascular predominance in the periphery of the nodule), further divided into complete or partial, intrano-

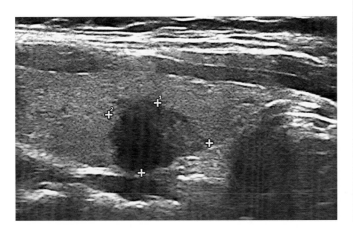

Fig. 11. Ultrasonographic appearance of a papillary thyroid carcinoma presenting as a hypoechoic lesion with irregular polylobulated borders in the posterior part of the thyroid lobe. Longitudinal scan.

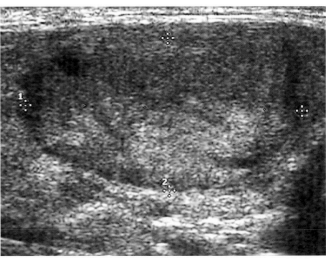

Fig. 12. Papillary thyroid carcinoma presenting an irregular, thick halo. Longitudinal scan.

dular (vascular predominance within the lesion) or peri-intranodular (flow in the periphery and within the nodule; fig. 13). The latter two can be further divided by power Doppler into two subtypes: moderate (moderate blood flow with a homogeneous structure and regular caliber of blood vessels) and increased (high blood flow with anarchical structure with a tortuous caliber of vessels). Data from the literature clearly indicate that the flow pattern must not be used in a differential diagnosis of thyroid cancer and that it should always be interpreted along with other US characteristics [19].

Finally, although the risk of malignancy does not change with the size of the lesion [20], US permits the precise measurement of the size of the thyroid nodule. Each lesion should be measured in all its three diameters, i.e. anteroposterior, transverse and longitudinal. Nodule growth is defined as a 20% increase in the nodule diameter (with a minimum increase in two dimensions of at least 2 mm) or a 50% increase in the nodule volume [11]. Most benign thyroid nodules grow with time; thus, a growing nodule does not necessarily indicate a tumor. A very rapid growth of a thyroid lesion, instead, should raise the suspicion of medullary or anaplastic thyroid carcinoma or thyroid lymphoma.

Benign Nodules

Benign thyroid nodules are a common finding comprising hyperplastic nodules and micro- or macrofollicular adenomas, and usually present with variable ultrasonographic features (online suppl. video 2). Benign nodules may also be found in the context of an autoimmune thyroiditis and, due to the heterogeneous echotexture of this condition, it may be challenging to detect true nodules. Real-time imaging in two planes along with Doppler studies may be necessary to differentiate pseudonodules from true nodules. The 'white knight' nodular pattern, a hyperechoic nodule with a background of hypoechogenicity, described in HT, is suggestive of benign disease, being thought to represent a benign regenerative nodule. The aggregation of more of these nodules, surrounded by a linear thin hypoechoic area, generates the so-called 'giraffe pattern' [21].

Thyroid Cancer

Thyroid cancer is represented by a heterogeneous group of malignancies, including differentiated thyroid carcinoma, medullary carcinoma, anaplastic carcinoma and thyroid lymphoma. Incidence, presentation, natural history, prognosis and treatment vary greatly among the different malignancies. According to the guidelines of the ATA, the primary role of US in thyroid cancer is to evaluate the characteristics and extension of the tumor beyond the thyroid capsule and to assess for cervical nodal metastases [22].

PTC represents 80% of all thyroid cancers and is often characterized by neck lymphatic spread. Multifocality is frequently due to the rich lymphatic network allowing tumor emboli to travel to other intrathyroidal sites. Nevertheless,

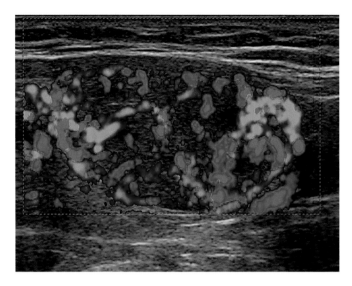

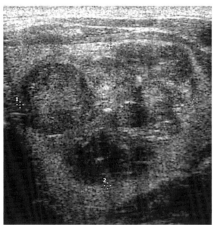

Fig. 13. Benign thyroid lesion presenting with blood flow in the periphery and within the nodule. Longitudinal scan.

Fig. 14. Ultrasonographic appearance of an FTC presenting as a rounded hypoechoic and heterogeneous lesion of the right thyroid lobe. Transverse scan.

classical PTC has an excellent prognosis, with a 10-year survival of 90%, worsening only in large tumors with gross extrathyroidal extension and distant metastasis, and in aggressive variants. Suspicious US features generally include an irregular or taller-than-wide shape, ill-defined or irregular borders and microcalcifications (fig. 11).

Follicular thyroid carcinoma (FTC) represents about 5–10% of thyroid cancers and usually presents as a solitary mass. In angioinvasive FTC, unlike PTC, hematogenous spread is more common than lymphatic spread, with distant metastases found in the lung, bone and brain. The FTC prognosis is worse than that of PTC, but is still favorable when nonangioinvasive. At US evaluation, FTC commonly presents as a large nodule with an irregular halo that may be isoechoic. Usually, in aggressive FTC, an inhomogeneous US pattern is observed due to its irregular growth and possible colliquation areas (fig. 14).

Hürthle cell carcinoma (HCC) represents less than 3% of thyroid cancers but Hürthle cells can also be observed in HT and benign thyroid nodules. The behavior of HCC is variable. The ultrasonographic appearance of HCC is similar to that of FTC, showing as an inhomogeneous, iso- to hypoechoic lesion.

Medullary thyroid carcinoma (MTC) arises from the parafollicular C cells, which secrete calcitonin. MTC represents roughly 4% of thyroid cancers. Approximately 25% of cases occur as part of an inherited genetic disorder, such as familial MTC, or the MEN2A and B syndromes. The re-

maining 75% are sporadic. MTC often presents as a firm, encapsulated mass, often with nodal metastases at presentation, and may show a heterogeneous sonographic appearance. Its US features are variable, being comparable to those of papillary carcinomas, follicular neoplasms or hyperplastic nodules (fig. 15).

Poorly differentiated thyroid carcinoma (PDTC) and anaplastic thyroid carcinoma (ATC) comprise only a small group of thyroid cancers but represent a disproportionate contribution to thyroid cancer mortality. PDTC may represent an intermediate entity in the progression to undifferentiated ATC, which typically presents as a rapidly growing mass in elderly individuals. Extrathyroidal extension, cervical lymphadenopathy and distant metastasis are the rule in this setting, with an extremely poor prognosis. At US, ATC usually appears as a typically large, invasive and rapidly enlarging mass involving and replacing thyroid parenchyma (fig. 16).

Primary thyroid lymphoma is a rare disease that can be confused with ATC. Patients often present with a rapidly enlarging neck mass causing dysphagia and hoarseness. Infiltration of lymphocytes is a prerequisite to the development of thyroid lymphoma [23]. There are two typical patterns: (i) a diffuse enlargement of a markedly hypoechoic thyroid gland, or (ii) nodular lymphoma with distinct borders between the tumor and the surrounding thyroid parenchyma. A differential diagnosis with HT may sometimes be difficult to achieve, and FNC or core-needle biopsy are often

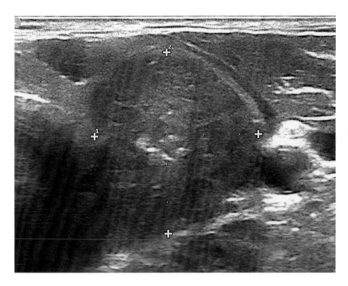

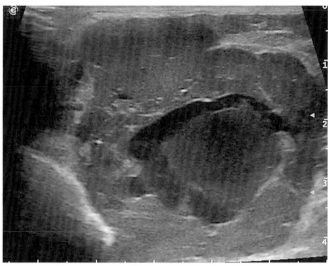

Fig. 15. Ultrasonographic appearance of an MTC presenting as a large hypoechoic mass with posterior irregular borders and internal coarse calcifications in the left thyroid lobe. Transverse scan.

Fig. 16. Ultrasonographic appearance of an anaplastic thyroid carcinoma, presenting as a large mass involving and replacing the left thyroid parenchyma. The lesion presents irregular margins and infiltrates subcutaneous tissues. Transverse scan.

17

18

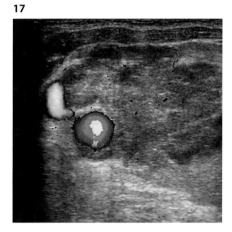

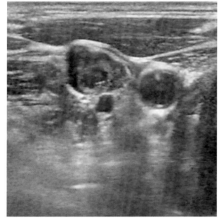

Fig. 17. Ultrasonographic appearance of a thyroid lymphoma presenting as a hypoechoic lesion involving the right thyroid lobe and encasing the homolateral carotid artery. Transverse scan.

Fig. 18. Ultrasonographic appearance of a metastatic lymph node of papillary thyroid carcinoma in the right level III, appearing with a rounded rather than oval shape, cystic changes and loss of the fatty hilum. Transverse scan.

needed. Thyroid lymphoma differs from aggressive thyroid carcinoma counterparts for its more homogenous appearance and lack of calcification, cystic degeneration and necrosis (fig. 17).

Once a thyroid neoplasm has been detected and evaluated, US is useful for preoperative evaluation of the contralateral lobe and cervical lymph nodes [22], and, in uncomplicated PTC, it may be all that is needed in the preoperative evaluation. Nevertheless, US may have some limitations in regional lymph node staging due to the difficulties in evaluation of the mediastinum and retropharyngeal regions. So-

nographic features that usually suggest metastatic nodes include loss of the fatty hilum, a rounded rather than oval shape, hypoechogenicity, cystic change, microcalcifications and increased vascularity [24] (fig. 18).

Elastography

Over the last few years US elastography (USE), a novel technology based on the elastic property of the tissue, has been added to the diagnostic armamentarium of US as an accurate, noninvasive predictor of thyroid malignancy. Currently, USE is not part of most ultrasound devices, being re-

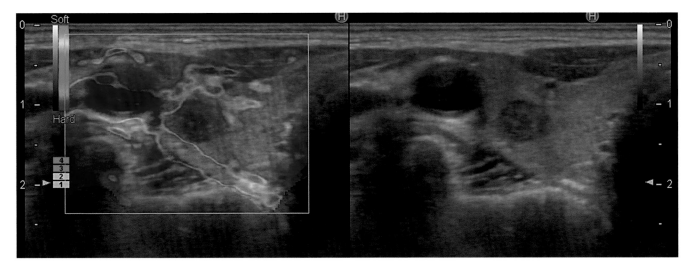

Fig. 19. Qualitative elastography appearance of a thyroid nodule appearing as a hypoechoic solid lesion in the right thyroid lobe (right side of the image). The same lesion appears completely blue (hard) at elastographic evaluation. Elastrographic stiffness suggests a higher risk of thyroid cancer. Transverse scan.

stricted to the more expensive varieties, and thus it cannot be performed routinely yet. As a consequence, USE has been considered as an ancillary technique to conventional US. Nevertheless, with regard to ultrasound imaging, USE is undeniably a major technological advancement and, if available, it may be a useful additional tool for the examiner. The technique is based on the principle that malignant lesions tend to be harder than benign ones. USE has been linked to an 'electronic palpation' in that it provides a reproducible stiffness estimation, also of otherwise not palpable lesions, overcoming the limits of clinical examination. USE may be qualitative on the basis of stiffness expression [25–27].

In qualitative USE an elasticity image is usually displayed over the B-mode image in a color scale depending on the magnitude of strain, usually red (soft tissue), green (intermediate degree of stiffness) and blue (firm, anelastic tissue). Based on the overall pattern the nodules can be immediately classified into different classes of firmness, with firm lesions more suspicious for thyroid cancer (fig. 19; online suppl. video 3). This classification may suffer from a certain degree of subjectivity in assigning the grade of elasticity [28]. In semiquantitative USE methods, the analysis provides numerical values that correspond to the ratios between the nodule and the healthy tissue at the same depth [26]. Several reports seem to confirm qualitative and semiquantitative USE as useful noninvasive tools for differential diagnosis [29], although, as recently reported [28], it seems to have lower sensitivity and specificity than previously

thought [29]. USE may also play a role in the differential diagnosis of indeterminate lesions [30] and in distinguishing nodules from pseudonodules in thyroiditis. Unfortunately, standard USE cannot be performed on partially cystic, calcific or coalescent nodules and its results should be interpreted with caution in some selected patient categories [31–34]. Shear wave USE, the newest and most promising quantitative elastographic method, seems to overcome these limitations, although larger prospective studies are needed to establish the diagnostic accuracy of this technique [35].

In summary, USE must not substitute conventional US, but it can be an important complement. In combination with US, USE could represent a useful, noninvasive tool in selecting thyroid nodules with a higher risk of malignancy. Table 1 presents an algorithm proposed for the differential diagnosis of thyroid lesions based on their ultrasonographic features.

Parathyroid Ultrasonography

Normal Anatomy

The anatomic location of the superior parathyroid glands is relatively constant; they typically reside on the dorsal part of the upper thyroid lobes at the level of the inferior border of the cricoid cartilage. The inferior parathyroid glands, instead, have a more variable location due to their embryo-

Table 1. Algorithm: US features and US classification system with five categories for a differential diagnosis of thyroid nodules [12]

Malignant US features (US-Mal)	Borderline US features (US-Bor)	Benign US features (US-Ben)
– Marked hypoechogenicity	– Hypoechogenicity	– Ovoid shape
– Spiculated margins	– Irregular shape	– Round shape
– Microlobulated margins	– Ill-defined margins	– Isoechogenicity
– Microcalcifications	– Irregular thick halo	– Hyperechogenicity
– Taller-than-wide shape	– Increased intranodular flow	– Well-defined margins
– Perithyroidal infiltration	– Increased peri-intranodular flow	– Regular margins
– Perithyroidal invasion	– Macrocalcifications	– Regular thin halo
– Metastatic lymphadenopathy	– Interrupted rim calcifications	– Perinodular vascularity
	– Elastographic hardness	– Spongiform appearance
		– Pure cystic lesion

Malignant: ≥3 US-Mal (regardless of the existence of US-Bor or US-Ben). Suspicious for malignancy: ≤2 US-Mal (regardless of the existence of US-Bor or US-Ben). Borderline: ≥1 US-Bor without US-Mal (regardless of the presence of US-Ben). Probably benign: ≥2 US-Ben (except spongiform appearance and pure cystic lesion), with no US-Mal and/or US-Bor. Benign: spongiform nodules, pure cystic lesions, without US-Mal and/or US-Bor.

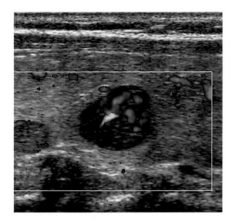

Fig. 20. Hypoechoic, vascularized parathyroid adenoma located within the left thyroid lobe. Longitudinal scan.

logic relationship to the thymus. They are usually located along the lateral lower pole of the thyroid gland but they can also be placed 1 cm below the lower thyroid lobe, or located anywhere between the angle of the mandible and the upper mediastinum. Unusual locations are the carotid bifurcation, within the carotid sheath and retropharyngeal. Finally, in approximately 2% of the general population, parathyroid tissue may also be found in thyroid parenchyma (fig. 20). Due to these anatomical variations their accurate localization may present some difficulties, but is crucial to the success of parathyroid surgery.

Parathyroid glands are very small, measuring approximately 6 mm in the craniocaudal and 3 mm in the transverse dimension. Therefore, in normal conditions, they are usually not identifiable by US. On the contrary, parathyroid adenomas are larger and more readily displayed on US imaging. When visualized, the size and number of the parathyroid glands should be documented, with size measurements preferably made in 3 dimensions. Unfortunately, the US identification of adenomatous parathyroid tissue may be difficult if the lesions are too small or placed in ectopic areas that are well-known blind spots for US, such as the retropharyngeal space, the mediastinum or in the depth of the neck. A 12- to 15-mHz linear probe is usually used in the study of parathyroid glands but sometimes the use of transducers with different penetrance may be necessary. Finally, US may contribute in the evaluation of patients with presumed parathyroid disease as guidance during fine-needle aspiration aimed at cyst aspiration, evaluation of parathormone levels in cyst fluid or cytologic examination.

Parathyroid Diseases
The ultrasonographic study of the parathyroid glands should be reserved strictly for localization purposes, after which proper diagnosis of primary hyperparathyroidism is made. Primary hyperparathyroidism is usually caused by a single parathyroid adenoma (90%) or multiglandular adenomatous disease (9%). Parathyroid carcinomas (1%) are very rare [36].

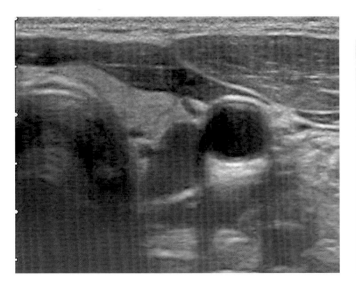

Fig. 21. Ultrasonographic appearance of a parathyroid adenoma appearing as a hypoechogenic lesion located closely to the posterior capsule of the thyroid gland. An indentation made by the parathyroid adenoma on the posterior capsule of the thyroid gland is clearly visible. Transverse scan.

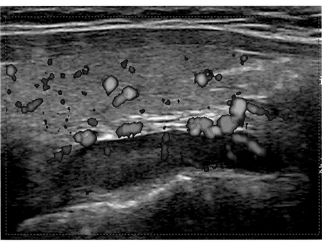

Fig. 22. Hypoechoic parathyroid adenoma located closely to the posterior capsule of the thyroid gland and presenting with an elongated shape. Longitudinal scan.

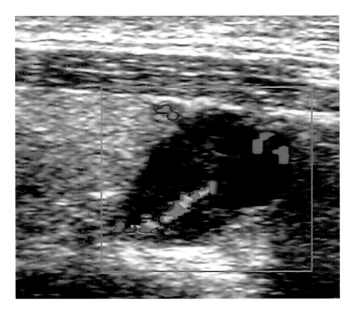

Fig. 23. Ultrasonographic appearance of a parathyroid adenoma. An extrathyroidal feeding artery entering at the parathyroid superior pole is clearly visible on Doppler evaluation. Longitudinal scan.

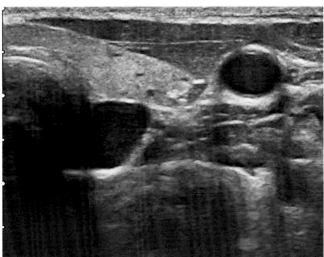

Fig. 24. Ultrasonographic appearance of a parathyroid cyst appearing as an anechoic lesion behind the left thyroid lobe, the typical position of the parathyroid gland. Transverse scan.

The most common sites of localization, such as the posterior margin of the thyroid capsule and the regions caudal to the thyroid lobes, should be inspected first. Maneuvers such as cough or deep breath can provide a transient glimpse of a mobile adenoma that is otherwise not visible. On US, a parathyroid adenoma tends to be round to ovoid, with low echogenicity in comparison with thyroid tissue. They are usually located in close relation to the posterior capsule of the thyroid gland. It is quite common to see an indentation made by the parathyroid adenoma on the posterior capsule of the thyroid gland, with a hyperechoic line separating the parathyroid and the thyroid glands representing the fibro-fatty capsule (fig. 21). Parathyroid adenomas are usually homogeneously hypoechoic with respect to the thyroid gland, but larger lesions may be more heterogeneous. The parathyroids may present variable shapes because they conform to the anatomical pressures of surrounding structures (fig. 22). When interrogated with Doppler, a typical adenoma often has a prominent extrathyroidal feeding artery entering at one pole (fig. 23), but may also present a diffuse flow within the adenoma. Generally, parathyroid adenomas are typically vascular when imaged with power Doppler. Finally, adenomas may have a cystic component or, sometimes, be completely cystic (fig. 24).

References

1 Dugar M, da Graca Bandeira A, Bruns J, Som PM: Unilateral hypopharyngitis, cellulitis, and a multinodular goiter: a triad of findings suggestive of acute suppurative thyroiditis. AJNR Am J Neuroradiol 2009;30:1944–1946.

2 Vulpoi C, Zbranca E, Preda C, Ungureanu MC: Contribution of ultrasonography in the evaluation of subacute thyroiditis. Rev Med Chir Soc Med Nat Iasi 2001;105:749–755.

3 Kang M, Ojili V, Khandelwal N, Bhansali A: Tuberculous abscess of the thyroid gland: a report of two cases. J Clin Ultrasound 2006;34:254–257.

4 Hayashi N, Tamaki N, Konishi J, Yonekura Y, Senda M, Kasagi K, Yamamoto K, Iida Y, Misaki T, Endo K: Sonography of Hashimoto's thyroiditis. J Clin Ultrasound 1986;14:123–126.

5 Yeh HC, Futterweit W, Gilbert P: Micronodulation: ultrasonographic sign of Hashimoto thyroiditis. J Ultrasound Med 1996;15:813–819.

6 Vitti P, Rago T, Mancusi F, Pallini S, Tonacchera M, Santini F, Chiovato L, Marcocci C, Pinchera A: Thyroid hypoechogenic pattern at ultrasonography as a tool for predicting recurrence of hyperthyroidism after medical treatment in patients with Graves disease. Acta Endocrinol 1992;126: 128–131.

7 Bogazzi F, Bartalena L, Brogioni S, Burelli A, Manetti L, Tanda ML, Gasperi M, Martino E: Thyroid vascularity and blood flow are not dependent on serum thyroid hormone levels: studies in vivo by color flow Doppler sonography. Eur J Endocrinol 1999;140:452–458.

8 Erdogan MF, Anil C, Cesur M, Baskal N, Erdogan G: Color flow Doppler sonography for the etiologic diagnosis of hyperthyroidism. Thyroid 2007;17: 223–231.

9 Ezzat S, Sarti DA, Cain DR, Braunstein GD: Thyroid incidentalomas: prevalence by palpation and ultrasonography. Arch Intern Med 1994;154: 1838–1840.

10 Gharib H, Papini E, Valcavi R, Baskin HJ, Crescenzi A, Dottorini ME, Duick DS, Guglielmi R, Hamilton CR Jr, Zeiger MA, Zini M; AACE/AME Task Force on Thyroid Nodules: American Association of Clinical Endocrinologists and Associazione Medici Endocrinologi medical guidelines for clinical practice for the diagnosis and management of thyroid nodules. Endocr Pract 2006;12: 63–102.

11 Gharib H, Papini E, Paschke R, Duick DS, Valcavi R, Hegedüs L, Vitti P; AACE/AME/ETA Task Force on Thyroid Nodules: American Association of Clinical Endocrinologists, Associazione Medici Endocrinologi, and European Thyroid Association medical guidelines for clinical practice for the diagnosis and management of thyroid nodules. Endocr Pract 2010;16(suppl 1):1–43.

12 Andrioli M, Carzaniga C, Persani L: Standardized ultrasound report for thyroid nodules: the endocrinologist's viewpoint. Eur Thyroid J 2013;2:37–48.

13 Cappelli C, Castellano M, Pirola I, Gandossi E, De Martino E, Cumetti D, Agosti B, Rosei EA: Thyroid nodule shape suggests malignancy. Eur J Endocrinol 2006;155:27–31.

14 Kim EK, Park CS, Chung WY, Oh KK, Kim DI, Lee JT, Yoo HS: New sonographic criteria for recommending fine-needle aspiration biopsy of nonpalpable solid nodules of the thyroid. AJR Am J Roentgenol 2002;178:687–691.

15 Moon WJ, Jung SL, Lee JH, Na DG, Baek JH, Lee YH, Kim J, Kim HS, Byun JS, Lee DH; Thyroid Study Group, Korean Society of Neuro- and Head and Neck Radiology: Benign and malignant thyroid nodules: US differentiation – multicenter retrospective study. Radiology 2008;247:762–770.

16 Nam-Goong IS, Kim HY, Gong G, Lee HK, Hong SJ, Kim WB, Shong YK: Ultrasonography-guided fine-needle aspiration of thyroid incidentaloma: correlation with pathological findings. Clin Endocrinol 2004;60:21–28.

17 Kim EK, Park CS, Chung WY, Oh KK, Kim DI, Lee JT, Yoo HS: New sonographic criteria for recommending fine-needle aspiration biopsy of nonpalpable solid nodules of the thyroid. AJR Am J Roentgenol 2002;178:687–691.

18 Papini E, Guglielmi R, Bianchini A, Crescenzi A, Taccogna S, Nardi F, Panunzi C, Rinaldi R, Toscano V, Pacella CM: Risk of malignancy in nonpalpable thyroid nodules: predictive value of ultrasound and color-Doppler features. J Clin Endocrinol Metab 2002;87:1941–1946.

19 Frates MC, Benson CB, Charboneau JW, Cibas ES, Clark OH, Coleman BG, Cronan JJ, Doubilet PM, Evans DB, Goellner JR, Hay ID, Hertzberg BS, Intenzo CM, Jeffrey RB, Langer JE, Larsen PR, Mandel SJ, Middleton WD, Reading CC, Sherman SI, Tessler FN; Society of Radiologists in Ultrasound: Management of thyroid nodules detected at US: Society of Radiologists in Ultrasound consensus conference statement. Radiology 2005;237:794–800.

20 Hegedüs L, Bonnema SJ, Bennedbaek FN: Management of simple nodular goiter: current status and future perspectives. Endocr Rev 2003;24:102–132.

21 Bonavita JA, Mayo J, Babb J, Bennett G, Oweity T, Macari M, Yee J: Pattern recognition of benign nodules at ultrasound of the thyroid: which nodule should be left alone? AJR Am J Roentgenol 2009;193:207–213.

22 Cooper DS, Doherty GM, Haugen BR, Kloos RT, Lee SL, Mandel SJ, Mazzaferri EL, McIver B, Pacini F, Schlumberger M, Sherman SI, Steward DL, Tuttle RM: Revised American Thyroid Association management guidelines for patients with thyroid nodules and differentiated thyroid cancer. Thyroid 2009;19:1167–1214.

23 Holm LE, Blomgren H, Lowhagen T: Cancer risks in patients with chronic lymphocytic thyroiditis. N Engl J Med 1985;312:601–604.

24 Frasoldati A, Valcavi R: Challenges in neck ultrasonography: lymphadenopathy and parathyroid glands. Endocr Pract 2004;10:261–268.

25 Trimboli P, Guglielmi R, Monti S, Misischi I, Graziano F, Nasrollah N, Amendola S, Morgante SN, Deiana MG, Valabrega S, Toscano V, Papini E: Ultrasound sensitivity for thyroid malignancy is increased by real-time elastography: a prospective multicenter study. J Clin Endocrinol Metab 2012; 97:4524–4530.

26 Cantisani V, D'Andrea V, Biancari F, Medvedyeva O, Di Segni M, Olive M, Patrizi P, Redler A, De Antoni E, Masciangelo R, Frezzotti F, Ricci P: Prospective evaluation of multiparametric ultrasound and quantitative elastosonography in the differential diagnosis of benign and malignant thyroid nodules: preliminary experience. Eur J Radiol 2012;81:2678–2683.

27 Sebag F, Vaillant-Lombard J, Berbis J, Griset V, Henry JF, Petit P, Oliver C: Shear wave elastography: a new ultrasound imaging mode for the differential diagnosis of benign and malignant thyroid nodules. J Clin Endocrinol Metab 2010;95: 5281–5288.

28 Unlütürk U, Erdogan MF, Demir O, Güllü S, Baskal N: Ultrasound elastography is not superior to grayscale ultrasound in predicting malignancy in thyroid nodules. Thyroid 2012;22:1031–1038.

29 Rago T, Santini F, Scutari M, Pinchera A, Vitti P: Elastography: new developments in ultrasound for predicting malignancy in thyroid nodules. J Clin Endocrinol Metab 2007;92:2917–2922.

30 Cantisani V, Ulisse S, Guaitoli E, De Vito C, Caruso R, Mocini R, D'Andrea V, Ascoli V, Antonaci A, Catalano C, Nardi F, Redler A, Ricci P, De Antoni E, Sorrenti S: Q-elastography in the presurgical diagnosis of thyroid nodules with indeterminate cytology. PLoS One 2012;7:e50725.

31 Andrioli M, Scacchi M, Carzaniga C, Vitale G, Moro M, Poggi L, Fatti LM, Cavagnini F: Thyroid nodules in acromegaly: the role of elastography. J Ultrasound 2010;13:90–97.

32 Scacchi M, Andrioli M, Carzaniga C, Vitale G, Moro M, Poggi L, Pecori Giraldi F, Fatti LM, Cavagnini F: Elastosonographic evaluation of thyroid nodules in acromegaly. Eur J Endocrinol 2009;161:607–613.

33 Andrioli M, Trimboli P, Amendola S, Valabrega S, Fukunari N, Mirella M, Persani L: Elastographic presentation of medullary thyroid carcinoma. Endocrine 2014;45:153–155.

34 Andrioli M, Persani L: Elastographic presentation of synchronous renal cell carcinoma metastasis to the thyroid gland. Endocrine 2014;47:336–337.

35 Sebag F, Vaillant-Lombard J, Berbis J, Griset V, Henry JF, Petit P, Oliver C: Shear wave elastography: a new ultrasound imaging mode for the differential diagnosis of benign and malignant thyroid nodules. J Clin Endocrinol Metab 2010;95: 5281–5288.

36 Ruda JM, Hollenbeak CS, Stack BC Jr: A systematic review of the diagnosis and treatment of primary hyperparathyroidism from 1995 to 2003. Otolaryngol Head Neck Surg 2005;132:359–372.

37 Köpf-Maier P: Wolf-Heidegger's Atlas of Human Anatomy, ed 6. Basel, Karger, 2005.

Massimiliano Andrioli, MD, PhD
EndocrinologiaOggi, Centro Medico
Viale Somalia 33
IT–00199 Rome (Italy)
E-Mail andrioli@endocrinologiaoggi.it

Buchfelder M, Guaraldi F (eds): Imaging in Endocrine Disorders.
Front Horm Res. Basel, Karger, 2016, vol 45, pp 16–23 (DOI: 10.1159/000442274)

Computed Tomography and Magnetic Resonance Imaging of the Thyroid and Parathyroid Glands

Rebekkah Warren Frunzac · Melanie Richards

Department of Surgery, Mayo Clinic, Rochester, Minn., USA

Abstract

Computed tomography (CT) and magnetic resonance imaging (MRI) are advanced imaging modalities that are not typically utilized as part of the initial evaluation of thyroid and parathyroid pathology. However, both modalities have applications in complex cases, particularly in the reoperative setting and in operative planning for initial or recurrent carcinomas. As part of a multimodal approach, CT and MRI can increase the successful preoperative localization of abnormal parathyroid glands. Newer imaging modalities, such as PET-CT and SPECT-CT in thyroid imaging, and 4D-CT in parathyroid imaging, can provide information on the anatomy as well as the function of pathologic tissues. Both modalities provide excellent assessment of the extent of disease, local invasion and distant metastases. Drawbacks include cost and availability, and these should be weighed against benefits in the context of the management of thyroid and parathyroid disease.

© 2016 S. Karger AG, Basel

Cross-sectional imaging with computed tomography (CT) and magnetic resonance imaging (MRI) has become a very important part of the modern physician's diagnostic arsenal. Both modalities are used to define anatomy, establish or narrow a differential diagnosis, and assess pathology. CT was first introduced in 1972 at the 32nd Congress of the British Institute of Radiology by an engineer named Godfrey Hounsfield [1]. This technology uses X-rays to obtain cross-sectional images of an object at different angles, allowing 3D image reconstruction. MRI relies on the nuclear magnetic resonance property of water molecules to define the water density of anatomic structures. This technology was first used in human anatomic imaging in 1977 [2]. CT and MRI are rarely routinely used as the initial imaging modality in thyroid or parathyroid disease, except in the case of 4D imaging for hyperparathyroidism. However, both modalities are used in the evaluation of complex thyroid and parathyroid anatomy and in operative planning.

Thyroid

Computed Tomography

CT imaging of the thyroid is largely limited to presurgical evaluation. CT is a widely available modality and provides excellent anatomic detail of structures in the head and neck. Specific scenarios in which CT is particularly useful include the evaluation of substernal goiter (fig. 1), locally invasive thyroid malignancy and metastatic disease [3]. In assessing thyroid pathology, CT should be performed without intravenous (IV) contrast material if possible for several reasons. First, due to the high concentration of iodine in the thyroid gland, it attenuates to a greater degree than surrounding structures, thus appearing brighter (80–100 Hounsfield units) [4], even in the absence of IV contrast. Second, CT IV contrast agents contain iodine and may lead to the suppression of iodine uptake into thyroid tissue, requiring a 4- to 6-week delay before radioiodine scintigraphy or therapy can be performed [5]. If high-resolution cross-sectional imaging must be performed concurrent with radioiodine administration, MRI can be used as an alternative to CT with iodinated IV contrast. Finally, administration of iodinated IV contrast may lead to a thyroid storm in patients with hyperthyroidism or thyrotoxicosis. Clinically, a thyroid storm can present as hyperpyrexia, tachycardia, decompensated heart failure with pulmonary edema and respiratory failure or cardiac arrest [6]. Although rare, there is a 10% mortality associated with thyroid storm and management should occur in an intensive care setting. The approach should be multimodal, including antipyrexia with cooling blankets and acetaminophen, β-blockade, inorganic iodine, antithyroid medications, and cardiac and respiratory support [7].

Magnetic Resonance Imaging
The indications for MRI of the head and neck in the evaluation of thyroid pathology are similar to those for CT scan. As mentioned previously, MRI can be used as an alternative to CT with iodinated contrast if radioiodine therapy or scintigraphy is to be undertaken. Multiplanar images should be obtained with multiple pulse sequences, including T1- and T2-weighted images [4]. On T2-weighted images, the thyroid gland appears hyperintense relative to the surrounding neck musculature. The normal thyroid enhances homogenously and heterogeneity can be seen in conditions such as multinodular goiter. Disease-containing lymph nodes often demonstrate hyperenhancement on T1-weighted images owing to the presence of colloid and thyroglobulin.

Benign Diseases
The normal thyroid is homogeneous in appearance and is located in the anterior neck. It comprises a left and right lobe measuring approximately 5 × 3 × 2 cm (L × W × D) connected by the thyroid isthmus. The isthmus usually overlies the trachea between the first and third tracheal rings, although it may be absent. In some patients a pyramidal lobe

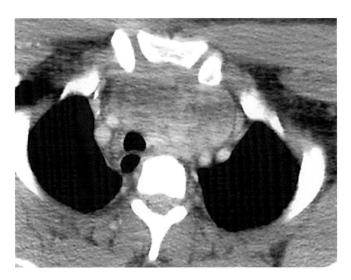

Fig. 1. CT imaging of a retrosternal goiter to identify the extent of tracheal compression and deviation.

may be present, extending cephalad from the isthmus toward the thyroid cartilage [see fig.1a in the chapter by Andrioli and Valcavi; this vol., p. 2]. CT imaging may be helpful in identifying ectopic thyroid tissue, which may be identified anywhere from the base of the tongue cranially, to the mediastinum caudally.

Multinodular Goiter
Ultrasound of the neck can provide highly detailed information about the presence of a multinodular goiter, including the size and extent of locoregional extension of the abnormal thyroid. However, at least 5% of patients with a multinodular goiter have retrosternal extension of thyroid tissue that cannot be fully characterized by ultrasound [8]. A chest X-ray may demonstrate a mediastinal mass or tracheal deviation, but the absence of these findings does not exclude significant, symptomatic disease [9]. Thus, a CT scan of the neck and chest is recommended as part of the preoperative evaluation for these patients (fig. 1, 2) [10]. A CT scan provides detailed information about the caudal extent of the goiter, its size and shape, and compression of local structures in the neck and chest. The likelihood of requiring an extracervical approach (median sternotomy or thoracotomy) for surgical excision of a retrosternal goiter is increased when the goiter extends below the level of the aortic arch, when it is in the posterior mediastinum, is dumbbell shaped or when the thoracic component is wider than the thoracic inlet [10].

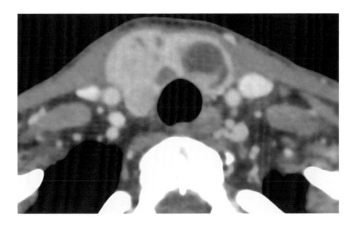

Fig. 2. CT of a huge goiter with hemorrhagic and cystic areas partially surrounding, but not compressing, the trachea.

Graves' Orbitopathy

Both CT and MRI can be used to evaluate orbital involvement in patients with Graves' disease. Spiral CT imaging yields excellent resolution of structures in the orbit, with the advantage that the bony and soft tissue components behave as a natural contrast medium for one another [11]. This allows imaging without the administration of IV iodinated contrast, which is contraindicated in Graves' disease. CT can be highly accurate for determining the volume of orbital tissues and etiology of decreased vision, particularly as a consequence of compression [12]. As such, this modality is used pre- and postoperatively in orbital decompression. Reconstruction in multiple dimensions helps to diminish artifacts from metal dental and jaw implants. Drawbacks of CT include radiation exposure to the lens and the inability to differentiate between active or acute disease and fibrotic end-stage disease.

MRI is the imaging modality of choice in Graves' orbitopathy [11]. On T2-weighted images it is possible to differentiate between active and quiescent or end-stage disease based on relaxation time [12]. Thus, this modality can be used functionally to monitor the response to therapy. Strong T2-weighted, fat-suppressed (turbo-inversion recovery-magnitude, TRIM) sequences have been useful in defining the degree of inflammation in extraocular muscles and can therefore be useful in differentiating between Graves' orbitopathy and other orbital pathologies, such as orbital myositis [11]. Images obtained with MRI demonstrate an excellent resolution of soft-tissue structures and can be used to accurately define the degree of orbital involvement, including optic nerve compression. It is important that both T1-

and T2-weighted images are obtained and gadolinium contrast can be used to further enhance the extraocular muscles and eyelid. MRI is more expensive and less widely available than CT. Additionally, it is less useful than CT for the evaluation of bony structures and is contraindicated in patients with implanted devices, such as nerve stimulators or pacemakers.

Thyroid Incidentalomas

Most thyroid nodules are nonpalpable lesions identified incidentally during imaging for unrelated conditions [3]. As a significant proportion of these lesions (approximately 10%) may contain carcinoma, it is recommended that patients with high-risk lesions undergo further evaluation, including examination by an experienced physician and thyroid ultrasonography, with or without fine-needle aspiration biopsy, as described in detail in the chapter by Andrioli and Valcavi [this vol., pp. 1–15].

Malignancy

Preoperative Planning

Once a thyroid malignancy has been identified, cross-sectional imaging may be useful in operative planning. Generally, for small, well-circumscribed tumors, high-resolution ultrasound of the neck provides adequate anatomic detail on which to make surgical decisions. However, extrathyroidal invasion represents a significant negative prognostic indicator in differentiated thyroid cancer [13] and detailed anatomic characterization with CT or MRI is necessary to define the extent of disease. Signs and symptoms of invasive thyroid malignancy include a fixed mass, dysphagia or shortness of breath. CT has been shown to be highly specific for the detection of invasion of the aerodigestive tract, vascular structures (common carotid artery and internal jugular vein) and the recurrently laryngeal nerve; however, the sensitivity of this modality ranges from 29 to 66% [14]. MRI may be superior to a CT scan for detecting tumor invasion of the aerodigestive tract. Wang et al. [15] demonstrated that MRI can be used to identify esophageal invasion with 91% accuracy when the outer layer is involved with tumor. Takashima et al. [16] demonstrated that tumor size and effacement of fatty tissues on MRI were highly predictive of recurrent laryngeal nerve invasion at the time of surgery. Only 38% of the patients in this study had clinical symptoms and 69% had abnormal findings at laryngoscopy.

Chest X-ray is frequently a part of the presurgical evaluation for patients undergoing a general anesthetic. For patients with thyroid cancer who have high-risk lesions (i.e.

age greater than 40 years, large tumors, local or lymphovascular invasion), chest X-ray can be considered part of the initial staging. Approximately 5–10% of patients with papillary thyroid cancer will present with distant metastases and approximately 50% of these are isolated to the lung [17]. Patients with abnormal chest X-ray or elevated thyroglobulin after thyroidectomy should undergo a whole-body radioiodine scan to evaluate the presence of residual local disease or distant metastases. If lung metastases are identified, CT of the chest can be used to plan the surgical resection, if indicated.

Patients with medullary thyroid cancer should be evaluated for the presence of RET proto-oncogene mutations prior to surgical intervention. It is recommended that these patients also undergo a CT scan of the chest and mediastinum in the presence of bulky local disease or significantly elevated serum calcitonin level (>400 pg/ml). All patients with RET mutations should undergo biochemical screening for pheochromocytoma (which occurs in half of patients with MEN2) and hyperparathyroidism. CT scan and MRI of the abdomen are both highly sensitive and specific for the localization of pheochromocytoma.

Poorly differentiated cancers of the thyroid, thyroid lymphoma and metastatic diseases to the thyroid are rare. Anaplastic thyroid cancer is a very aggressive malignancy with a poor prognosis and life expectancy measured in terms of weeks to months [4]. Cross-sectional imaging is used to determine the extent of disease, but surgery is generally limited to palliative resection because a mortality benefit is rarely achieved. Anaplastic thyroid cancer demonstrates a heterogeneous signal on T1- and T2-weighted MRI images, indicative of hemorrhage and necrosis [12]. In contrast, thyroid lymphoma is usually associated with a history of long-standing goiter. Lesions are generally homogeneous by MRI and slightly hyperintense relative to healthy thyroids on T2-weighted images. It may be difficult to distinguish lymphoma from thyroiditis in patients with a history of Hashimoto's disease, despite the use of cross-sectional imaging [4].

Recurrent Thyroid Carcinoma
Hybrid functional imaging modalities such as PET-CT (positron emission tomography-CT) and SPECT-CT (single-photon emission CT combined with high-resolution CT) may prove useful in cases where recurrent thyroid carcinoma is suspected, but lesions are not identified by ultrasound, conventional CT/MRI or a radioiodine whole-body scan [18]. A PET scan with 2-deoxy-2-fluoro-D-glucose (FDG) is widely used in the evaluation of nonthyroid malignancies and, occasionally, metabolically active thyroid nodules may be identified incidentally. These nodules have a 30–50% risk of being malignant, so further evaluation with thyroid ultrasound and FNA biopsy is usually recommended [19]. However, in the localization of locoregional recurrence of thyroid cancer, a PET scan alone offers minimal benefit relative to high-resolution ultrasonography [20]. PET-CT with FDG offered a positive predictive value of approximately 95% and negative predictive value of 65% in patients who underwent surveillance for recurrent differentiated thyroid cancer in a study by Razfar et al. [21]. In this study, the likelihood of a positive FDG PET-CT scan was significantly increased when the serum thyroglobulin level was greater than 10 ng/ml; thus, the authors recommend avoiding this modality in patients with serum thyroglobulin below 10 ng/ml.

PET-CT can also be performed using [124]I as the radionuclide. In imaging for localization of recurrent or metastatic differentiated thyroid cancer, [124]I PET-CT offered little advantage over a ^{131}I whole-body scan or FDG PET-CT [19]. However, the usefulness of this technology has been demonstrated in obtaining high-resolution dosimetry calculations for therapeutic radioiodine administration [22].

Alternative radiopharmaceuticals for use in PET-CT imaging have been investigated for the localization of medullary thyroid cancers, which do not concentrate iodine. These include ^{68}Ga-DOTATOC and ^{18}F-DOPA [19]. Unfortunately, these diagnostic tools have not been refined to the point that they offer a significant advantage over other currently available imaging modalities.

SPECT-CT with ^{131}I is another high-resolution hybrid imaging modality that combines conventional CT with ^{131}I radionuclide scintigraphy. This modality offers increased spatial resolution and differentiation of physiologic versus pathologic focal radionuclide update relative to planar imaging for differentiated thyroid cancer [23]. [131]I SPECT-CT can also be used for dosimetry measurements. However, due to its increased cost and limited availability, widespread use of this technology is not currently recommended.

Parathyroid

Overproduction of parathyroid hormone is largely the consequence of benign disease restricted to one hypercellular parathyroid gland (primary hyperparathyroidism) [3]. In approximately 15% of patients with primary hyperparathy-

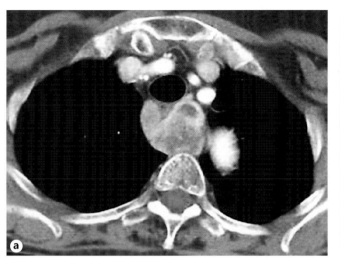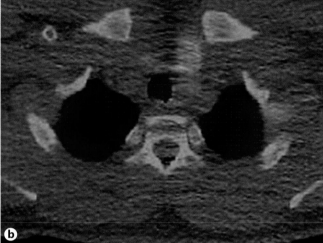

Fig. 3. A CT (**a**) and sestamibi SPECT-CT (**b**) fusion study to anatomically locate a parathyroid gland in the left thyroid-thymic tract.

roidism, two or more glands will be involved. Secondary hyperparathyroidism is a condition associated with a stimulus, such as chronic renal insufficiency, and is generally characterized by 4-gland hyperplasia. Tertiary hyperparathyroidism reflects a state of irreversible parathyroid autonomy that occurs in patients with prior secondary hyperparathyroidism, even after resolution of the inciting stimulus, for example after renal allograft for chronic renal insufficiency. Parathyroid malignancy is exceedingly rare, occurring in less than 1% of patients with primary hyperparathyroidism [24].

Historically, primary hyperparathyroidism was managed surgically with 4-gland exploration. However, improved imaging techniques are now available for preoperative localization of abnormal glands, allowing for directed exploration via a minimally invasive approach. In combination with intraoperative parathyroid hormone level monitoring, preoperative localization has resulted in reductions to operative times, hospital lengths of stay, risk of recurrent laryngeal nerve injury and permanent hypoparathyroidism [25]. A radionuclide sestamibi (fig. 3) scan and ultrasound of the neck are generally considered the primary imaging modalities for localization of hyperfunctional parathyroid glands. However, CT and MRI are also useful in parathyroid localization, particularly in cases of negative sestamibi imaging or persistent hyperparathyroidism after initial parathyroid exploration [25].

Computed Tomography
Due to the complex anatomy of the neck and the small and nonspecific appearance of abnormal parathyroid glands on CT imaging, it is not recommended that CT be used as the sole imaging modality in parathyroid localization [25]. CT is useful in imaging anatomic regions not amenable to ultrasonography, such as the mediastinum and tracheoesophageal groove. IV iodinated contrast should be used when possible to improve enhancement of hyperfunctioning parathyroid glands [24]. Findings can be compared to results obtained by sestamibi radionuclide scanning or ultrasonography in order to improve the precision of localization. Contrast-enhanced CT is also recommended as part of a multi-imaging approach to evaluation of initial or recurrent parathyroid carcinoma [25].

More recently, the 4D-CT technique has been applied to parathyroid imaging. This technique is performed using a protocol similar to CT angiography [25], with acquisition of precontrast, postcontrast and washout images. Parathyroid tissue demonstrates low attenuation on the noncontrast images and peak enhancement on the arterial phase, with washout between the arterial and delayed phases (fig. 4a, b, fig. 5) [26]. In contrast, lymph nodes do not show arterial phase enhancement [27]. Sections of approximately 1.25 mm are acquired in the axial plane, with computer-generated sagittal and coronal reconstructions [28]. During the arterial and delayed phases, images are obtained from the angle of the mandible through the level of the carina to aid in identification of ectopic parathyroid tissue, including

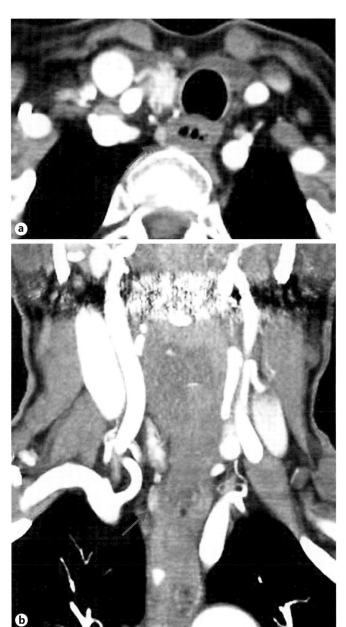

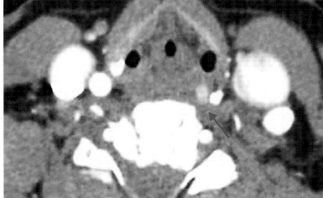

Fig. 5. 4D-CT imaging arterial phase study of an undescended left superior parathyroid gland located adjacent to the piriform sinus.

Fig. 4. a, b 4D-CT imaging showing arterial phase uptake of a right superior parathyroid gland posterior to the tracheoesophageal groove.

glands located within the carotid sheath, thyroid capsule and mediastinum (fig. 4, 5). Using 4D-CT, Rodgers et al. [29] reported lateralization of parathyroid adenoma (fig. 3) to the correct side with 88% sensitivity and to the correct gland with 70% sensitivity. In the same study, 4D-CT offered a distinct advantage over sestamibi imaging in the de-

tection of multigland disease. Mortenson et al. [30] reported a high degree of success in the preoperative identification of abnormal parathyroid glands in the setting of reoperative intervention for primary hyperparathyroidism. For these reasons, some centers have begun to utilize 4D-CT as the initial imaging modality for parathyroid localization in the setting of hyperparathyroidism [31]. 4D-CT is associated with a lower cost than sestamibi scintigraphy with SPECT, but higher radiation exposure and should be used with caution in children and young adults who may be at increased risk for development of future thyroid carcinoma.

Magnetic Resonance Imaging
MRI has been described in the initial evaluation of primary hyperparathyroidism, persistent, postoperative hyperparathyroidism and parathyroid carcinoma. Hypercellular parathyroid glands appear hypointense on T1 sequences, with strong contrast enhancement and a hyperintense signal on T2-weighted images [32]. Normal parathyroid glands are very difficult to visualize by MRI. Like CT, MRI may be more useful than ultrasound for imaging abnormal parathyroids in anatomic regions that are difficult to assess, such as the mediastinum and tracheoesophageal groove [33]. Gotway et al. [34] reported a sensitivity of 82% and positive predictive value of 89% in the detection of abnormal parathyroid glands using MRI. The presence of multinodular goiter was associated with both false positive and false negative studies. The detection of ectopic parathyroid adenomas was excellent, with 94% of these glands being identified. Like CT, MRI is recommended as part of a multimodal approach

to operative planning for initial or recurrent parathyroid carcinoma [25]. MRI may provide better anatomic detail than a CT scan in cases of reoperation where the presence of metal clips may lead to artifacts.

Conclusion

Although CT and MRI are not generally recommended as first-line imaging modalities for assessing thyroid and parathyroid pathology, both modalities have applications in complex cases, particularly in the reoperative setting and in operative planning for initial or recurrent carcinomas. As part of a multimodal approach, CT and MRI can increase the successful preoperative localization of abnormal parathyroid glands. Newer imaging modalities, such as PET-CT and SPECT-CT in thyroid imaging and 4D-CT in parathyroid imaging can provide information on anatomy, as well as the function of pathologic tissues. Both modalities provide excellent assessment of the extent of disease, local invasion and distant metastases. Drawbacks include cost and availability, and these should be weighed against benefits in the context of the management of thyroid and parathyroid disease.

References

1 Beckmann EC: CT scanning the early days. Br J Radiol 2006;79:5–8.
2 Ai T, Morelli JN, Hu X, Hao D, Goerner FL, Ager B, Runge VM: A historical overview of magnetic resonance imaging, focusing on technological innovations. Invest Radiol 2012;47:725–741.
3 Vazquez BJ, Richards ML: Imaging of the thyroid and parathyroid glands. Surg Clin North Am 2011;91:15–32.
4 Loevner LA, Kaplan SL, Cunnane ME, Moonis G: Cross-sectional imaging of the thyroid gland. Neuroimaging Clin N Am 2008;18:445–461.
5 Hessel A, Chalian AA, Clayman GL: Surgical management of recurrent thyroid cancer. Neuroimaging Clin N Am 2008;18:517–525.
6 Alkhuja S, Pyram R, Odeyemi O: In the eye of the storm: iodinated contrast medium induced thyroid storm presenting as cardiopulmonary arrest. Heart Lung 2013;42:267–269.
7 Bahn RS, Burch HB, Cooper DS, Garber JR, Greenlee MC, Klein I, Laurgberg P, McDougall IR, Montori VM, Rivkees SA, Ross DS, Sosa JA, Stan MN; American Thyroid Association; America Association of Clinical Endocrinologists: Hyperthyroidism and other causes of thyrotoxicosis: management guidelines of the American Thyroid Association and American Association of Clinical Endocrinologists. Endocr Pract 2011;17:456–520.
8 Mercante G, Gabrielli E, Pedroni C, Formisano D, Bertolini L, Nicoli F, Valcavi R, Barbieri V: CT cross-sectional imaging classification system for substernal goiter based on risk factors for an extracervical surgical approach. Head Neck 2011;33:792–799.
9 Randolph GW, Shin JJ, Grillo HC, Mathisen D, Katlic MR, Kamani D, Zurakowski D: The surgical management of goiter: part II. Surgical treatment and results. Laryngoscope 2011;121:68–76.
10 Qureishi A, Garas G, Tolley N, Palazzo F, Athanasiou T, Zacharakis E. Can pre-operative computed tomography predict the need for a thoracic approach for removal of retrosternal goitre? Int J Surg 2013;11:203–208.

11 Kirsch E, Hammer B, von Arx G: Graves' orbitopathy: current imaging procedures. Swiss Med Wkly 2009;139:618–623.
12 Aiken AH: Imaging of thyroid cancer. Semin Ultrasound CT MR 2012;33:138–149.
13 Hotomi M, Sugitani I, Toda K, Kawabata K, Fujimoto Y: A novel definition of extrathyroidal invasion for patients with papillary thyroid carcinoma for predicting prognosis. World J Surg 2012;36:1231–1240.
14 Seo YL, Yoon DY, Lim KJ, Cha JH, Yun EJ, Choi CS, Bae SH: Locally advanced thyroid cancer: can CT help in prediction of extrathyroidal invasion to adjacent structures? AJR Am J Roentgenol 2010;195:W240–W244.
15 Wang J, Takashima S, Matsushita T, Takayama F, Kobayashi T, Kadoya M: Esophageal invasion by thyroid carcinomas: prediction using magnetic resonance imaging. J Comput Assist Tomogr 2003;27:18–25.
16 Takashima S, Takayama F, Wang J, Kobayashi S, Kadoya M: Using MR imaging to predict invasion of the recurrent laryngeal nerve by thyroid carcinoma. AJR Am J Roentgenol 2003;180:837–842.
17 Saindane AM: Pitfalls in the staging of cancer of thyroid. Neuroimaging Clin N Am 2013;23:123–145.
18 Makeieff M, Burcia V, Raingeard I, Eberle MC, Cartier C, Garrel R, Crampette L, Guerrier B: Positron emission tomography-computed tomography evaluation for recurrent differentiated thyroid carcinoma. Eur Ann Otorhinolaryngol Head Neck Dis 2012;129:251–256.
19 Mosci C, Iagaru A: PET/CT imaging of thyroid cancer. Clin Nucl Med 2011;36:e180–e185.
20 Grant CS, Thompson GB, Farley DR, Richards ML, Mullan BP, Hay ID: The value of positron emission tomography in the surgical management of recurrent papillary thyroid carcinoma. World J Surg 2008;32:708–715.

21 Razfar A, Branstetter BF 4th, Christopoulos A, Lebeau SO, Hodak SP, Heron DE, Escott EJ, Ferris RL: Clinical usefulness of positron emission tomography-computed tomography in recurrent thyroid carcinoma. Arch Otolaryngol Head Neck Surg 2010;136:120–125.
22 Sgouros G, Kolbert KS, Sheikh A, Pentlow KS, Mun EF, Barth A, Robbins RJ, Larson SM: Patient-specific dosimetry for ^{131}I thyroid cancer therapy using ^{124}I PET and 3-dimensional-internal dosimetry (3D-ID) software. J Nucl Med 2004;45:1366–1372.
23 Barwick TD, Dhawan RT, Lewington V: Role of SPECT/CT in differentiated thyroid cancer. Nucl Med Commun 2012;33:787–798.
24 Kunstman JW, Kirsch JD, Mahajan A, Udelsman R: Clinical review: parathyroid localization and implications for clinical management. J Clin Endocrinol Metab 2013;98:902–912.
25 Fakhran S, Branstetter BF 4th, Pryma DA: Parathyroid imaging. Neuroimaging Clin N Am 2008;18:537–549.
26 Hoang JK, Sung WK, Bahl M, Phillips CD: How to perform parathyroid 4D CT: tips and traps for technique and interpretation. Radiology 2014;270:15–24.
27 Ellika S, Patel S, Aho T, Marin H: Preoperative localization of parathyroid adenomas using 4-dimensional computed tomography: a pictorial essay. Can Assoc Radiol J 2013;64:258–268.
28 Hunter GJ, Schellingerhout D, Vu TH, Perrier ND, Hamberg LM: Accuracy of four-dimensional CT for the localization of abnormal parathyroid glands in patients with primary hyperparathyroidism. Radiology 2012;264:789–795.
29 Rodgers SE, Hunter GJ, Hamberg LM, Schellingerhout D, Doherty DB, Ayers GD, Shapiro SE, Edeiken BS, Truong MT, Evans DB, Lee JE, Perrier ND: Improved preoperative planning for directed parathyroidectomy with 4-dimensional computed tomography. Surgery 2006;140:932–940.

30 Mortenson MM, Evans DB, Lee JE, Hunter GJ, Shellingerhout D, Vu T, Edeiken BS, Feng L, Perrier ND: Parathyroid exploration in the reoperative neck: improved preoperative localization with 4D-computed tomography. J Am Coll Surg 2008; 206:888–895.

31 Starker LF, Mahajan A, Bjorklund P, Sze G, Udelsman R, Carling T: 4D parathyroid CT as the initial localization study for patients with de novo primary hyperparathyroidism. Ann Surg Oncol 2011; 18:1723–1728.

32 Phillips CD, Shatzkes DR: Imaging of the parathyroid glands. Semin Ultrasound CT MR 2012;33: 123–129.

33 Kang YS, Rosen K, Clark OH, Higgins CB: Localization of abnormal parathyroid glands of the mediastinum with MR imaging. Radiology 1993;189: 137–141.

34 Gotway MB, Reddy GP, Webb WR, Morita ET, Clark OH, Higgins CB: Comparison between MR imaging and ^{99m}Tc MIBI scintigraphy in the evaluation of recurrent of persistent hyperparathyroidism. Radiology 2001;218:783–790.

Melanie Richards, MD
Department of Surgery, Mayo Clinic
200 First Street SW
Rochester, MN 55905 (USA)
E-Mail richards.melanie@mayo.edu

Buchfelder M, Guaraldi F (eds): Imaging in Endocrine Disorders.
Front Horm Res. Basel, Karger, 2016, vol 45, pp 24–36 (DOI: 10.1159/000442275)

Role of Nuclear Medicine in the Diagnosis of Benign Thyroid Diseases

Sara Garberoglio[a] · Ornella Testori[b]

[a]Servizio di Endocrinologia, Ospedale Privato Sedes Sapientiae, Turin, and [b]Reparto di Medicina Nucleare, Azienda Ospedaliera Nazionale SS Antonio e Biagio e Cesare Arrigo di Alessandria, Alessandria, Italy

Abstract

A deep understanding of thyroid pathophysiology is the basis for diagnosing and treating benign thyroid diseases with radioactive materials, known as radiopharmaceuticals, which are introduced into the body by injection or orally. After the radiotracer administration, the patient becomes the emitting source, and several devices have been studied to detect and capture these emissions (gamma or beta-negative) and transform them into photons, parametric images, numbers and molecular information. Thyroid scintigraphy is the only technique that allows the assessment of thyroid regional function and, therefore, the detection of areas of autonomously functioning thyroid nodules. Scintigraphy visualizes the distribution of active thyroid tissue and displays the differential accumulation of radionuclides in the investigated cells, thus providing a functional map. Moreover, this technique is a fundamental tool in the clinical and surgical management of thyroid diseases, including: single thyroid nodules with a suppressed thyroid-stimulating hormone level, for which fine-needle aspiration biopsy (FNAB) is used to identify hot nodules; multinodular goiters, especially larger ones, to identify cold or indeterminate areas requiring FNAB and hot areas that do not need cytologic evaluation, and to evaluate mediastinal extension; the diagnosis of ectopic thyroid tissue; subclinical hyperthyroidism to identify occult hyperfunctioning tissue; follicular lesions to identify a functioning cellular adenoma that could be benign, although such nodules are mostly cold on scintigraphy; to distinguish low-uptake from high-uptake thyrotoxicosis, and to determine eligibility for radioiodine therapy.

© 2016 S. Karger AG, Basel

The thyroid gland is uniquely able to take up iodine, an essential component of its hormones, from the environment and to concentrate it thousands of times. This phenomenon allowed the use of iodine isotopes in the diagnosis of thyroid diseases as early as about 70 years ago, although the mechanism of iodine uptake at the molecular level was not carefully examined until the late twentieth century. In 1939, a group of scientists from the University of Berkeley documented the uptake of radioactive iodine in human thyroid for the first time. This led to the first therapeutic radioiodine applications in patients with hyperthyroidism and thyroid cancer [1–3].

Nowadays, we know that the uptake of iodine in the thyroid gland is attributed to the sodium-iodide symporter (NIS) [1], described in 1993 by Kaminsky et al. [4]. The uptake of iodine by the thyroid cells is still widely used in the evaluation of thyroid function by means of a radioiodine uptake test and thyroid scintigraphy [1, 5, 6].

Clinical practice in thyroid benign diseases should be based on international guidelines. The most prominent and recent of these (2010) resulted from a consensus among the AACE (American Association of Clinical Endocrinologist), AME (Associazione Medici Endocrinologi, the Italian Association of Endocrinologists), ETA (European Thyroid Association) and other leading endocrinologists in the field of thyroid diseases.

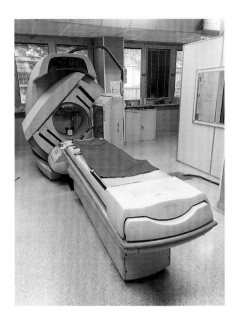

Fig. 1. SPECT scanner (image courtesy of Division of Nuclear Medicine, Azienda Ospedaliera Città della Salute e della Scienza of Turin, Turin, Italy).

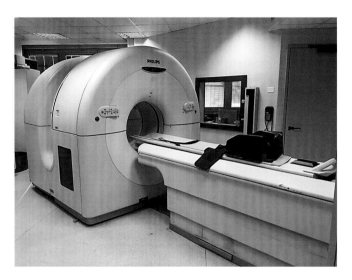

Fig. 2. PET-CT scanner (image courtesy of Division of Nuclear Medicine, Azienda Ospedaliera Città della Salute e della Scienza of Turin, Turin, Italy).

The AACE protocol for the standardized production of clinical practice guidelines followed to rate the evidence level of each reference (on a scale of 1–4) and to link the guidelines to the strength of recommendations on the basis of grade designations from A (action based on strong evidence) through to D (action not based on any evidence or not recommended). The best evidence level (BEL), corresponding to the best conclusive evidence found, accompanies the recommendation grade. Some recommendations were upgraded or downgraded on the basis of expert opinion [7, 8].

Nuclear Medicine: Radiopharmacology and Methods

A deep understanding of thyroid pathophysiology is the basis for diagnosing and treating benign thyroid diseases with radioactive materials, known as radiopharmaceuticals, which are introduced into the body by injection or swallowing. In the body, the radioactive tracers are able to trace the fate of the nonradioactive analogue substances – with whom they share mechanical, chemical or biological properties – and finally bind the receptors with high sensitivity and without perturbing body homeostasis. At the same time, being radioactive, radioactive tracers can be easily detected. Several radiopharmaceuticals can be used, and different devices have been studied to record their emissions.

Devices

Following radiotracer administration the patient becomes the emitting source. Several devices have been studied to detect and capture these emissions (gamma, beta-negative, beta-positive) and transform them into photons, parametric images, numbers and molecular information, including:
- rectilinear scanner, the oldest imaging device, no longer used;
- gamma camera planar scanner, the most commonly used nuclear medicine device for the diagnosis of benign thyroid disease as it can give segmental 2D images, whole-body reconstructions and dynamic acquisitions;
- SPECT scanner, a 3D tomographic device that uses gamma camera data from many projections, reconstructed in different planes (fig. 1); it can be CT-aided;
- PET-CT scanner, CT-aided positron emission tomography (PET; fig. 2);

– uptake probe with a multichannel analyzer for gamma emission quantitation.

Nuclear medicine images can be superimposed with tomographic imaging (CT) or magnetic resonance imaging to produce special views in a practice known as image fusion or coregistration. These views allow the information from two different exams to be correlated and interpreted in one image, leading to more precise information and accurate diagnoses.

Radiopharmaceuticals

The most used radiopharmaceuticals in diagnostic thyroid imaging are radioiodines (^{123}I, ^{131}I) and technetium pertechnetate (technetium-99m; ^{99m}Tc). They can be administered intravenously, which is more suitable for uptake measurements, or orally. Each of these imaging agents has some advantage and disadvantages.

Technetium-99m

^{99m}Tc is usually administered intravenously in the form of ^{99m}TcO$_4$Na (sodium pertechnetate) obtained from a molybdenum-technetium generator. The advantages of ^{99m}Tc include the high availability in nuclear medicine departments, the low energy of the gamma photons (140 keV) and the relatively short half-life (6 h). These characteristics make it possible to use much higher activity than ^{131}I at a lower cost, to register more accurate images in a shorter acquisition time and (last but not least) with an absorbed dose much lower than with the diagnostic ^{131}I activity [1, 9, 10].

^{99m}Tc is iodomimetic which means that it is transported and captured into thyroid cells in a similar way as the isotopes of iodine, i.e. by the means of NIS. The maximal accumulation of ^{99m}Tc-pertechnetate is obtained 15–20 min after intravenous administration. In this initial phase, the increase of ^{99m}Tc activity in the thyroid runs parallel to the increase of activity of intravenous ^{123}I. The percentage of ^{99m}Tc accumulated in thyrocytes reflects the dynamics of the absorption of iodine to the thyroid tissue. After 15–30 min, however, the curve of the thyroid ^{99m}Tc activity reaches a plateau and then decreases, while the uptake of iodine is still increasing. This results from the fact that the ^{99m}Tc-pertechnetate is not subject to organification (as in the case of iodine), and is washed out from the thyrocytes.

Measurement of Technetium Uptake

In some centers great attention is given to the evaluation of ^{99m}Tc uptake in the thyroid. The concept of this measurement is based on the assumption that the uptake of ^{99m}Tc by thyrocytes takes place using the same mechanism as with iodine. Under the conditions of euthyroidism, with normal iodine intake, the maximum uptake of ^{99m}Tc is 0.5–2.0% of the administered activity. As in the case of iodine uptake, this percentage is lower in hypothyroidism, iodine contamination and subacute thyroiditis, while it is higher in Graves' disease and in iodine deficiency. This measurement is simple and is performed as a supplement of thyroid scintigraphy by comparing the number of counts in the thyroid with the number of counts above the syringe containing the ^{99m}Tc-pertechnetate prior to injection (both corrected by background subtraction); more precise information is given by uptake probes [1, 9, 10].

Iodine Isotopes: ^{123}I and ^{131}I

^{123}I is a pure gamma emitter with relatively low energy (159 keV) and a short half-life (13 h) of gamma photons; the physical properties are largely similar to ^{99m}Tc. The advantage of ^{123}I is the higher specificity and persistence of accumulation in the thyroid due to the organification that allows later acquisitions and careful assessment of iodine kinetics in the thyroid tissue. Compared with ^{99m}Tc, ^{123}I provides more detailed images with a clear demarcation of the thyroid tissue from surrounding tissues, consequently allowing a better visualization of retrosternal thyroid tissue and of the thyroid gland when thyroid uptake is low. Moreover, the real iodine turnover in the thyroid can be assessed, while ^{99m}Tc uptake is a surrogate parameter. However, ^{123}I availability is low because it is produced using a cyclotron and has high costs, so it is not available in all institutions for routine use [1, 7, 10–12].

^{131}I is the most commonly used radioactive isotope of iodine, it emits beta and gamma radiations with a half-life of 8.1 days. Its gamma rays, used for diagnostic purposes, have higher energy than ^{99m}Tc and ^{123}I (364 keV). As a result, ^{131}I scintigraphy should be limited to:
– the monitoring of treatment in patients with differentiated thyroid cancer;
– the imaging of ectopic thyroid (i.e. retrosternal or lingual thyroid, and stuma ovarii);
– dosimetric pretreatment evaluations;
– kinetic studies in dishormonogenetic pathologies (see the next chapter) [1, 6, 9, 10].

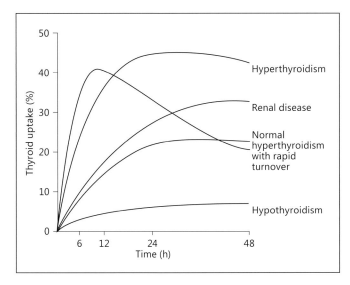

Fig. 3. Measurement of iodine uptake; RAIU in health and disease. Examples of thyroidal RAIU curves under various pathological conditions. Note the prolonged uptake in renal disease due to decreased urinary excretion of the isotope and the early decline in thyroidal radioiodine content in some patients with thyrotoxicosis associated with a small but rapidly overturning intrathyroidal iodine pool (from www.thyroidmanager.org/chapter/evaluation-of-thyroid-function-in-health-and-disease/).

Measurement of Iodine Uptake

The iodine uptake test (RAIU; fig. 3) is performed using a gamma camera or a gamma probe positioned at a fixed distance from the patient's neck. Measurements are performed at various intervals after oral administration of 1–3.7 MBq (30–100 µCi) of ^{131}I. Measures in the first 24 h are essential for the assessment of the maximal iodine accumulation in the thyroid. Therefore, for practical reasons, measurements are often performed at 1, 2, 6 and 24 h after administration of the diagnostic amount of ^{131}I. The test is mainly performed in patients planned for radioiodine treatment due to hyperthyroidism. For dosimetric purposes, it is essential to know the residence time of ^{131}I in the thyroid tissue, so measurements are performed on several consecutive days [1, 9].

Iodine uptake is a parameter with a relatively high variability. On average, in euthyroid patients the uptake is 25–50% 24 h after the administration of the diagnostic activity. It may be higher in hyperthyroidism and lower in hypothyroidism. Apart from the thyroid functional status, many other (mostly iatrogenic) factors may influence the level of thyroid iodine uptake [1].

Thyroid Scintigraphy

Thyroid scintigraphy is the only technique that allows the assessment of thyroid regional function and detection of areas of autonomously functioning thyroid nodules (AFTNs) [7, 10]. Scintigraphy visualizes the distribution of active thyroid tissue and displays the differential accumulation of radionuclides in the investigated cells, thus providing a functional map [1, 9]. Moreover, this technique is a fundamental tool in the clinical and surgical management of thyroid diseases [6].

The most used radionuclides in scintigraphy, according to the AACE/AME/ETA guidelines, are ^{123}I or ^{99m}Tc (grade B; BEL 3). ^{131}I thyroid uptake is not recommended for routine diagnostic use unless low-uptake thyrotoxicosis is suspected (grade A; BEL 3) or for dosimetric appraisal before therapy with ^{131}I (fig. 4a, b).

At a fixed interval (usually 15–120 min) after iodine administration, the patient is placed in a sitting or reclining position to obtain planar images. Anatomical landmarks are achieved by placing a marker over the sternal notch.

While interpreting a thyroid scintigraphy the physician should be aware of possible pitfalls as a considerable number of cases of unexpected radioiodine uptake have been reported [1, 9, 10, 13]. Although the exact mechanisms are not fully understood, several hypothesis have been postulated, including:

- functional NIS expression in normal tissues, including thymus, breast, salivary glands, gastrointestinal tract, or various benign and malignant tumors;
- metabolism of radioiodinated thyroid hormones;
- retention or contamination by radioiodinated body fluids (i.e. saliva, tears, blood, urine, exudate, transudate, gastric and mucosal secretions, etc.);
- retention and uptake of radioiodine in inflamed tissues;
- thyroid metastasis.

Moreover, activity in vascular structures can give a poor image quality when uptake is low, which is why ^{123}I scintiscans have a higher diagnostic power than ^{99m}Tc [7]. The physician must also be aware of concomitant conditions that can affect diagnosis [1], including:

- history of thyroid disease;
- ultrasound (US) image or report;
- current thyroid-stimulating hormone (TSH) levels;
- therapies, in particular thyroid hormones, antithyroid drugs and iodine-containing agents (amiodarone, disinfectant and expectorant drugs).

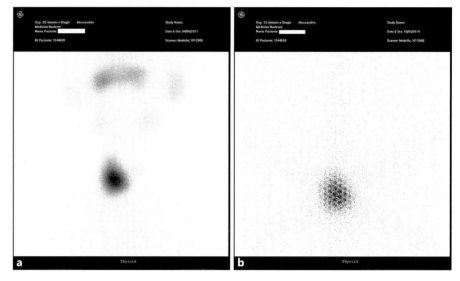

Fig. 4. AFTN ^{99m}Tc scintiscan (**a**), ^{131}I scintiscan (**b**). Image courtesy of Dr. A. Muni, Service of Nuclear Medicine, Alessandria Hospital, Alessandria, Italy.

The report of a thyroid scan should contain:
– the location of thyroid tissue (normal, ectopic, retrosternal goiter);
– the structure and size of the gland (symmetry of the lobes, eventually pyramidal lobe) – it should be noted that scintigraphy is not able to accurately determine the diameters of the thyroid lobes, especially in the sagittal axis (thickness); therefore, the description of size should be limited to reporting a clear deviation from normal;
– the tracer distribution in the thyroid, foci of increased or decreased tracer accumulation (warm, hot or cold nodules), correlating with the physical examination of the neck [1];
– an appraisal of the thyroid to background ratio – a depressed ratio is the functional image of depressed thyroid uptake or of depressed renal function;
– an appraisal of the thyroid to salivary gland ratio – the normal ratio is about 3:1; if less, it can be due to iodine contamination, hypotrophy or inflammation.

Other Thyroid Examinations and Tests

^{99m}Tc-MIBI Scintigraphy

There have been some reports of the utility of thyroid imaging using methoxyisobutylisonitrile (^{99m}Tc-MIBI) in the past decades. Uptake of this tracer in the mitochondria of cancer cells is associated with an increased number and activity of mitochondria, as well as with increased perfusion of the lesion. It has been suggested that the ^{99m}Tc-MIBI scan should be used in cases of inconclusive biopsy and/or cold nodule. Clinical trials have not yielded conclusive results and, therefore, this method was not included in the guidelines of the management of thyroid nodular disease. There are, however, data indicating that a negative scintigraphy using ^{99m}Tc-MIBI practically excludes malignancy [1].

Positron Emission Tomography with ^{18}F-FDG

PET with ^{18}F-FDG is widely employed in the diagnosis of advanced differentiated thyroid carcinoma. The diagnosis of benign thyroid disease using PET is not recommended routinely, but there are clinical situations in which a thyroid problem is detected incidentally on a PET/CT scan performed for other reasons. The normal thyroid does not utilize glucose. ^{18}F-FDG uptake in the thyroid gland is observed in approximately 2% of PET studies [1, 14, 15]. It can be either focal or diffuse. Retrospective studies performed on thousands of PET and PET/CT images showed that the probability of thyroid cancer in cases of incidentally detected focal metabolic activity in the thyroid (so-called incidentalomas) varies from 27 to 47% [1, 16] (fig. 5). On the other hand, diffuse, moderate accumulation of ^{18}F-FDG in the entire gland indicates an inflammatory process, usually associated with chronic Hashimoto thyroiditis [1].

In summary, according to the AACE/AME/ETA guidelines, incidentalomas detected by PET with ^{18}F-FDG should undergo US evaluation plus US-guided fine-needle aspiration biopsy (FNAB) because of the high risk of malignancy (grade C; BEL 3), while in cases of diffuse ^{18}F-FDG uptake, TSH and thyroid antibody (AbTPO, AbTg) measurements

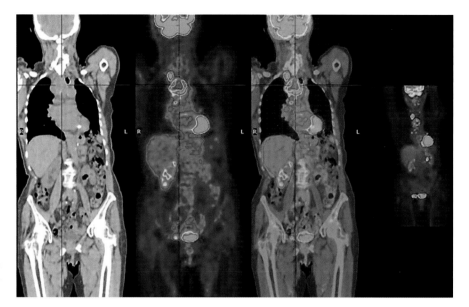

Fig. 5. PET imaging, coronal slices. Thyroid incidentaloma of the right lobe, 'hot' on an 18F-FDG scan performed for another cause. Image courtesy of Dr. A. Muni, Service of Nuclear Medicine, Alessandria Hospital, Alessandria, Italy.

are recommended [1, 7]. A scan with 18F-FDG is recommended in advanced differentiated thyroid carcinoma (lesions positive to FDG and negative to iodine predict a poor outcome) [17].

Suppression Thyroid Scintigraphy
The aim of a suppression scan is to visualize autonomous thyroid tissue, i.e. functioning independently of the hypothalamic-pituitary-thyroid axis. This test was widely employed in earlier decades before the ultrasensitive TSH (1986). It involves the performance of thyroid scintigraphy with a radioiodine uptake measurement before and after the administration of triiodothyronine or thyroxine preparation for 7–14 days; the recommended daily dose is 80 μg of L-triiodothyronine or 150 μg of levothyroxine.

In a normal gland, administered thyroid hormone decreases the radioactive iodine accumulation by at least 50%. No change or a reduction of iodine uptake of less than 30% indicates the autonomous process. This test can also be done by measuring 99mTc uptake instead of iodine. An autonomous nodule that is warm at the baseline image converts to a hot nodule as the surrounding normal tissue becomes suppressed. Therefore, in some centers, a suppression test is also used in preparation for radioiodine treatment of a nontoxic nodular goiter [1, 9, 10].

Potassium Perchlorate Test
The potassium perchlorate test is used to evaluate disorders of iodine organification. In normal conditions after the in-

flux into the cell via NIS, the iodide ions are rapidly oxidized by thyroid peroxidase and are subsequently incorporated into tyrosyl residues of thyroglobulin. This process takes no more than 2–3 h [1, 10]. In the case of an organification defect (peroxidase defect in Pendred syndrome), free iodine, which has not been organified, is washed out from the cell. Potassium perchlorate inhibits the NIS activity, reducing the flow of iodide into the cell. Thus, in cases of deficient peroxidase, the content of iodine in the thyroid gland is reduced after administration of perchlorate because of iodine washout. The test consists of iodine uptake measurement 2–3 h after intravenous injection of 123I or oral administration of 131I, followed by a subsequent measurement 2 h after oral administration of potassium or sodium perchlorate. A decrease in iodine uptake by 20% confirms the organification defect. In healthy subjects iodine uptake after administration of perchlorate should not be reduced [1, 9].

Diagnostic Provisional Dosimetry
Dosimetry in nuclear medicine is the measurement and calculation of the absorbed dose in tissues resulting from the exposure to indirect and direct ionizing radiation after the incorporation of radionuclides. The dose is reported in gray units (Gy) for mass. The radiation dose refers to the amount of energy deposited in matter and its biological effect on living tissue, and should not be confused with activity, measured in units of Curie or Becquerel. Incorporation of a radionuclide will give a dose which is dependent on the activity, time of exposure and energy of the

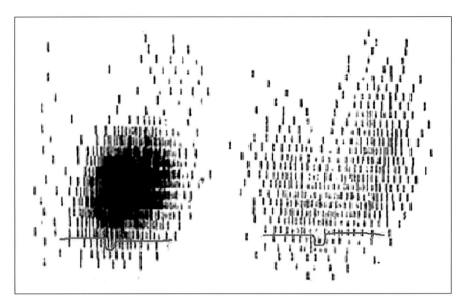

Fig. 6. AFTNs before (left) and 1 year after ^{131}I therapy (right). After treatment, the abnormal focal accumulation in the left lobe was decreased and the extranodal uptake was no longer inhibited. Image courtesy of Dr. A. Muni, Service of Nuclear Medicine, Alessandria Hospital, Alessandria, Italy.

radiation emitted. The dose equivalent is then dependent upon the additional assignment of weighting factors describing biological effects for different kinds of radiation on different organs (www.dm.usda.gov/ohsec/rsd/dosimetry.htm). Dosimetry is employed in order to give a dose as low as reasonably achievable in diagnostic and therapeutic nuclear medicine (ALARA: as low as reasonably achievable) [18].

Radioiodine is indicated for the treatment of hyperthyroidism attributable to a hyperfunctioning nodule or a toxic multinodular goiter (MNG) [7, 19]. The aims of radioiodine treatment are the ablation of the autonomously functioning areas, the achievement of euthyroidism in MGN and the reduction of goiter size [7, 19]. Indications are a hyperfunctioning and/or symptomatic goiter, previous thyroid surgery or surgical risk (grade B; BEL 2; fig. 6).

AFTNs are usually more radioresistant than toxic diffuse goiters and higher radiation activities may be needed for successful treatment, especially in countries with iodization programs leading to decreased uptake of radioactive iodine [7, 20, 21]. Radioiodine therapy normalizes thyroid function in 85–100% of patients with hyperfunctioning thyroid nodules or toxic MNGs [7, 21]. After treatment, the thyroid volume generally decreases substantially (median decrease 35% at 3 months and 45% at 24 months) [7]. Radioiodine treatment is generally effective and safe. Although some investigators have indicated that radioiodine treatment may be associated with an increased cardiovascular and cancer mortality, other large-scale epidemiologic studies have dem-

onstrated discordant results [7]. After ablation of the autonomous tissue, most patients become euthyroid because of residual normal thyroid tissue, which is no longer suppressed. Nevertheless, depending on the amount of radioiodine used, follow-up of thyroid function and the possible presence of autoimmune thyroiditis, postradioiodine hypothyroidism may develop in up to 60% after 20 years [7, 22]. In up to 5% of patients immunogenic hyperthyroidism may result from radioiodine treatment of toxic or nontoxic nodular goiter because of induction of TSH-receptor antibodies (TRAbs) [7]. This typically occurs 3–6 months after radioiodine treatment and could be due to initially undetectable TRAbs in Graves' disease [7]. Radioiodine treatment is best suited for small- to medium-sized benign goiters, for patients previously treated surgically, for those with serious comorbidities or for patients refusing surgery [7, 23].

Ablative approaches using radioiodine are effective for the treatment of Graves' disease, but their ophthalmologic and biological autoimmune responses remain controversial. Therefore, it is not proposed as a first-line treatment, but it can be the choice when hyperthyroidism is not controlled or recurs after initial antithyroid drug treatment, and when surgery is contraindicated or refused [24, 25].

Therapeutic dosing of radioiodine remains controversial, and fixed and calculated activities have been proposed. The fixed activity implies the risk of over- or undertreatment: the first induces useless hyperradiation to normal tissues and should be avoided; the second fails to cure hyperthyroidisms, which impairs health, creates disability and, occasionally, poses a risk to life as the disorder should be eliminated as soon as possible. Calculated activity needs US estimation of volume (corrected by scintigraphic assessment of the functional areas), and measurements of the maximum thyroid uptake and of the mean residence time. These measurements are not time or cost consuming, and assure healing in 86% of patients at the first administration cycle, avoiding overtreatment [26].

Benign Thyroid Diseases and Indications for Nuclear Medicine Tests

Thyroid Embryology, Anatomy and Physiology

The vascular thyroid gland develops from the ventral wall of the pharynx and grows caudally from the base of the tongue (the foramen cecum) to approximately the level of the cricoid cartilage at the base of the neck. The thyroglossal duct usually obliterates during fetal development. A narrow isthmus connects the lower thirds of the two lobes. A pyramidal lobe, representing the caudal end of the thyroglossal duct, is sometimes present, extending from the isthmus or the medial portion of one of the lobes superiorly [6].

Thyroid Dysgenesis

Thyroid scintigraphy is a tool to evaluate congenital hypothyroidism. Early treatment of congenital hypothyroidism is necessary for normal development and intelligence. Therefore, heel stick blood screening for abnormal plasma levels of T4 and/or TSH is performed. Neonates with abnormal hormone levels can have thyroid imaging to establish the etiology. There are three typical abnormal scintigraphic patterns:

- visualization of ectopic tissue;
- lack of visualization of the gland;
- markedly increased trapping in the normal thyroid location due to dyshormonogenesis.

Lack of visualization of the gland is the most common pattern. In the majority of cases it indicates agenesis, although it can be detected in transient hypothyroidism secondary to maternal antibodies or mild dyshormonogenesis. Occasionally, thyroid imaging is normal, implying a false positive blood test and prompting reevaluation [1, 6, 27].

Moreover, scintigraphic imaging allows the detection of ectopic thyroid tissue. The thyroid gland sometimes fails to descend completely resulting in rests of tissue along its course. This can result in a lingual thyroid, a prominent pyramidal lobe or other ectopic tissue. Midline ectopic activity usually represents a lingual thyroid rest. Rarely, the thyroid gland can descend beyond its normal location, finally residing in the chest [6].

A rare form of ectopy is struma ovarii, a monodermal teratoma that contains mostly thyroid tissue and may cause hyperthyroidism. In this case the thyroid can be easily detected by US, while it is silent in scintigraphy because the uptake is blocked.

Dysfunctional Thyroid Disorders

Nuclear medicine can be used for the evaluation of hyperthyroidism and thyrotoxicosis. The term 'thyrotoxicosis' refers to a clinical state that results from high thyroid hormone action in tissues, generally due to high tissue thyroid hormone levels, with different possible etiologies, manifestations and potential therapies [8]. In general, thyrotoxicosis can occur if:

- the thyroid is inappropriately stimulated by trophic factors;
- there is a constitutive activation of thyroid hormone synthesis and secretion leading to autonomous release of excess thyroid hormone;
- thyroid stores of preformed hormone are passively released in excessive amounts, owing to autoimmune, infectious, chemical or mechanical insult;
- there is exposure to extrathyroidal sources of thyroid hormone, either endogenous (struma ovarii, metastatic differentiated thyroid cancer, subacute thyroiditis) or exogenous (factitious thyrotoxicosis) [8].

Quantitative ^{99m}Tc scintigraphy (the calculation of technetium thyroid uptake under suppression) is a sensitive and specific technique for the diagnosis and quantitation of thyroid autonomy and is a reliable predictor of hyperthyroidism in the setting of euthyroid autonomy [7, 10]. Many clinical forms characterized by both hyperthyroidism and thyrotoxicosis or just by thyrotoxicosis can be distinguished.

In the first scenario, a thyrotoxicosis may be associated with thyroid hyperfunction, with a normal or elevated radioiodine uptake over the neck, in the following conditions [8]:

- toxic diffuse goiter (Graves' disease);
- toxic MNG;
- toxic adenoma;
- trophoblastic disease;
- TSH-producing pituitary adenomas;

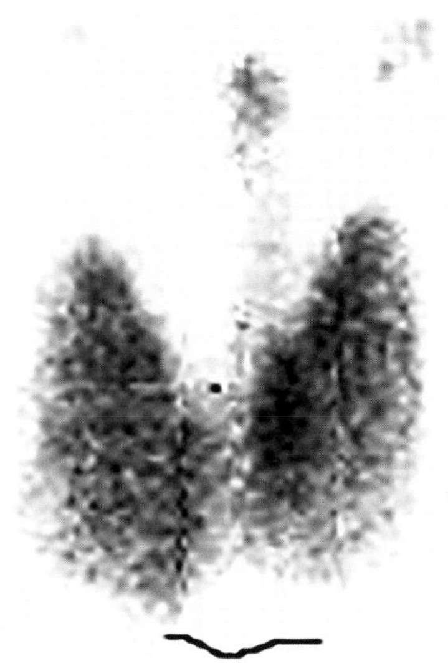

Fig. 7. Toxic MNG with depressed uptake due to excessive iodine supply. Image courtesy of Dr. A. Muni, Service of Nuclear Medicine, Alessandria Hospital, Alessandria, Italy.
Fig. 8. Graves' disease with an enlarged gland and increased trapping and visualization of the pyramidal lobe. Image courtesy of Dr. A. Muni, Service of Nuclear Medicine, Alessandria Hospital, Alessandria, Italy.

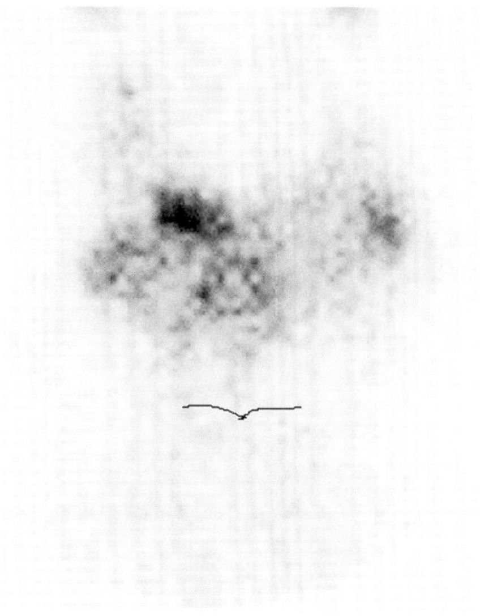

– resistance to thyroid hormone (T3 receptor mutation).

In the second scenario, a thyrotoxicosis without thyroid hyperfunction associated with a near-absent radioiodine uptake over the neck is related to the following diseases [8]:
– painless (silent) thyroiditis;
– amiodarone-induced thyroiditis;
– subacute (granulomatous, de Quervain's) thyroiditis;
– iatrogenic thyrotoxicosis;
– factitious ingestion of thyroid hormone;
– struma ovarii;
– acute thyroiditis;
– extensive metastases from follicular thyroid cancer.

In cases of nodular hyperthyroidism the execution of scintigraphy is indicated. In cases of nonnodular hyperthyroidism the scintigraphy can be useful to discriminate between hyperthyroidism with low or high uptake, and to evaluate the dosimetric parameters and eligibility to therapy with ^{131}I.

The differential diagnosis of thyrotoxicosis can quickly be narrowed with ^{99m}Tc imaging; a 'cold' or poorly visualized gland is most likely iatrogenic or subacute/silent thyroiditis, multinodular localization is most likely toxic MNG (fig. 7) and a diffusely 'hot' gland is most likely Graves' disease [6] (fig. 8).

The diagnosis of Graves' disease does not exclude the presence of thyroid nodules. Hyperthyroidism of autoimmune origin with the presence of focal lesions, cold at ^{99m}Tc, is known as Marine-Lenhart syndrome (fig. 9). Thyroid scintigraphy in this syndrome is of particular value since the risk of thyroid cancer is higher than in a cold nodule without autoimmune thyroid disease – the cancer risk is estimated to be 15–19% [1]. In addition, thyroid cancer coexisting with Graves' disease is clinically more aggressive and requiring of more complex management [1, 28].

In countries without dietary iodine deficiency, as in the USA and in northern Europe, Graves' disease (toxic diffuse goiter) represents the most common cause of hyperthyroidism. It is an autoimmune disorder in which thyrotropin receptor antibodies (TRAbs) stimulate the TSH receptor, increasing thyroid hormone production.

Instead, the natural history of nodular thyroid disease includes growth of established nodules, new nodule formation and the development of autonomy over time [6, 8]. Hormone production may progress from subclinical to overt hyperthyroidism, and the administration of pharmacological amounts of iodine to such patients may result in iodine-induced hyperthyroidism [8]. Thyroid hormones are elevated, suppressing TSH, and the RAIU is elevated. It is important to obtain the TSH level because early Hashimoto's thyroiditis could also demonstrate an increased RAIU, mimicking Graves' disease, but in Hashimoto's disease TSH is increased. Hashimoto's disease could also sometimes demonstrate thyroid hormone release secondary to inflammation ('hashitoxicosis'), with inhibited TSH. In this scenario, the RAIU is usually decreased, as it is in the late stages of Hashimoto's thyroiditis, secondary to gland destruction [6].

Although toxic nodular goiter is less common than Graves' disease in young people, its prevalence increases

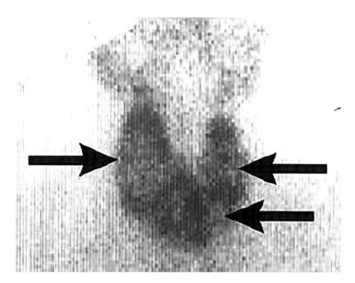

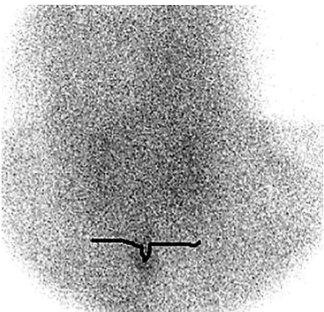

Fig. 9. Marine-Lenhart syndrome. The anterior ⁹⁹ᵐTc-pertechnetate image shows an enlarged thyroid with diffusely increased radiotracer trapping, as in Graves' disease. However, within the gland are distinct cold nodules (arrows). Reproduced from Intenzo et al. [31].

Fig. 10. Subacute thyroiditis. Image courtesy of Dr. A. Muni, Service of Nuclear Medicine, Alessandria Hospital, Alessandria, Italy.

with age and in the presence of iodine deficiency. Therefore, toxic nodular goiter is actually more common than Graves' disease in older patients living in areas with iodine deficiency [8].

Several varieties of thyroiditis can present with thyrotoxicosis, including postpartum thyroiditis, painless thyroiditis, drug-induced thyroiditis, subacute thyroiditis, traumatic thyroiditis and acute thyroiditis. In general, thyroid dysfunction caused by thyroiditis is less severe than that seen with other forms of endogenous thyrotoxicosis; the RAIU is universally low during the thyrotoxic stage, owing to the leaking of thyroid hormone with suppression of serum TSH concentrations [8].

The diagnosis of subacute thyroiditis in a thyrotoxic patient should be based on clinical history, physical examination and the RAIU (fig. 10). Subacute thyroiditis, which probably is secondary to viral illness, presents with moderate-to-severe pain in the thyroid, often radiating to the mastoids, ears, jaw or throat. Patients may have malaise, low-grade fever and fatigue in addition to the symptoms of thyrotoxicosis. The thyroid is firm and painful to palpation. In addition to laboratory evidence of thyrotoxicosis, the erythrocyte sedimentation rate or C-reactive protein is elevated and mild anemia is common. Thyroid ultrasonography shows diffuse heterogeneity and decreased or normal color-flow Doppler, rather than the enhanced flow characteristic

of Graves' disease [8]. The associated inflammatory process usually has a thyrotoxic phase with low RAIU, often followed by short euthyroid and hypothyroid phases, before recovery. During the hypothyroid phase uptake could be mildly increased, although the gland has not yet regained its efficient hormonogenesis function. A similar triphasic response of thyroid function can be seen with silent (lymphocytic) thyroiditis and postpartum thyroiditis. Postpartum thyroiditis, usually considered a subtype of silent thyroiditis, occurs in 5–10% of pregnancies [1, 6].

Low RAIU is also seen in thyroid hormone ingestion, excess dietary iodine, recent administration of iodinated contrast media, some medications and cosmetics. These can easily be distinguished from subacute or silent thyroiditis because they are biochemically euthyroid or hypothyroid. Amiodarone contains 75 mg of iodine per 200-mg tablet. Amiodarone can cause either hyperthyroidism in patients with preexisting thyroiditis or type I or type II thyrotoxicosis. Type I thyrotoxicosis is caused by excess thyroid hormone synthesis from the high iodine levels. Type II thyrotoxicosis is similar to the destructive release of hormone in subacute thyroiditis. The thyroid scan and uptake will be low in all situations because of the high iodine content of amiodarone [1, 6, 8]. Absent uptake in the neck in a patient with thyrotoxicosis can also be seen with struma ovarii and metastatic follicular thyroid carcinoma [6, 27].

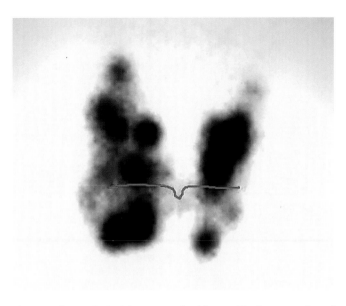

Fig. 11. A large MNG with warm and cold areas. The lower portion of the gland penetrates into the superior mediastinum. Image courtesy of Dr. A. Muni, Head Nuclear Medicine at Alessandria Hospital, Italy.

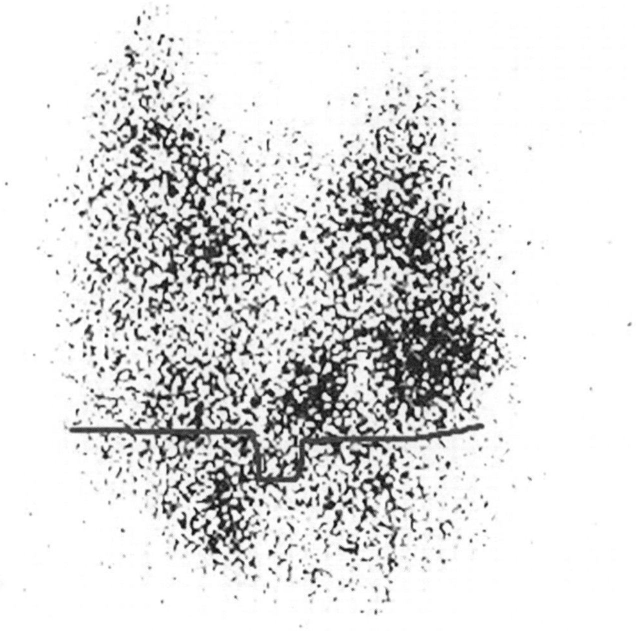

Fig. 12. ^{99m}Tc thyroid scintiscan of a retrosternal goiter. The depressed thyroid to background ratio and the depressed thyroid to salivary gland ratio are due to an excessive iodine supply. Image courtesy of Dr. A. Muni, Head Nuclear Medicine at Alessandria Hospital, Italy.

Nodular Thyroid Diseases

According to the AACE/AME/ETA guidelines scintigraphy is recommended in all cases of thyroid nodule or MNG if the TSH level is below the lower limit of the reference range or if ectopic thyroid tissue or a retrosternal goiter is suspected (grade B; BEL 3; fig. 11, 12). In iodine-deficient regions a scintigraphy should be considered to exclude autonomy of a thyroid nodule or MNG, even if TSH is normal (grade C; BEL 3). On the basis of the pattern of radionuclide uptake, nodules may be classified as hyperfunctioning ('hot'), hypofunctioning ('cold') or indeterminate [7, 10]. Hot nodules almost never represent clinically significant malignant lesions, whereas cold or indeterminate nodules have a reported malignancy risk of 3–15% [7, 29]. As most thyroid lesions are cold or indeterminate, and only a minority of them are malignant, the predictive value of hypofunctioning or indeterminate nodules for the presence of malignant involvement is low [7]. The diagnostic specificity is further decreased in small lesions (<1 cm) that are below the resolution threshold of scintigraphy [7, 10, 30]. The role of scintigraphy in the diagnostic workup of thyroid nodules is limited in countries with iodine-rich diets, in which serum TSH measurement and thyroid US can correctly diagnose autonomous nodules in most patients [7, 30] and FNAB facilitates accurate diagnosis of a malignant lesion [7]. Moreover, because the resolution of US is con-

siderably greater than that of scintigraphy, radionuclide scanning has little place in the topographic assessment of nodular goiter and no place in the measurement of thyroid nodules. However, in areas with iodine deficiency, thyroid scintigraphy is used as part of the evaluation of patients with MNG [7, 10] because it provides useful information on the functional characterization of thyroid nodules. It allows the early diagnosis of thyroid autonomy and prioritization of cold and indeterminate nodules in MNGs for FNAB [7, 10]. In patients from these regions, the serum TSH may remain unsuppressed even if autonomy is present because of the low proliferation rate of thyroid epithelial cells and the low synthesis rate of thyroid hormones by iodine-depleted thyroid glands [7]. Moreover, in the early phases of autonomy, the bulk of autonomous tissue may be insufficient to suppress the TSH level [7, 10, 27]. The early recognition of autonomous nodules, before they induce the suppression of TSH, enables early treatment to avoid thyroid growth and progression toward manifest hyperthyroidism [7]. Furthermore, in iodine-deficient euthyroid goiters, microscopic areas of hot thyroid tissue contain constitutively activating TSH receptor mutations, which increase the risk of iodine-induced hyperthyroidism [7]. Thyroid scintigraphy should be performed in all patients with nodular goiter undergoing treatment with radioiodine, since it allows the identification of the anatomical distribution of active thyroid tissue, which is important in the selection of therapeutic ^{131}I activity [1].

The scintigraphy allows the assessment of the extension of mediastinal or retrosternal goiter if US is unable to evaluate the lower pole of thyroid gland. Mediastinal masses on chest radiography and CT scan are often substernal goiters. [123]I or ^{131}I are the preferred agent for the characterization of such lesions because of their higher target-to-background ratio, greater tissue specificity and decreased blood pool activity as compared with [99m]Tc [1, 6, 7].

Thyroid Scintigraphy Indications: Summary
Thyroid scintigraphy is indicated in the following settings [1, 6, 7]:
1 – single thyroid nodules with a suppressed TSH level, FNAB is not necessary for hot nodules;
– MNGs, even without suppressed TSH;
– to identify cold or indeterminate areas for FNAB biopsy and hot areas that do not need cytologic evaluation;
2 – large MNGs, especially with substernal extension;
– diagnosis of ectopic thyroid tissue;
– subclinical hyperthyroidism, to identify occult hyperfunctioning tissue;
– follicular lesions, to identify a functioning cellular adenoma that could be benign; however, such nodules are mostly cold on scintigraphy;
– to distinguish low-uptake from high-uptake thyrotoxicosis;
– to determine eligibility for radioiodine therapy.

Acknowledgements

The authors are very grateful to Dr. A. Muni (Head of Nuclear Medicine Unit, Alessandria Hospital, Italy) for image permissions, and to Dr. R. Rossetto Giaccherino (Division of Endocrinology, Diabetes and Metabolism, Città della Salute e della Scienza University Hospital of Turin, Turin, Italy) for her precious support and supervision.

References

1 Czepczynski R: Nuclear medicine in the diagnosis of benign thyroid diseases. Nuclear Med Rev 2012; 15:113–119.

2 Becker DV, Sawin CT: Radioiodine and thyroid disease: the beginning. Semin Nucl Med 1996;26: 155–164.

3 Keston AS, Ball RP, Frantz VK, Palmer WW: Storage of radioactive iodine in a metastasis from thyroid carcinoma. Science 1942;2466:362–363.

4 Kaminsky SM, Levy O, Salvador C, Dai G, Carrasco N: The Na+/I-symporter of the thyroid gland. Soc Gen Physiol Ser 1993;48:251–262.

5 Chung JK: Sodium iodide symporter: its role in nuclear medicine. J Nucl Med 2002;43:1188–1200.

6 Smith JR, Oates E: Radionuclide imaging of the thyroid gland: patterns, pearls, and pitfalls. Clin Nucl Med 2004;29:181–193.

7 Gharib H, Papini E, Paschke R, Duick D, Valcavi R, Hegedüs L, Vitti P: American Association of Clinical Endocrinologists, Associazione Medici Endocrinologi and European Thyroid Association medical guidelines for clinical practice for the diagnosis and management of thyroid nodules. Endocr Pract 2010;16(suppl 1):1–43.

8 Bahn RS, Burch HB, Cooper DS, Garber JR, Greenlee MC, Klein I, Laurberg P, McDougall IR, Montori VM, Rivkees SA, Ross DS, Sosa JA, Stan MN; American Thyroid Association; American Association of Clinical Endocrinologists: Hyperthyroidism and other causes of thyrotoxicosis: management guidelines of the American Thyroid Association and American Association of Clinical Endocrinologists. Endocr Pract 2011;17:456–520.

9 Pfannenstiel P, Hotze LA, Saller B: Schilddrüsenerkrankungen: Diagnose und Therapie. Berliner Med Verlagsanstalt 1997;86–94.

10 Meller J, Becker W: The continuing importance of thyroid scintigraphy in the era of high-resolution ultrasound. Eur J Nucl Med 2002;29(suppl 2):S425–S438.

11 American Thyroid Association (ATA) Guidelines Taskforce on Thyroid Nodules and Differentiated Thyroid Cancer; Cooper DS, Doherty GM, Haugen BR, Kloos RT, Lee SL, Mandel SJ, Mazzaferri EL, McIver B, Pacini F, Schlumberger M, Sherman SI, Steward DL, Tuttle RM: Revised American Thyroid Association management guidelines for patients with thyroid nodules and differentiated thyroid cancer. Thyroid 2009;19:1167–1214.

12 Mansi L, Moncayo R, Cuccurullo V, Dottorini ME, Rambaldi PF: Nuclear medicine in diagnosis, staging and follow-up of thyroid cancer. Q J Nucl Med Mol Imaging 2004;48:82–95.

13 Oh JR, Ahn BC: False-positive uptake on radioiodine whole-body scintigraphy: physiologic and pathologic variants unrelated to thyroid cancer. Am J Nucl Med Mol Imaging 2012;3:362–385.

14 Kresnik E, Gallowitsch HJ, Mikosch P, Stettner H, Igerc I, Gomez I, Kumnig G, Lind P: Fluorine-18-fluorodeoxyglucose positron emission tomography in the preoperative assessment of thyroid nodules in an endemic goiter area. Surgery 2003; 133:294–299.

15 Smith RB, Robinson RA, Hoffman HT, Graham MM: Preoperative FDG-PET imaging to assess the malignant potential of follicular neo- plasms of the thyroid. Otolaryngol Head Neck Surg 2008; 138:101–106.

16 King DL, Stack BC Jr, Spring PM, Walker R, Bodenner DL: Incidence of thyroid carcinoma in fluorodeoxyglucose positron emission tomography-positive thyroid incidentalomas. Otolaryngol Head Neck Surg 2007;137:400–404.

17 Treglia G, Muoio B, Giovanella L, Salvatori M: The role of positron emission tomography and positron emission tomography/computed tomography in thyroid tumours: an overview. Eur Arch Oto-rhinolaryngol 2013;270:1783–1787.

18 Webster EW, et al: A Primer on Low Level Ionizing Radiations and its Biological Effect. AAPM Report 18. New York, American Association of Physicists in Medicine, 1986.

19 Meier DA, Brill DR, Becker DV, Clarke SE, Silberstein EB, Royal HD, Balon HR; Society of Nuclear Medicine: Procedure guideline for therapy of thyroid disease with [131]Iodine. J Nucl Med 2002;43: 856–861.

20 Hegedus L, Bonnema SJ, Bennedbaek FN: Management of simple nodular goiter: current status and future perspectives. Endocr Rev 2003;24:102–132.

21 Reiners C, Schneider P: Radioiodine therapy of thyroid autonomy. Eur J Nucl Med Mol Imaging 2002;29(suppl 2):S471–S478.

22 Ceccarelli C, Bencivelli W, Vitti P, Grasso L, Pinchera A: Outcome of radioiodine-131 therapy in hyperfunctioning thyroid nodules: a 20 years' retrospective study. Clin Endocrinol (Oxf) 2005; 62:331–335.

23 Weetman AP: Radioiodine treatment for benign thyroid disease. Clin Endocrinol (Oxf) 2007;66: 757–764.

24 Nwatsock JF, Taieb D, Tessonnier L, Mancini J, Dong-A-Zok F, Mundler O: Radioiodine thyroid ablation in Graves' hyperthyroidism: merits and pitfalls. World J Nucl Med 2012;11:7–11.

25 Stokkel MP, Handkiewicz Junak D, Lassmann M, Dietlein M, Luster M: EANM procedure guidelines for therapy of benign thyroid disease. Eur J Nucl Med Mol Imaging 2010;37:2218–2228.

26 Sisson JC, Avram AM, Rubello D, Gross MD: Radioiodine treatment of hyperthyroidism: fixed or calculated doses; intelligent design or science? Eur J Nucl Med Mol Imaging 2007;34:1129–1130.

27 Sarkar SD: Benign thyroid disease: what is the role of nuclear medicine? Semin Nucl Med 2006;36: 185–193.

28 David Charkes N: Graves' disease with functioning nodules (Marine-Lenhart syndrome). J Nucl Med 1972;13:885–892.

29 Slowinska-Klencka D, Klencki M, Sporny S, Lewinski A: Fine-needle aspiration biopsy of the thyroid in an area of endemic goiter: influence of restored sufficient iodine supplementation on the clinical significance of cytological results. Eur J Endocrinol 2002;146:19–26.

30 Meier DA, Kaplan MM: Radioiodine uptake and thyroid scinitiscanning. Endocrinol Metab Clin North Am 2001;30:291–313.

31 Intenzo M, et al: Scintigraphic manifestations of thyrotoxicosis. RadioGraphics 2003;23:857–869

Sara Garberoglio, MD
Servizio di Endocrinologia
Ospedale Privato Sedes Sapientiae
Via Giorgio Bidone 31
IT–10125 Turin (Italy)
E-Mail saragarberoglio@gmail.com

Buchfelder M, Guaraldi F (eds): Imaging in Endocrine Disorders.
Front Horm Res. Basel, Karger, 2016, vol 45, pp 37–45 (DOI: 10.1159/000442276)

Hybrid Molecular Imaging in Differentiated Thyroid Carcinoma

Daniela Schmidt · Torsten Kuwert

Nuklearmedizinische Klinik, Universitätsklinikum Erlangen, Erlangen, Germany

Abstract

Radioactive isotopes of radioiodine are frequently used in differentiated thyroid carcinoma (DTC) both for diagnosis and therapy. Their accumulation in thyroid cancer tissue is dependent on the expression and activity of the sodium-iodide symporter (NIS). Scintigraphic imaging using either planar or single-photon emission computed tomography (SPECT) cameras allows the visualization of their distribution within the human body. Due to only a poor visualization of morphology by these techniques, their diagnostic accuracy is, however, limited. This limitation is overcome when hybrid systems integrating a SPECT camera with an X-ray CT scanner are used. Roughly one third of patients with diagnostically unclear foci of radioiodine accumulation will benefit from the use of SPECT/CT, also in terms of therapeutic management. SPECT/CT has, therefore, become the gold standard of nuclear imaging in DTC. NIS expression may be absent in DTC. In this case, the glucose transporters are usually upregulated. Therefore, PET/CT using ^{18}F-deoxyglucose can be used to diagnose and localize tumor recurrence as a prerequisite to, in particular, surgical intervention.

© 2016 S. Karger AG, Basel

The incidence of differentiated thyroid carcinoma (DTC) approximates 1 in 10,000 [for reviews and guidelines, see 1–3]. According to their histological appearances, DTCs can be subdivided into the papillary and follicular type, together with some rarer entities, such as the oncocytic variant. DTCs usually retain some properties of their mother cells, such as the ability to produce the protein thyroglobulin (TG) or to accumulate iodine. Their proliferation rate is, in general, comparatively slow. Nevertheless, dedifferentiation of DTCs may occur, leading to a loss of their radioiodine-accumulating capacity and to faster growth.

Surgical removal of the primary as well as of metastases is the first treatment option in all DTCs. In all patients except those with low-stage papillary DTC, total thyroidectomy is mandatory. Following surgery, radioablation of thyroid remnants using the radioactive iodine isotope ^{131}I is usually performed, at least in patients with higher tumor stages or in whom metastases are suspected. In DTCs, ^{131}I may also be used to destroy tumor deposits later in the course of the disease. Radiation therapy and chemotherapy only have a palliative role in thyroid neoplasms. The therapeutic potential of small-molecule inhibitors of signal transduction cascades is just being explored and, therefore, to date there is no standard treatment of thyroid neoplasms [for a review, see 4].

After thyroidectomy and radioablation, DTC patients are followed up by cervical ultrasound and by measurement of the serum value of TG. TG is secreted into the bloodstream by normal and neoplastic thyroid cells and is a highly sensitive tumor marker for DTC, in particular after removal of the thyroid gland. High serum levels of thyroid-stimulating hormone (TSH) increase TG secretion, so that TG measurement is more sensitive for the detection of tumor tissue in hypothyreosis or after intramuscular injection of recombinant human TSH [5]. Furthermore, radioiodine scans using diagnostic doses of radioiodine are also part of the routine follow-up, as will be described in more detail below. X-ray CT (computerized tomography) as well as MRI (magnetic resonance imaging) of the neck are usually not performed in DTC follow-up due to their limited accuracy in differentiating benign from malignant cervical lymph nodes and scar tissue from local recurrences. As in other tumors, these modalities are, nevertheless, indicated to diagnose distant metastases, e.g. in the lung or the skeleton.

The mean survival of DTC patients is longer than that of subjects afflicted by most other cancers [1]. As in other tumors, a higher tumor stage as well as the presence of distant and/or regional metastases is associated with a worsening prognosis [1]. In addition, the loss of differentiated features and, in particular, that of the capacity of iodine accumulation may complicate the course of disease. Accurate information on these prognostic variables early after diagnosis is essential to individually plan patient management since patients at high risk of recurrence require more intensive follow-up than those at low risk [3].

The Use of Radioiodine in Thyroid Carcinomas

Iodine is a building block of the thyroid hormones. Thyroid tissue, therefore, has the capacity to concentrate this element. The molecule mediating this accumulation is a protein cotransporting iodine and sodium – the sodium-iodide symporter (NIS) [6]. NIS is also expressed by DTCs, but usually not by anaplastic or medullary thyroid carcinomas. However, NIS expression in DTCs may vary, with dedifferentiation of these tumors reducing its density in tumor tissue [7].

NIS expression is regulated by TSH via the action of the adenylate cyclase and protein kinase A [8]. Therefore, all procedures using radioactive isotopes of iodine for diagnosis and therapy of DTC are performed at high TSH levels. This may be obtained by leaving DTC patients off medication with thyroid hormone after a total thyroidectomy or by intramuscular injection of recombinant human TSH prior to administration of the radiopharmaceutical.

Several radioactive isotopes of iodine emit radiation suitable for medical purposes and, in particular, scintigraphy: ^{124}I is a positron emitter and may thus be used in PET (positron emission tomography). Although promising clinical results have been obtained with this tracer [9], the comparatively high costs of PET limit its widespread use. ^{123}I is a pure gamma emitter. Its 160-keV photons are eminently suitable for conventional gamma camera imaging, including single-photon emission computed tomography (SPECT) [10]. Due to the high energy of the 364-keV photons emitted by ^{131}I, the quality of gamma camera images of ^{131}I distribution is inferior to those depicting ^{123}I uptake. ^{123}I is, however, more expensive than ^{131}I, which is the most frequently used isotope of iodine in nuclear medicine. ^{131}I is the only isotope of iodine currently used for therapy. Its radioactive decay also produces electrons, the energy of which is deposited within 1 mm of their arisal within the tissue concentrating this radiopharmaceutical.

In DTC, there are two therapeutic indications for applying ^{131}I [3]: First, ^{131}I is used directly after total thyroidectomy to eliminate remaining nonneoplastic tissue left by the surgeon. The second indication for the therapeutic use of ^{131}I is the treatment of radioiodine-accumulating metastases.

After therapeutic application of ^{131}I, its distribution in the human body is usually visualized by scintigraphy in order to gain information on the metastatic spread of the tumor. ^{131}I may also be given at lower doses to the patient, for diagnostic purposes only [for a review, see 3]. This is usually performed 6–12 months after radioablation to evaluate its success, regularly in the follow-up of patients at high risk of recurrence, and when during follow-up the suspicion of recurrence arises, e.g. at high or rising serum TG levels. In patients with low risk of recurrence and without evidence of relapse, radioiodine scintigraphy is not indicated; some controversy exists with regard to its role in the follow-up of patients with intermediate risk.

With radioiodine scintigraphy, DTC tissue is identified by its ability to accumulate radioiodine. Radioiodine is not only accumulated by tissue of thyroid origin [for a review,

Table 1. False negative findings on planar whole-body radioiodine scans in DTC [adapted from 23]

Mechanism	Typical examples
[131]I uptake adjacent to and undistinguishable from the site of physiological tracer accumulation[1]	LNM in the neck mistaken for thyroid remnant, pelvic metastases mistaken for uptake in the bladder, abdominal filiae confounded with physiological intestinal uptake
No NIS expression[2]	Metastasis of Hürthle cell carcinoma, dedifferentiated tumor
Partial volume effect due to a small focus size[2]	Microscopic LNM

[1] In most instances, the option to exactly localize and further characterize the focus of ^{131}I uptake on the CT images provided by SPECT/CT is helpful in establishing the correct diagnosis.
[2] These false negative findings will not be elucidated by SPECT/CT.

Table 2. False positive findings on planar whole-body radioiodine scans in DTC [adapted from 11]

Mechanism	Typical examples
[131]I uptake in ectopic thyroid tissue	Pyramidal lobe, struma ovarii
Skin contamination	Urine, sweat
Physiological ^{131}I uptake mistaken for tumor	Bowel activity, breast uptake
[131]I uptake in abnormalities of organs physiologically concentrating iodine	Meckel's diverticulum, asymmetrical salivary glands, renal cysts
Increased blood volume or NIS expression in inflammatory or neoplastic foci	Rheumatoid arthritis, mucocele, lung cancer, meningioma
Unexplained	Thymic uptake in children

In most instances, the option to exactly localize and further characterize the focus of ^{131}I uptake on the CT images provided by SPECT/CT is helpful in establishing the correct diagnosis.

see 11] – the salivary glands, the mucosae of the mouth, pharynx and stomach, the lactating breast as well as the hyperplastic thymus also express NIS. Furthermore, radioiodine is excreted via the kidneys and the liver. Therefore, the ureters, the bladder, and the intestines may also exhibit radioiodine uptake. False negative results of radioiodine imaging may, therefore, occur when foci of radioiodine accumulation is falsely attributed to uptake in one of the organs physiologically concentrating radioiodine (table 1). This is the rule in scintigraphic images obtained at radioablation of thyroid remnants performed directly after thyroidectomy. On these images, radioiodine uptake in cervical lymph node metastases (LNM) usually cannot be reliably distinguished from that in benign thyroid remnants. A further cause of false negative findings on radioiodine scans is the absence of the NIS in thyroid tumor tissue, as already mentioned above.

Due to these false negatives, the sensitivity of planar radioiodine scanning for detecting DTC metastases is somewhat limited and has been reported to range between 45 and 75% when using an elevation of the serum TG value as the gold standard [for a review, see 12]. However, radioiodine-positive but TG-negative metastases have been reported in the literature [13, 14], meaning the validity of this gold standard could be questioned. The sensitivity of radioiodine scintigraphy increases with the dose of radioiodine administered.

False positive results of radioiodine imaging may occur when radioiodine uptake in the organs physiologically concentrating radioiodine is mistaken for tumor deposits (table 2). This may, in particular, be the case when these exhibit anatomical variants or anomalies caused by disease. Typical examples of this mechanism are renal cysts or Meckel's diverticula. Rarely, radioiodine uptake may also be found in tumors of nonthyroid origin or in inflammatory foci. These may, therefore, also account for false positive findings.

Publications reporting the specificity of planar radioiodine scanning for staging DTC are scarce since it is difficult to establish an independent gold standard in representative groups of patients. Specificity is, nevertheless, believed to be higher than sensitivity [12].

Single-Photon Emission Computed Tomography/ Computed Tomography in Differentiated Thyroid Carcinoma

Scintigraphic images of the distribution of radioiodine in the human body are poor in anatomical landmarks. This leads to problems in their interpretation. These may be overcome when registering the molecular maps of NIS expression pixel-wise to image datasets from imaging modalities better suited to visualizing morphology than radioiodine scanning, such as CT or MRI. Obviously, this is only possible when the distribution of radioiodine within the patient's body is three-dimensionally represented. In the case of ^{131}I scintigraphy, this is achieved by using SPECT. Earlier attempts at image registration had to rely on software-based techniques to align independently acquired image datasets. Yamamoto et al. [15]. used this approach and reported a significant increase in the diagnostic accuracy of DTC.

The anatomical accuracy of software-based registration of independently acquired image datasets is limited by the scarcity of common anatomical landmarks between ^{131}I-SPECT and CT/MRI. Differences in patient positioning may also contribute to its lack of precision. A further disadvantage of software-based fusion is its high logistical demand – two examinations have to be scheduled instead of only one and the independently acquired image datasets have to be brought together in one viewing console for their joint interpretation.

These limitations can be overcome by hybrid cameras that integrate a nuclear medical detector unit with a CT or MRI scanner in one gantry. With these types of systems the two datasets are acquired directly after another with the patient in the same position on the examination bed. In the case of the neck, the average SPECT/CT misalignment was reported to be 0.57 + 0.20 cm [16].

In 1999, the first systems combining a dual-headed SPECT camera with a low-dose nonspiral CT scanner in one gantry became commercially available. This was followed by the development of hybrid cameras equipped by multislice spiral-CT devices in 2004. Currently, an array of SPECT/CT systems incorporating CT scanners of nearly every performance level have entered the marketplace [for reviews, see 17–19]. The clinical value of SPECT/CT in general and in DTC has recently been reviewed [20–24].

SPECT/CT allows the exact localization of foci of radioiodine uptake and thus has the potential to differentiate reliably between uptake in metastases of thyroid cancer and that in organs physiologically accumulating this tracer.

In 2004, the first evidence on the clinical value of SPECT/CT in DTC was published. Tharp et al. [25] reported a 57% increment in the diagnostic accuracy of ^{131}I-SPECT/CT compared to planar imaging in a group of 71 DTC patients from two institutions in whom on the whole 96 image datasets had been obtained.

The majority of the evidence available to date has addressed the potential role of ^{131}I-SPECT/CT in patients studied at radioablation [26–30]. With the exception of the paper by Wong et al. [27], the patients included in these studies were examined after oral application of a therapeutic dose of [131]I. These publications reported that the lesion-related increment in diagnostic accuracy varies between 31 and 47.6%. The benefit of SPECT/CT in this patient group is mainly due to its ability to better localize cervical foci of radioiodine uptake with regard to the thyroid bed. SPECT/CT thus enables a differentiation between thyroid remnants and LNM, which is not possible on planar images due to a lack of anatomical landmarks (fig. 1; online suppl. video 1; see www.karger.com/doi/10.1159/000442276 for all online suppl. material). However, there are two limitations of SPECT/CT in this regard. LNM in the central compartment of the neck may falsely be interpreted as thyroid remnants. Since the SPECT/CT criterion used in all studies for the diagnosis of LNM is their location outside this compartment, central foci of uptake are usually attributed to thyroid remnants. Furthermore, microscopic disease may also escape detection by hybrid imaging.

Common to all studies on the value of SPECT/CT performed at radioablation is the lack of an independent gold standard. Techniques of structural imaging are not accurate in this clinical setting for two reasons: directly after thyroid surgery, reactively enlarged lymph nodes may be present; furthermore, LNM are frequently small and may measure well below 1 cm in diameter so that they elude detection by

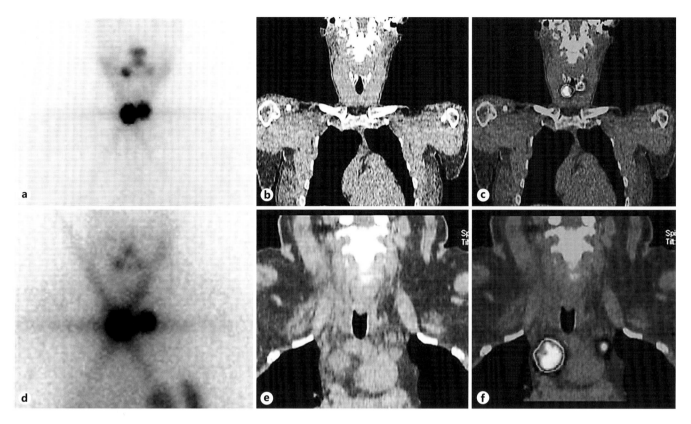

Fig. 1. Images **a–c** and **d–f** were obtained in 2 patients with papillary DTC, respectively, at radioiodine ablation performed 4 weeks after total thyroidectomy. Planar ^{131}I scintigraphies (**a**, **d**) disclose two foci of radioiodine accumulation in each subject. **a–c** SPECT/CT fusion image (**c**) and low-dose CT (**b**) help localize these foci to the thyroid bed, allowing a diagnosis of benign thyroid remnants in this patient. **d–f** The foci of radioiodine uptake correspond to mediastinal LNM well visible on the low-dose CT image (**e**).

these techniques. Reoperation of the neck is usually not indicated directly after radioablation since the latter may eliminate the metastases in the months to come, thus making additional surgery superfluous. Clearly, the performance of neck dissections is not feasible for purely scientific purposes. To date, therefore, all the papers published lack comparison to histopathology.

The impact of SPECT/CT on patient management was also analyzed in two of the above-cited papers. Schmidt et al. [28] could show that SPECT/CT leads to a revision of nodal stage in roughly 25% of all DTC patients studied. Their data were in the meantime reproduced in a more homogeneous and larger group of 151 patients with a T1 papillary carcinoma pooled from two institutions [30], including 96 patients affected by microcarcinomas. Since lymph node involvement is an independent prognostic variable in papillary DTC and also in microcarcinomas, the results from SPECT/CT alter the strategy of follow-up in a quarter of DTC patients.

The considerably higher accuracy of SPECT/CT in detecting cervical LNM at radioablation opens further questions with regard to patient management. In particular, the question arises as to how the LNM diagnosed by SPECT/CT should be treated. A publication reporting follow-up in patients studied by SPECT/CT at radioablation has recently been published. Schmidt et al. [31] could demonstrate that 18 out of 22 radioiodine-positive metastases were no longer detected 5 months after radioablation of thyroid remnants. This observation argues against surgical intervention at least in all patients with a SPECT/CT diagnosis of LNM at radioablation. In 3 patients of the group studied, four radioiodine-positive LNMs had persisted. The number of lesions included in this study is definitely too small to identify the variables governing the effect of radioiodine given for radioablation of thyroid remnants on LNM. Nevertheless, it should be noted that 17 out of 18 LNMs eliminated by radioiodine were smaller

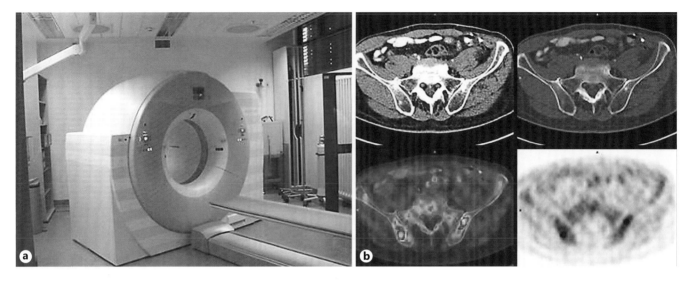

Fig. 2. A PET/CT camera (**a**) allows the visualization of regional glucose metabolism together with CT morphology (**b**).

than 0.9 ml, whereas this was the case for only one of the persisting foci.

Only 1 out of 61 patients staged as negative also by SPECT/CT in the study published by Schmidt et al. [31] had developed a hitherto undetected radioiodine-positive cervical foci on follow-up. Wong et al. [27] and Aide et al. [29] have also reported a high negative predictive value of SPECT/CT performed at radioablation with regard to tumor persistence and therapy success in their subjects. These data suggest that SPECT/CT may also be used to stratify patients with regard to the risk of recurrence or tumor persistence, thus allowing better tailoring of follow-up.

SPECT/CT was also reported to be of considerable benefit also at follow-up of DTC patients, i.e. several months after radioablation. The incremental diagnostic value was 67.8 and 73.9%, respectively, in two studies that predominantly addressed this clinical setting [32, 33]. On a patient basis, this improvement in diagnostic accuracy led to a change in therapeutic strategy in 47.1% of the patients with locally advanced or metastatic disease reported by Chen et al. [32]. Spanu et al. [33] reported a modification in therapeutic management caused by SPECT/CT in 35.6% of cases with SPECT/CT proof of malignant lesions, and of 20.3% of patients with a SPECT/CT diagnosis of benign disease. Menges et al. [34] pointed out that, in particular, patients with foci outside the thyroid bed benefitted from SPECT/CT.

SPECT/CT offers the option of attenuation correction of SPECT images [for a review, see 19]. Furthermore, the CT information on the size of a lesion of interest could also be used to correct SPECT images for partial volume artifacts. By integrating these corrections into up-to-date iterative reconstruction software, quantitation of tissue radioactivity concentration in terms of absolute values seems possible and has been demonstrated in phantom measurements [35, 36] and in patients [37]. This is true at least when tracers labelled by ^{99m}Tc are used. Papers proving this assumption for the high-energy photons of ^{131}I are, however, still missing. Nevertheless, at least two publications have already used SPECT/CT for dosimetry of radioiodine therapy [38, 39]. The accuracy of this approach and its possible impact on the dosage of ^{131}I given for therapeutic purposes remain to be investigated, but are highly interesting issues.

Position Emission Tomography/Computed Tomography in Differentiated Thyroid Carcinoma

PET/CT is the second hybrid imaging system established in nuclear medicine (fig. 2). It combines a PET camera with a multislice spiral-CT in one gantry.

In the case of dedifferentiation, DTC and its deposits may lose NIS expression and thus the ability to concentrate radioiodine. In their pioneering study, Feine et al. [40] have shown that in these cases an upregulation of the key proteins of glucose metabolism may occur so that PET with

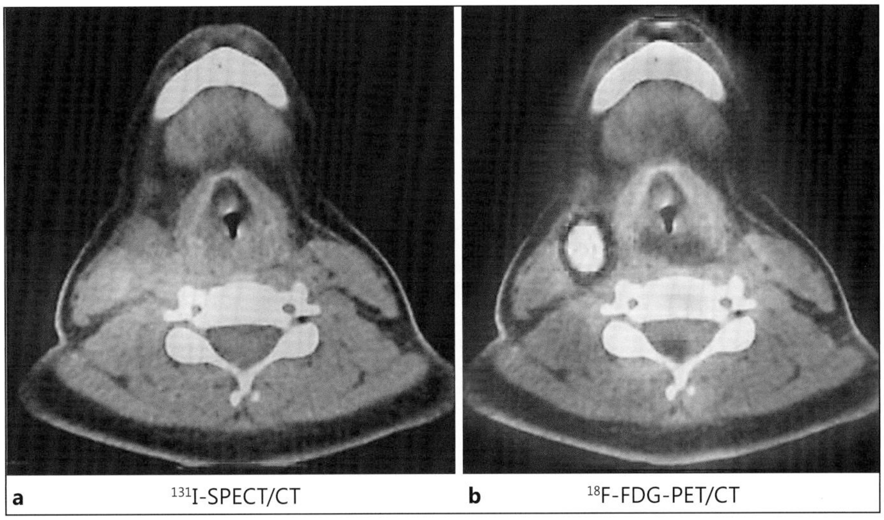

Fig. 3. a ^{131}I-SPECT/CT fusion image obtained in a 15-year-old female with a pT3mpN1 papillary DTC. **b** ^{18}F-FDG-PET fusion image obtained in the same patient and in the same week. The patient had an elevated TG serum concentration. By PET, an FDG-avid lymph node metastasis is visualized that has no radioiodine accumulation.

^{131}I-SPECT/CT a

^{18}F-FDG-PET/CT b

^{18}F-deoxyglucose (FDG) may be used for diagnosis [41, 42]. Figure 3 illustrates this so-called 'flip-flop' phenomenon. The molecular mechanisms responsible for this constellation are largely unknown, although it can be speculated that alterations in signal transduction pathways caused by oncogenes might play a pertinent role [43]. Patients harboring FDG-positive metastases (see online suppl. videos 2 and 3) have been shown to have a worse prognosis compared to those FDG negative [44]. Furthermore, FDG-positive metastases are more frequently found in patients with histological proof of dedifferentiation of the primary compared to those with well-differentiated DTC.

Conforming to a guideline issued by the Society of Nuclear Medicine [45], FDG-PET/CT has to be considered in patients without pathological iodine-positive foci, but elevated serum TG values. In this setting, in about one third of patients, FDG-avid metastases can be detected [46]. The probability of their detection rises with increasing serum TG levels, being highest at TG values >21 ng/dl and very low at TG levels <2 ng/dl in the study by Mosci and Iagaru [42]. As demonstrated for SPECT, combining PET with CT gives more accurate results [47].

Emerging evidence indicates that FDG-PET/CT might also be useful for preoperative staging in high-risk patients with aggressive DTC, in the case of negative whole-body iodine scans and positive anti-TG antibodies, and for prognostication and determination of the disease extent in high-risk groups [41]. Furthermore, also patients with Hurthle cell carcinoma or with poorly differentiated thyroid carcinoma can benefit from the use of FDG-PET/CT at the beginning of treatment.

The use of radiopharmaceuticals tracing DTC expression of the somatostatin receptors or the DOPA-decarboxylase such as ^{68}Ga-DOTATATE or ^{18}F-DOPA is only rarely indicated in DTC. Somatostatin receptor imaging can be useful in those cases in whom, due to a lack of other therapeutic options, radioreceptor therapy is considered.

Conclusions

Using PET and SPECT, NIS and GLUT expression can be visualized in vivo with high accuracy in DTC. Combining these molecular imaging techniques with CT has greatly increased their diagnostic accuracy.

References

1 Schlumberger M, Pacini F: Thyroid Tumors. Paris, Editions Nucléon, 2003.

2 Pacini F, Schlumberger M, Dralle H, Elisei R, Smit JW, Wiersinga W; European Thyroid Cancer Task Force: European consensus for the management of patients with differentiated thyroid carcinoma of the follicular epithelium. Eur J Endocrinol 2006;154:787–803.

3 Cooper DS, Doherty GM, Haugen BR, Kloos RT, Lee SL, Mandel SJ, Mazzaferri EL, McIver B, Pacini F, Schlumberger M, Sherman SI, Steward DL, Tuttle RM: Revised American Thyroid Association management guidelines for patients with thyroid nodules and differentiated thyroid cancer. Thyroid 2009;19:1167–1214.

4 Santoro M, Carlomagno F: Drug insight: small-molecule inhibitors of protein kinases in the treatment of thyroid cancer. Nat Clin Pract Endocrinol Metab 2006;2:42–52.

5 Weintraub BD, Szkudlinski MW: Development and in vitro characterization of human recombinant thyrotropin. Thyroid 1999;9:447–450.

6 Dai G, Levy O, Carrasco N: Cloning and characterization of the thyroid iodide transporter. Nature 1996;379:458–460.

7 Castro MR, Bergert ER, Goellner JR, Hay ID, Morris JC: Immunohistochemical analysis of sodium iodide symporter expression in metastatic differentiated thyroid cancer: correlation with radioiodine uptake. J Clin Endocrinol Metab 2001;86:5627–5632.

8 Bläser D, Maschauer S, Kuwert T, Prante O: In vitro studies on the signal transduction of thyroidal uptake of ^{18}F-FDG and ^{131}I-iodide. J Nucl Med 2006;47:1382–1388.

9 Freudenberg LS, Antoch G, Frilling A, Jentzen W, Rosenbaum SJ, Kühl H, Bockisch A, Görges R: Combined metabolic and morphologic imaging in thyroid carcinoma patients with elevated serum thyroglobulin and negative cervical ultrasonography: role of ^{124}I-PET/CT and FDG-PET. Eur J Nucl Med Mol Imaging 2008;35:950–957.

10 Ali N, Sebastian C, Foley RR, Murray I, Canizales AL, Jenkins PJ, Drake WM, Plowman PN, Besser GM, Chew SL, Grossman AB, Monson JP, Britton KE: The management of differentiated thyroid cancer using ^{123}I for imaging to assess the need for ^{131}I therapy. Nucl Med Commun 2006;27:165–169.

11 Shapiro B, Rufini V, Jarwan A, Geatti O, Kearfott KJ, Fig. LM, Kirkwood ID, Gross MD: Artifacts, anatomical and physiological variants, and unrelated diseases that might cause false-positive whole-body ^{131}I scans in patients with thyroid cancer. Semin Nucl Med 2000;30:115–132.

12 Lind P, Kohlfürst S: Respective roles of thyroglobulin, radioiodine imaging, and positron emission tomography in the assessment of thyroid cancer. Semin Nucl Med 2006;36:194–205.

13 Ma C, Kuang A, Xie J, Ma T: Possible explanations for patients with discordant findings of serum thyroglobulin and ^{131}I whole-body scanning. J Nucl Med 2005;46:1473–1480.

14 Caballero-Calabuig E, Cano-Terol C, Sopena-Monforte R, Reyes-Ojeda D, Abreu-Sánchez P, Ferrer-Rebolleda J, Sopena-Novales P, Plancha-Mansanet C, Félix-Fontestad J: Influence of the thyroid remnant in the elevation of the serum thyroglobulin after thyroidectomy in differentiated thyroid carcinoma: importance of the diagnostic iodine total-body scanning. Eur J Nucl Med Mol Imaging 2008;35:1449–1456.

15 Yamamoto Y, Nishiyama Y, Monden T, Matsumura Y, Satoh K, Ohkawa M: Clinical usefulness of fusion of ^{131}I SPECT and CT images in patients with differentiated thyroid carcinoma. J Nucl Med 2003;44:1905–1910.

16 Bennewitz C, Kuwert T, Han J, Ritt P, Hahn D, Thimister W, Hornegger J, Uder M, Schmidt D: Computer-aided evaluation of the anatomical accuracy of hybrid SPECT/spiral-CT imaging of lesions localized in the neck and upper abdomen. Nucl Med Commun 2012;331153–1159.

17 Seo Y, Mari C, Hasegawa BH: Technological development and advances in single-photon emission computed tomography/computed tomography. Semin Nucl Med 2008;38:177–198.

18 Patton JA, Townsend DW, Hutton BF: Hybrid imaging technology: from dreams and visions to clinical devices. Semin Nucl Med 2009;39:247–263.

19 Ritt P, Vija H, Hornegger J, Kuwert T: Absolute quantification in SPECT. Eur J Nucl Med Mol Imaging 2011;38(suppl 1):S69–S77.

20 Even-Sapir E, Keidar Z, Bar-Shalom R: Hybrid imaging (SPECT/CT and PET/CT) – improving the diagnostic accuracy of functional/metabolic and anatomic imaging. Semin Nucl Med 2009;39:264–275.

21 Bockisch A, Freudenberg LS, Schmidt D, Kuwert T: Hybrid imaging by SPECT/CT and PET/CT: proven outcomes in cancer imaging. Semin Nucl Med 2009;39:276–289.

22 Mariani G, Bruselli L, Kuwert T, Kim EE, Flotats A, Israel O, Dondi M, Watanabe N: A review on the clinical uses of SPECT/CT. Eur J Nucl Med Mol Imaging 2010;37:1959–1985.

23 Menges M, Uder M, Kuwert T, Schmidt D: ^{131}I SPECT/CT in the follow-up of patients with differentiated thyroid carcinoma. Clin Nucl Med 2012;37:555–560.

24 Avram AM: Radioiodine scintigraphy with SPECT/CT: an important diagnostic tool for thyroid cancer staging and risk stratification. J Nucl Med 2012;53:754–764.

25 Tharp K, Israel O, Hausmann J, Bettman L, Martin WH, Daitzchman M, Sandler MP, Delbeke D: Impact of ^{131}I-SPECT/CT images obtained with an integrated system in the follow-up of patients with thyroid carcinoma. Eur J Nucl Med Mol Imaging 2004;31:1435–1442.

26 Ruf J, Lehmkuhl L, Bertram H, Sandrock D, Amthauer H, Humplik B, Ludwig Munz D, Felix R: Impact of SPECT and integrated low-dose CT after radioiodine therapy on the management of patients with thyroid carcinoma. Nucl Med Commun 2004;25:1177–1182.

27 Wong KK, Zarzhevsky N, Cahill JM, Frey KA, Avram AM: Incremental value of diagnostic ^{131}I SPECT/CT fusion imaging in the evaluation of differentiated thyroid carcinoma. AJR Am J Roentgenol 2008;191:1785–1794.

28 Schmidt D, Szikszai A, Linke R, Bautz W, Kuwert T: Impact of ^{131}I SPECT/spiral CT on nodal staging of differentiated thyroid carcinoma at the first radioablation. J Nucl Med 2009;50:18–23.

29 Aide N, Heutte N, Rame J-P, Rousseau E, Loiseau C, Henry-Amar M, Bardet S: Clinical relevance of single-photon emission computed tomography/computed tomography of the neck and thorax in postablation ^{131}I scintigraphy for thyroid cancer. J Clin Endocrinol Metab 2009;94:2075–2084.

30 Mustafa M, Kuwert T, Weber K, Knesewitsch P, Negele T, Haug A, Linke R, Bartenstein P, Schmidt D: Regional lymph node involvement in T1 papillary thyroid carcinoma: a bicentric prospective SPECT/CT study. Eur J Nucl Med Mol Imaging 2010;37:1462–1466.

31 Schmidt D, Linke R, Uder M, Kuwert T: Five months' follow-up of patients with and without iodine-positive lymph node metastases of thyroid carcinoma as disclosed by ^{131}I-SPECT/CT at the first radioablation. Eur J Nucl Med Mol Imaging 2010;37:699–705.

32 Chen L, Luo Q, Shen Y, Yu Y, Yuan Z, Lu H, Zhu R: Incremental value of ^{131}I SPECT/CT in the management of patients with differentiated thyroid carcinoma. J Nucl Med 2008;49:1952–1957.

33 Spanu A, Solinas ME, Chessa F, Sanna D, Nuvoli S, Madeddu G: ^{131}I SPECT/CT in the follow-up of differentiated thyroid carcinoma: incremental value versus planar imaging. J Nucl Med 2009;50:184–190.

34 Menges M, Uder M, Kuwert T, Schmidt D: ^{131}I SPECT/CT in the follow-up of patients with differentiated thyroid carcinoma. Clin Nucl Med 2012;37:555–560.

35 Vandervoort E, Celler A, Harrop R: Implementation of an iterative scatter correction, the influence of attenuation map quality and their effect on absolute quantitation in SPECT. Phys Med Biol 2007;52:1527–1545.

36 Shcherbinin S, Celler A, Belhocine T, Vanderwerf R, Driedger A: Accuracy of quantitative reconstructions in SPECT/CT imaging. Phys Med Biol 2008;53:4595–4604.

37 Zeintl J, Vija AH, Yahil A, Hornegger J, Kuwert T: Quantitative accuracy of clinical ^{99m}Tc SPECT/CT using ordered-subset expectation maximization with 3-dimensional resolution recovery, attenuation, and scatter correction. J Nucl Med 2010;51:921–928.

38 Song H, He B, Prideaux A, He B, Frey EC, Ladenson PW, Wahl RL, Sgouros G: Lung dosimetry for radioiodine treatment planning in the case of diffuse lung metastases. J Nucl Med 2006;47:1985–1994.

39 Sisson JC, Dewaraja YK, Wizauer EJ, Giordano TJ, Avram AM: Thyroid carcinoma metastasis to skull with infringement of the brain: treatment with radioiodine. Thyroid 2009;19:297–303.

40 Feine U, Lietzenmayer R, Hanke JP, Held J, Wöhrle H, Müller-Schauenburg W: Fluorine-18-FDG and iodine-131 uptake in thyroid cancer. J Nucl Med 1996;37:1468–1472.

41 Palaniswamy SS, Subramanyam P: Diagnostic utility of PET/CT in thyroid malignancies: an update. Ann Nucl Med 2013;27:681–693.

42 Mosci C, Iagaru A: PET/CT imaging of thyroid cancer. Clin Nucl Med 2011;36:e180–e185.

43 Reinfelder J, Maschauer S, Foss CA, Nimmagadda S, Fremont V, Wolf V, Weintraub BD, Pomper MG, Szkudlinski MW, Kuwert T, Prante O: Effects of recombinant human thyroid-stimulating hormone superagonists on thyroidal uptake of ^{18}F-fluorodeoxyglucose and radioiodide. Thyroid 2011;21:783–792.

44 Schlüter B, Bohuslavizki KH, Beyer W, Plotkin M, Buchert R, Clausen M: Impact of FDG PET on patients with differentiated thyroid cancer who present with elevated thyroglobulin and negative ^{131}I scan. J Nucl Med 2001;42:71–76.

45 Fletcher JW, Djulbegovic B, Soares HP, Siegel BA, Lowe VJ, Lyman GH, Coleman RE, Wahl R, Paschold JC, Avril N, Einhorn LH, Suh WW, Samson D, Delbeke D, Gorman M, Shields AF: Recommendations on the use of ^{18}F-FDG PET in oncology. J Nucl Med 2008;49:480–508.

46 Grünwald F, Kälicke T, Feine U, Lietzenmayer R, Scheidhauer K, Dietlein M, Schober O, Lerch H, Brandt-Mainz K, Burchert W, Hiltermann G, Cremerius U, Biersack HJ: Fluorine-18 fluorodeoxyglucose positron emission tomography in thyroid cancer: results of a multicentre study. Eur J Nucl Med 1999;26:1547–1552.

47 Palmedo H, Bucerius J, Joe A, Strunk H, Hortling N, Meyka S, Roedel R, Wolff M, Wardelmann E, Biersack HJ, Jaeger U: Integrated PET/CT in differentiated thyroid cancer: diagnostic accuracy and impact on patient management. J Nucl Med 2006;47:616–624.

Prof. Dr. Torsten Kuwert, MD
Nuklearmedizinische Klinik
Universitätsklinikum Erlangen
Ulmenweg 18
DE–91054 Erlangen (Germany)
E-Mail torsten.kuwert@uk-erlangen.de

Buchfelder M, Guaraldi F (eds): Imaging in Endocrine Disorders.
Front Horm Res. Basel, Karger, 2016, vol 45, pp 46–54 (DOI: 10.1159/000442277)

Endoscopic Ultrasound in Endocrinology: Imaging of the Adrenals and the Endocrine Pancreas

Peter Herbert Kann

Endokrinologie & Diabetologie, Zentrum für Innere Medizin, Universitätsklinikum Marburg (UKGM), Marburg, Germany

Abstract

Endoscopic ultrasound (EUS) imaging of adrenal glands and its application to diagnostic procedures of adrenal diseases has been reported since 1998. It can be considered a relevant advantage in the field of adrenal diseases. Indeed, EUS allows the detection of adrenal lesions (even very small ones) and their characterization, the assessment of malignancy criteria, the early detection of neoplastic recurrences, the preoperative identification of morphologically healthy parts of the glands, the differentiation of extra-adrenal from adrenal tumors, and of the pathological entities associated with adrenal insufficiency, and the fine-needle aspiration biopsy (EUS-FNA) of suspicious lesions. At the same time, its clinical relevance depends on the experience of the endosonographer. Moreover, EUS is also by far the best and most sensitive imaging technique to detect and assess the follow-up of pancreatic manifestation of MEN1 disease. It furthermore enables the preoperatively localization of insulinomas and critical structures in their neighborhood, and may be relevant in planning surgical strategy. A positive EUS in a case of insulinoma furthermore confirms the endocrine diagnosis, especially considering the differential diagnosis of hypoglycemia factitia by oral antidiabetics. It can be supplemented by EUS-FNA. Again, it has to be considered that EUS may reveal false positive and false negative results, and the quality of the findings largely depends on the endosonographer's skills and experience. The most important technical details together with the advantages and limitations of EUS, and the pathognomonic characteristic of benign and malignant disorders of the adrenals and pancreas are presented here. © 2016 S. Karger AG, Basel

Following earlier reports of imaging the left adrenal using endoscopic ultrasound (EUS) [1], imaging of both adrenal glands and its systematic use in diagnostic procedures of adrenal diseases was reported for the first time in 1998 [2–4]. In these first days, however, the technical quality of imaging was still not really satisfactory. Compared to the already established EUS of the pancreas [5–7], EUS of the adrenals was developed later as initial imaging of the right adrenal gland was found to be difficult and problematic [8].

In the meantime, a great deal of experience in performing EUS imaging of the adrenals and the value of this diagnostic technique has been gained [9–12]. Imaging as well as exact identification of healthy, i.e. morphologically normal, tissue of the adrenals has markedly improved. In particular, modification of the imaging technique of the right adrenal gland was substantial in this process, currently allowing imaging in almost every patient without a history of gastroduodenopancreatic surgery [13]. EUS differentiates between the adrenal medulla and cortex, and identifies very small tumors and atrophic adrenals, as a manifestation of autoimmune Addison's disease.

As already mentioned, EUS of the pancreas was established more than 20 years ago. It soon became obvious that besides the imaging of inflammation and adenocarcinomas, EUS may be valuable in the diagnosis of other endocrine pancreatic diseases [5–7, 14–17].

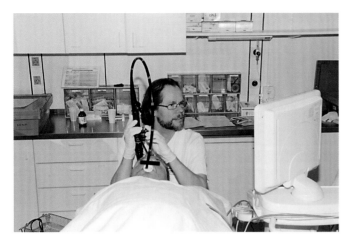

Fig. 1. EUS imaging of the left adrenal and the pancreas. The endosonographer is sitting in an overhead position, the patient is lying in a supine position.

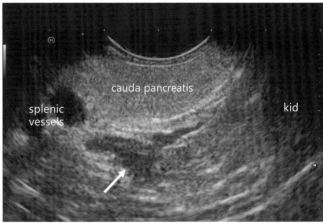

Fig. 2. EUS imaging of a normal left adrenal (arrow). The medulla (bright) and cortex (dark) can be differentiated by echogenicity. Landmarks include the cranial pole of the left kidney (kid), the distal pancreatic tail and the splenic vessels.

Technical Details

EUS imaging of the adrenals is performed using an endosonoscope with a longitudinal ultrasound transducer. The adrenals can be visualized by sector scanning, whereby switching the frequency from 7.5 to 5 MHz is sometimes useful in improving the imaging of the right gland, which is frequently further away from the transducer than the left adrenal. Furthermore, this technical device also provides the option of EUS-guided fine-needle aspiration (EUS-FNA) biopsy of adrenal masses (especially in the left gland) in the small subgroup of patients who may benefit from a cytological/histopathological diagnosis [11, 18].

After local anesthesia of the pharynx with a spray, the endosonoscope is inserted into the patient while lying on their left side. Since imaging of the adrenals often deals with the detection or exclusion of very small morphological changes, sufficient sedation is mandatory. At our center, after intravenous injection of atropine (0.125–0.5 mg), premedication is usually carried out with pethidine (25–50 mg) and diazepam (5–20 mg).

In order to facilitate the imaging procedure the endosonographer now changes position and sits in an overhead position to the patient who is now lying in a supine position (fig. 1). Imaging of the left adrenal is easily performed from the proximal stomach. The transducer is directed craniocaudally and the sound direction dorsally. Landmarks for the correct identification of the left adrenal are the cranial

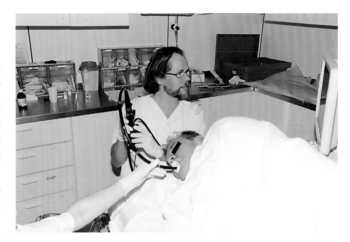

Fig. 3. EUS imaging of the right adrenal gland. The endosonographer is sitting in an overhead position, the patient is lying on his right side.

pole of the left kidney, the distal pancreatic tail and the splenic vessels (fig. 2). Imaging of the right adrenal presents no problems in patients without a history of gastroduodenopancreatic surgery when using the right approach. Under optical control, the transducer has to be placed in the antrum just in front of the pylorus after which the patient must turn to lie on their right side (fig. 3). The transducer is now flexed totally towards the right side, so that the tip of the endosonoscope is behind the angulus. With the transducer in this position, the endosonoscope is carefully retracted until the landmarks – cranial pole of the right kidney, inferior caval vein and caudal parts of the liver – can be identified. Thereafter, the right adrenal gland can be imaged behind the inferior caval vein (fig. 4).

EUS imaging of the pancreas can be performed using different endosonoscopes. Circular transducers as well as longitudinal scanners can be used. The pancreatic body and tail are usually imaged from the stomach. The head and the processus uncinatus can be considered from the antrum, the duodenal bulb, and the descending and the horizontal part of the duodenum [4–6, 17]. Personal experience has revealed that EUS of the pancreas with the patient in a supine position may reduce the probability of missing small pancreatic lesions (fig. 1). Definitive diagnosis of a pancreatic neuroendocrine tumor (NET) may be revealed by EUS-FNA [19–21].

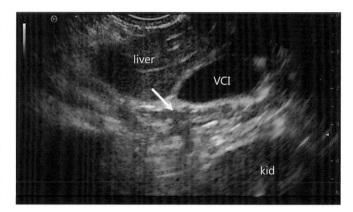

Fig. 4. EUS imaging of a normal right adrenal gland (arrow). The medulla (bright) and cortex (dark) can be differentiated by echogenicity. Landmarks include the cranial pole of the right kidney (kid), the inferior caval vein (VCI) and caudal portion of the liver.

Resolution

EUS allows in vivo separation of the signals generated by the adrenal medulla (hyperechoic) and the cortex (hypoechoic). Tumors and nodules with a diameter as low as 2–3 mm can be identified [10]. Using EUS, pancreatic tumors also with a minimum diameter of 2–3 mm can be detected [5, 22].

Indications and Typical Findings

Based on the knowledge available today, the following constellations can be considered as valid indications for EUS of the adrenal glands.

Detection of Small Adrenal Tumors
EUS of the adrenals enables the detection of morphological abnormalities, such as nodular formations down to a diameter of about 3 mm, e.g. in adrenal manifestations of MEN1 disease. There is some evidence that EUS of the adrenals may even be superior to MRI and/or CT when focusing on small adrenal tumors and taking postoperative histology as the gold standard – for example in primary aldosteronism (see below) [4, 9, 23]. However, this needs to be established in larger cohorts and confirmed by other investigators.

Characterization of Adrenal Masses
In the case of ACTH-independent Cushing's syndrome, a solitary adenoma of an adrenal gland can easily be charac-terized by identification of a capsule, interruption/abruption of the medullary echo and different echogenicity. In some cases, a different perfusion pattern may be detected by color-coded duplex EUS [24]. Differentiation from diffuse and nodular hyperplasia is easily possible [10].

The diagnosis of primary aldosteronism is still a very crucial issue. The problems associated with screening and confirmation testing will not be discussed in detail in this context. However, it should be pointed out that EUS enables the identification of a unilateral adenoma even in cases where CT and MRI are negative and selective venous sampling was unsuccessful – which is not rarely the case [23]. Important diagnostic criteria for Conn's adenoma (aldosterone-producing adenoma) seem to be a tumor diameter <2 cm, a round or oval shape of the hypoechoic mass, detection of a capsular bordering the normal adrenal tissue, and the termination of the signal generated by the adrenal medulla at the tumor capsule (fig. 5). Bilateral adrenal hyperplasia can also be imaged and differentiated between a diffuse type and nodular morphology [10]. The exact differential diagnosis is of high clinical relevance, as in the first case surgery is indicated, and in the second case medical treatment is recommended.

To date, EUS of the adrenals in the diagnosis of Conn's adenoma is not a routine diagnostic approach and has not been addressed in guidelines on primary aldosteronism, probably because it has unfortunately not been established in the majority of endocrine centers worldwide.

If the adrenals are enlarged, it is also possible to identify lipid-containing tumors, such as adrenal myelolipoma, due to the high echogenicity (fig. 6).

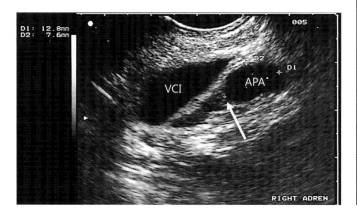 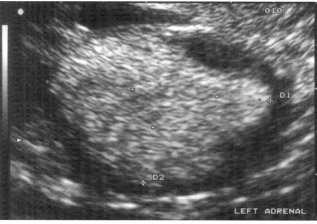

Fig. 5. EUS of a typical aldosterone-producing (Conn's) adenoma (APA) within the right adrenal gland, 12.8 × 7.6 mm. The adenoma is hypoechoic compared to the other parts of the adrenal cortex, and a capsule can be seen. The echo of the adrenal medulla stops at the tumor capsule (arrow). VCI = Inferior caval vein.

Fig. 6. EUS of a typical myelolipoma. The tumor is clearly hyperechoic due to its lipid content and surrounded by normal adrenal cortex tissue (hypoechoic).

Assessing Criteria of Malignancy in Adrenal Tumors
When planning the surgical strategy for adrenal masses, the preoperative detection of criteria for malignancy may be clinically relevant as in these cases endocrinologists and endocrine surgeons might consider endoscopic resection to be the wrong approach. Adrenocortical carcinomas are generally heterogeneous in their echocomplex pattern, but malignant and benign pheochromocytomas can present the same characteristics. Thus, heterogeneity of an adrenal tumor is not a clear criterion for malignancy.

The relevance of EUS is to show or exclude the infiltration of neighboring organs and to detect effusion – suggestive criteria for malignancy. Other clear criteria for malignancy include the detection of local or regional lymph node metastases and vascular invasion [10].

Adrenal metastases are typically large and hypoechoic, and clear identification and histopathological differentiation can be obtained by EUS-FNA [25].

Assessing the Growth Velocity of Adrenal Tumors
EUS is suitable for the follow-up of adrenal tumors that have been characterized as hormonal inactive and are not suspected to be malignant. In general, it can be offered as an alternative to MRI or CT.

EUS has been shown to be more sensitive in detecting adrenal involvement in MEN1 than CT [26]. A recent study on adrenal masses in MEN1 showed that in adulthood these tumors tend to remain morphologically stable over a long time period [27]. EUS follow-up studies enable the detection of atypically growing adrenal tumors in MEN1, as the adrenals can easily be considered during the periodically recommended EUS for studying pancreatic lesions in these patients (see below).

Early Detection of Recurrence of Malignant Adrenal Tumors
In postoperative care of adrenocortical carcinomas and pheochromocytomas, EUS enables the detection of small recurrences in the tumor area and in neighboring regions.

Preoperative Identification of Morphologically Normal Parts of the Adrenals
Bilateral adrenal masses are detected in some cases. This may be in genetically determined diseases such as multiple endocrine neoplasia type 2a and b [28] and von Hippel Lindau's disease, for example, and also in other situations such as ACTH-independent endogenous hypercortisolism (fig. 7a–c). It may be important to know preoperatively whether there are morphologically completely normal parts of an adrenal gland that can be left in situ in order to avoid lifelong replacement therapy with adrenal steroid hormones in these patients.

Differentiation of Extra-Adrenal from Adrenal Tumors
Using conventional ultrasound, CT and MRI, it may be difficult to consider whether a tumor is really an adrenal mass or

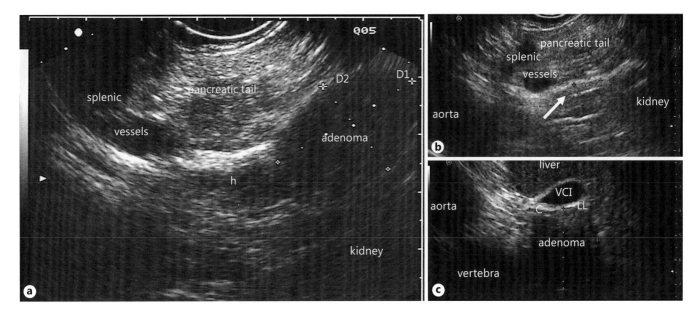

Fig. 7. A 60-year-old female patient suffering from ACTH-independent endogenous hypercortisolism (Cushing's syndrome). Imaging revealed bilateral adrenal masses and adenomas were suspected on both sides. By selective venous catheterization, the left adrenal gland was identified to be the source of cortisol secretion. By preoperative EUS, besides characterization of an adenoma, a morphologically healthy part (h) of the left adrenal could be identified (**a**) which could be left in situ by the surgeon (selective adenomectomy) and could be imaged by EUS postoperatively (arrow; **b**). This strategy was considered useful since it remained questionable whether it might become necessary to remove the contralateral hormonally inactive adenoma (diameter 33 mm) and possibly also the entire right adrenal gland (**c**) in the future. C = Corpus; LL = lateral limb; VCI = inferior caval vein.

just located adjacent to the adrenal gland. This question occurs in pheochromocytomas/paragangliomas [29] as well as in other situations. In such cases EUS may be helpful (fig. 8).

Differentiation of Different Entities of Adrenal Insufficiency
Different diseases causing adrenocortical insufficiency have typical morphologies that can be detected by EUS. Addison's disease shows a marked atrophy of the adrenal glands (fig. 9), while organ calcifications are suggestive for adrenal insufficiency following adrenal tuberculosis.

Endoscopic Ultrasound-Guided Fine-Needle Adrenal Aspiration Biopsy
EUS easily enables guided FNAs of the left adrenal gland [30, 31] (fig. 10). On the right side, the tumor needs to be quite large to make transduodenal EUS-FNA possible [32, 33]. Frequently, CT-guided biopsy is a preferential alternative in such cases. Nevertheless, transcaval EUS-FNA of right adrenal lesions has been recently reported [34].

In most cases, it is possible to reach a definitive diagnosis by EUS-FNA biopsy [18, 11, 35]. The following statements can be formulated regarding the indication for FNA biopsy of the

adrenal glands [11]: (1) biopsy of an adrenal mass enables differentiation between adrenal tissue and nonadrenal tissue, i.e. in particular detection of metastases and/or lymphomas; (2) differentiation between adrenocortical adenoma and adrenocortical carcinoma is not possible with FNA, thus, this is not an indication for biopsy; (3) because of complications reported in the literature caused by mechanical manipulations of pheochromocytomas [36], FNA of adrenal masses should not be performed if pheochromocytoma has not been excluded.

MEN1 Disease with Pancreatic Involvement
The diagnostic value of EUS in the management of patients with MEN1 disease has emerged during the last decade. We have learned that the measurement of tumor diameter in pancreatic NETs is effectively reproducible [37]. We have further gained information about the natural dynamics of tumor growth and development which enables us to identify lesions with an abnormal and thus suspicious growth pattern [38–40]. A 'normal' growth velocity has been calculated as an increase in the largest tumor diameter of 1–2% per month. About every 2 years a new pancreatic lesion may be detected in a normal course of the disease. EUS has been

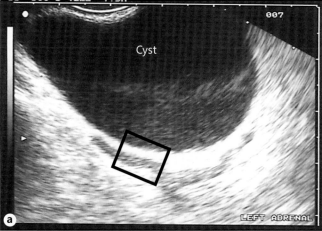

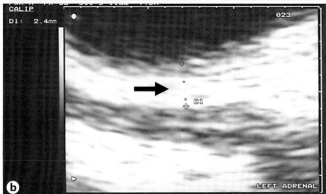

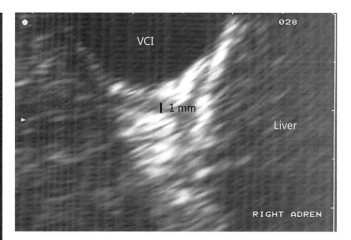

Fig. 9. Marked atrophy of the adrenals can be observed in autoimmune Addison's disease (here, the right adrenal). Their thickness is here only 1 mm. Similar findings may be expected in adrenomyeloneuropathy/adrenoleukodystrophy. VCI = Inferior caval vein.

Fig. 8. a A 48-year-old female patient with an incidental diagnosis of a cystic adrenal mass. **b** By EUS, a 2.4-mm lamella between the lesion and the adrenal could be identified (arrow). Thus, the diagnosis was of an extra-adrenal cystic lesion with a sedimentation phenomenon. It was assumed that this might be a posttraumatic remnant after a motorcycle accident some years ago. Follow-up and no surgical treatment was recommended. Nevertheless, the patient insisted on an operation as she now reported local pain in this location. Histopathological analysis revealed a rare diagnosis: a bronchogenic cyst with circumscribed gastric mucosal metaplasia.

shown to be much more sensitive in detecting pancreatic NETs in MEN1 than other imaging methods: the detection rate in lesions <15 mm is about 10-fold higher than by CT, MRI and somatostatin receptor scintigraphy [38]. EUS has been shown to provide the highest preoperative sensitivity compared to other imaging methods [41].

Insulinoma

The diagnostic process in suspected insulinomas is primarily based on endocrine standard test procedures, especially the fasting test [42, 43]. Imaging is not a first-line tool in the diagnosis of insulinomas, but is rather used to localize the source of pathological insulin secretion and to plan the surgical strategy [44–47]. By analyzing the topography of the tumor and surrounding critical anatomical structures carefully, the surgeon may have a reliable basis on which to consider whether minimal invasive surgery may be the appropriate way to cure the patient [22]. Sometimes, in a case with unclear findings in the fasting test, missing toxicology and suspected hypoglycemia factitia, it may be very important that EUS-FNA reveals a doubtless diagnosis.

Insulinomas – like pancreatic NETs in general – usually appear hypoechoic (fig. 11), but can also be isoechoic with a small halo to the surrounding pancreas, completely isoechoic, and, in rare cases, hyperechoic. 'Invisible insulinomas' seem to occur in about 10% of cases. The risk of missing an insulinoma because it has the same echogenicity as the surrounding healthy pancreatic tissue seems to be predominantly relevant in slim, young female patients that per se have a quite hypoechoic pancreas [48]. However, the most important determining factor in reaching a correct diagnosis by EUS seems to be the individual experience of the endosonographer with the given method and indication [49].

An additional problem seems to be the correct position of the patient. There are so far no data on this question available in the literature. However, investigating the patient lying on his or her left side may be problematic, although this is practiced in numerous centers. The crucial point seems to be that the transducer slips over the pan-

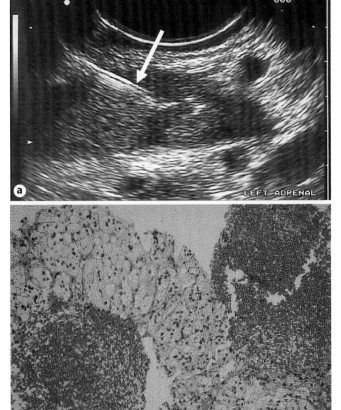

Fig. 10. a EUS-FNA of a small left adrenal mass in a 55-year-old male patient with a history of malignant melanoma and suspected adrenal metastasis. b Histopathological analysis revealed normal adrenal tissue. There was no evidence for malignancy. Thus, the final diagnosis was adrenal hyperplasia as confirmed by fine-needle biopsy.

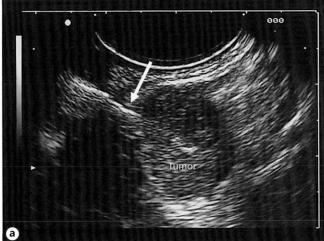

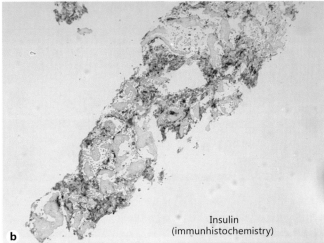

Fig. 11. A 27-year-old male patient with recurrent symptomatic hypoglycemic episodes following physical activity. A fasting test revealed borderline results; toxicology was negative. a EUS detected a 14-mm hypoechoic tumor in the pancreatic tail which was proven to be an insulinoma by EUS-FNA. b Histological analysis revealed NET cells positive for insulin by immunohistochemistry. The tissue sample was obtained by a needle biopsy.

creas to a more lateral position, meaning small tumors may be missed. Our experience shows that a negative EUS performed elsewhere may become positive if the patient lies in a supine position. Analysis of the EUS features may yield evidence to help determine whether the tumor is more likely benign or malignant [5]. If angioinvasion is proven by EUS, this has to be taken as a clear sign of malignancy.

In summary, despite the methodical limitations responsible for false negative results (and, in rare cases, false positive results, see below), EUS enables the identification and correct localization of an insulinoma in about 80–90% of patients. Today, EUS has the best diagnostic performance in the localization of insulinoma compared to CT and MRI [50, 51, 33]. However, its current predominant relevance

seems to be the identification of patients that may qualify for minimal invasive surgery [22].

Other Indications and Problems

All other morphological abnormalities of the pancreas may be imaged by EUS. Hypoechoic lesions that show a clear border and are not heterogeneous may be NETs. Diagnosis can be verified by EUS-FNA.

Gastrinomas may lie in the pancreas, but more frequently occur in the duodenal wall and may be very small. EUS has been shown to be unreliable in the diagnosis of gastrinomas, especially when using a longitudinal scanner for the duodenum [52].

An undisputed problem in EUS imaging of the pancreas is false positive findings, which have also been documented in the literature [6]. It has been suggested to name them PNUDs (pancreatic nodules of unknown dignity). Single cases which have been treated surgically showed that such nodular regions in the pancreas may be completely normal pancreatic tissue by histological analysis, probably ectopic tissue of the ventral primordium, which frequently appears hypoechoic. In our experience, an intrapancreatic accessory spleen can also be identified as the histological substrate of a PNUD. Such unclear nodular regions in the pancreas may be detected in about 1% of all EUS procedures of the pancreas [6]. EUS-FNA may be helpful for a differential diagnosis.

Conclusion

In some European centers, EUS of the adrenals has developed from an experimental procedure into an established diagnostic standard procedure. We can conclude that EUS performed by an experienced investigator after sufficient premedication is a harmless procedure for the patient [53]. The complication rate is comparable to that of a conventional gastroscopy, there is no exposure to radiation and no need to apply contrast media. The diagnostic value and clinical impact are high, and the procedure is not very expensive. For all these reasons, EUS can be considered to be a relevant advantage in diagnosing and differentiating adrenal diseases, although the clinical relevance of EUS findings largely depends on the personal experience of the endosonographer, as well as procedure indications.

It should be considered mandatory to provide an EUS performed by a highly qualified and experienced endosonographer in centers where patients with pancreatic NETs are diagnosed and treated by surgery. Today, the adequate care of patients suffering from MEN1 disease is no longer imaginable without performing EUS at regular intervals [39]. EUS does not only play a relevant role in diagnosing insulinomas, but is especially helpful in planning the surgical strategy.

References

1 Chang KJ, Erickson RA, Nguyen P: Endoscopic ultrasound (EUS) and EUS-guided fine-needle aspiration of the left adrenal gland. Gastrointest Endosc 1996;44:568–572.

2 Kann P, Bittinger F, Hengstermann C, Engelbach M, Beyer J: Endosonographische Darstellung der Nebennieren: Eine neue Methode. Ultraschall Med 1998;19:4–9.

3 Kann P, Bittinger F, Hengstermann C, Engelbach M, Beyer J: Endosonography of the adrenal glands: normal size – pathological findings. Exp Clin Endocrinol Diabetes 1998;106:123–129.

4 Kann P, Heintz A, Bittinger F, Herber S, Kunt T, Beyer J: Endosonograpie bei kleinen Nebennierenraumforderungen: Morphologischer Nachweis der mikro- und makronodulären Nebennierenrindenhyperplasie in vivo als Ursache einer autonomen Sekretion von Steroidhormonen. Tumordiagn Ther 1999;20:135–143.

5 Kann P, Bittinger F, Engelbach M, Bohner S, Weis A, Beyer J: Endosonography of insulin-secreting and clinically non-functioning neuroendocrine tumors of the pancreas: criteria for benignancy and malignancy. Eur J Med Res 2001;6:385–390.

6 Kann PH, Wirkus B, Keth A, Goitom K: Pitfalls in endosonographic imaging of suspected insulinomas: pancreatic nodules of unknown dignity. Eur J Endocrinol 2003;148:531–534.

7 Müller MF, Meyerberger C, Bertschinger P, Schaer R, Marincek B: Pancreatic tumors: evaluation with endoscopic US, CT, and MR imaging. Radiology 1994;190:745–751.

8 Dietrich CF, Wehrmann T, Hoffmann C, Herrmann G, Caspary WF, Seifert H: Detection of the adrenal glands by endoscopic or transabdominal ultrasound. Endoscopy 1997;29:859–864.

9 Kann P, Heintz A, Bittinger F, Kessler S, Forst T, Weis A, Beyer J: Bildgebende Diagnostik der Nebennieren: neue Aspekte durch die Einführung der Endosonographie. Minimal Inv Chir 2000;9:58–61.

10 Kann PH: Endoscopic ultrasound imaging of the adrenals. Endoscopy 2005;37:244–253.

11 Meyer S, Bittinger F, Keth A, von Mach MA, Kann P: Endosonographically controlled transluminal fine needle aspiration biopsy: diagnostic quality by cytologic and histopathologic classification. Dtsch Med Wochenschr 2003;128:1585–1591.

12 Rösch T, Will U, Chang KJ (eds): Longitudinal Endosonography – Atlas and Manual for Use in the Upper Gastrointestinal Tract. Berlin, Springer, 2001.

13 Uemura S, Yasuda I, Kato T, Doi S, Kawaguchi J, Yamauchi T, Kaneko Y, Ohnishi R, Suzuki T, Yasuda S, Sano K, Moriwaki H: Preoperative routine evaluation of bilateral adrenal glands by endoscopic ultrasound and fine-needle aspiration in patients with potentially resectable lung cancer. Endoscopy 2013;45:195–201.

14 Auernhammer CJ, Engelhardt D, Göke B: Primary hyperparathyroidism, adrenal tumors and neuroendocrine tumors of the pancreas – clinical diagnosis and imaging requirements (in German). Radiologe 2003;43:265–274.

15 Dadan J, Wojskowicz P, Wojskowicz A: Neuroendocrine tumors of the pancreas. Wiad Lek 2008;61:43–47.

16 Fischer L, Mehrabi A, Büchler MW: Neuroendocrine tumors of the duodenum and pancreas: surgical strategy. Chirurg 2011;82:583–590.

17 Krstić M, Sumarac M, Diklić A, Tatić S, Pavlović A, Tomić D, Micić D, Kendereski A, Milinić N, Petakov M: Endoscopic ultrasonography (EUS) in preoperative localization of neuroendocrine tumors (NET) of the pancreas. Acta Chir Iugosl 2005;52:97–100.

18 Chhieng DC, Jhala D, Jhala N, Eltoum I, Chen VK, Vickers S, Heslin MJ, Wilcox CM, Eloubeidi MA: Endoscopic ultrasound-guided fine-needle aspiration biopsy: a study of 103 cases. Cancer 2002;96:232–239.

19 Chang F, Chandra A, Culora G, Mahadeva U, Meenan J, Herbert A: Cytologic diagnosis of pancreatic endocrine tumors by endoscopic ultrasound-guided fine-needle aspiration: a review. Diagn Cytopathol 2006;34:649–658.

20 Chatzipantelis P, Salla C, Konstantinou P, Karoumpalis I, Sakellariou S, Doumani I: Endoscopic ultrasound-guided fine-needle aspiration cytology of pancreatic neuroendocrine tumors: a study of 48 cases. Cancer 2008;114:255–262.

21 Gornals J, Varas M, Catalá I, Maisterra S, Pons C, Bargalló D, Serrano T, Fabregat J: Definitive diagnosis of neuroendocrine tumors using fine-needle aspiration-puncture guided by endoscopic ultrasonography. Rev Esp Enferm Dig 2011;103:123–128.

22 Kann PH, Rothmund M, Zielke A: Endoscopic ultrasound imaging of insulinomas: limitations and clinical relevance. Exp Clin Endocrinol Diabetes 2005;113:471–474.

23 Roggenland D, Schneider S, Klein HH, Kann PH: Endosonographie – eine zusätzliche diagnostische Möglichkeit bei der Differenzierung der beiden häufigsten Formen des primären Hyperaldosteronismus. Med Klin 2006;101:65–68.

24 Meyer S, von Mach MA, Ivan D, Schäfer S, Habbe N, Kann B, Kann PH: Color-coded duplex endoscopic ultrasound of the adrenals. J Endocrinol Invest 2008;31:882–887.

25 van der Bruggen W, Arens AI, van der Drift MA, de Geus-Oei LF, Gotthardt M, Oyen WJ: Referred shoulder pain in a patient with small cell lung cancer: adrenal gland metastases. Neth J Med 2013;71:203–206.

26 Waldmann J, Bartsch DK, Kann PH, Fendrich V, Rothmund M, Langer P: Adrenal involvement in multiple endocrine neoplasia type 1: results of 7 years prospective screening. Langenbecks Arch Surg 2007;392:437–443.

27 Schaefer S, Shipotko M, Ivan D, Klose K-J, Waldmann J, Langer P, Meyer S, Kann PH: Natural course of small adrenal lesions in multiple endocrine neoplasia type 1 (MEN1): an endoscopic ultrasound (EUS) imaging study. Eur J Endocrinol 2008;158:699–704.

28 Rinke A, Galan SR, Fendrich V, Kann PH, Bartsch DK, Gress TM: Hereditary neuroendocrine tumors: multiple endocrine neoplasia type 1 and 2 (in German). Internist 2012;53:400–407.

29 Kann PH, Wirkus B, Behr Th, Klose K-J, Meyer S: Endosonographic imaging of benign and malignant pheochromocytomas. J Clin Endocrinol Metab 2004;89:1694–1697.

30 Ang TL, Chua TS, Fock KM, Tee AK, Teo EK, Mancer K: EUS-FNA of the left adrenal gland is safe and useful. Ann Acad Med Singapore 2007; 36:954–957.

31 Schuurbiers OC, Tournoy KG, Schoppers HJ, Dijkman BG, Timmers HJ, de Geus-Oei LF, Grefte JM, Rabe KF, Dekhuijzen PN, van der Heijden HF, Annema JT: EUS-FNA for the detection of left adrenal metastasis in patients with lung cancer. Lung Cancer 2011;73:310–315.

32 Eloubeidi MA, Morgan DE, Cerfolio RJ, Eltoum IA: Transduodenal EUS-guided FNA of the right adrenal gland. Gastrointest Endosc 2008;67:522–527.

33 Sharma R, Ou S, Ullah A, Kaul V: Endoscopic ultrasound (EUS)-guided fine needle aspiration (FNA) of the right adrenal gland. Endoscopy 2012; 44(suppl 2):E385–E386.

34 Lococo F, Attili F, Meacci E, Petrone G, Inzani F, Granone P, Costamagna G, Larghi A: Transcaval endoscopic ultrasound-guided fine needle aspiration of a right adrenal lesion. Endoscopy 2013; 45(suppl 2):E201–E202.

35 Vilmann P: Endoscopic ultrasound-guided fine-needle biopsy in Europe. Endoscopy 1998;30 (suppl 1):A161–A162.

36 Casola G, Nicolet V, van Sonnenberg E, Withers C, Bretagnolle M, Saba RM, Bret PM: Unsuspected pheochromocytoma: risk of blood-pressure alterations during percutaneous adrenal biopsy. Radiology 1986;159:733–735.

37 Kann PH, Kann B, Fassbender WJ, Forst T, Bartsch DK, Langer P: Small neuroendocrine pancreatic tumors in multiple endocrine neoplasia type 1 (MEN1): least significant change of tumor diameter as determined by endoscopic ultrasound (EUS) imaging. Exp Clin Endocrinol Diabetes 2006;114:361–365.

38 Kann PH, Balakina E, Ivan D, Bartsch DK, Meyer S, Klose K-J, Behr T, Langer P: Natural course of small, asymptomatic neuroendocrine pancreatic tumours in multiple endocrine neoplasia type 1: an endoscopic ultrasound imaging study. Endocr Relat Cancer 2006;13:1195–1202.

39 Waldmann J, Habbe N, Fendrich V, Slater EP, Kann PH, Rothmund M, Langer P: Fast-growing pancreatic neuroendocrine carcinoma in a patient with multiple endocrine neoplasia type 1: a case report. J Med Case Rep 2008;2:354–361.

40 Zimmer T, Scherubl H, Faiss S, Stolzel U, Riecken EO, Wiedenmann B: Endoscopic ultrasonography of neuroendocrine tumours. Digestion 2000; 62(suppl 1):45–50.

41 Lewis MA, Thompson GB, Young WF Jr: Preoperative assessment of the pancreas in multiple endocrine neoplasia type 1. World J Surg 2012;36: 1375–1381.

42 Hirshberg B, Livi A, Bartlett DL, Libutti SK, Alexander HR, Doppman JL, Skarulis MC, Gorden P: Forty-eight-hour fast: the diagnostic test for insulinoma. J Clin Endocrinol Metab 2000;85:3222–3226.

43 Okabayashi T, Shima Y, Sumiyoshi T, Kozuki A, Ito S, Ogawa Y, Kobayashi M, Hanazaki K: Diagnosis and management of insulinoma. World J Gastroenterol 2013;19:829–837.

44 Besim H, Korkmaz A, Hamamcy O, Karaahmetoglu S: Review of eight cases of insulinoma. East Afr Med J 2002;79:368–372.

45 Böttger T, Junginger T, Beyer J, Duber C: Diagnosis of the origin and therapy of organic hyperinsulinism. Med Klin 1995;90:688–692.

46 Lippert H, Wolff H, Kuhn F: Diagnosis and therapy of hyperinsulinism (in German). Langenbecks Arch Chir Suppl II Verh Dtsch Ges Chir 1990: 1007–1008.

47 Nesje LB, Varhaug JE, Husebye ES, Odegaard S: Endoscopic ultrasonography for preoperative diagnosis and localization of insulinomas. Scand J Gastroenterol 2002;37:732–737.

48 Kann PH, Ivan D, Pfützner A, Forst T, Langer P, Schaefer S: Preoperative diagnosis of insulinoma: low body mass index, young age and female gender are associated with negative imaging by endoscopic ultrasound. Eur J Endocrinol 2007;157: 209–213.

49 Fendrich V, Bartsch DK, Langer P, Zielke A, Rothmund M: Diagnosis and surgical treatment of insulinoma – experiences in 40 cases. Dtsch Med Wochenschr 2004;129:941–946.

50 Ardengh JC, Rosenbaum P, Ganc AJ, Goldenberg A, Lobo EJ, Malheiros CA, Rahal F, Ferrari AP: Role of EUS in the preoperative localization of insulinomas compared with spiral CT. Gastrointest Endosc 2000;51:552–555.

51 Joseph AJ, Kapoor N, Simon EG, Chacko A, Thomas EM, Eapen A, Abraham DT, Jacob PM, Paul T, Rajaratnam S, Thomas N: Endoscopic ultrasonography – a sensitive tool in the preoperative localization of insulinoma. Endocr Pract 2013; 19:602–608.

52 Kann PH: The value of endoscopic ultrasound in localizing gastrinoma. Wien Klin Wochenschr 2007;119:585–587.

53 Weis A, Hengstermann C, Beyer J, Kann P: Endosonographic imaging of the adrenal glands and the endocrine pancreas: patient's subjective experiences. Exp Clin Endocr Diab 2000;108(suppl 1):146.

Univ.- Prof. Dr. med. Dr. phil. Peter Herbert Kann, MA
Endokrinologie & Diabetologie, Zentrum für Innere Medizin
Zentrum für In-Vitro-Diagnostik – Endokrinologie
Philipps-Universität/Universitätsklinikum Marburg (UKGM)
Baldinger Strasse, DE–35033 Marburg (Germany)
E-Mail kannp@med.uni-marburg.de

Buchfelder M, Guaraldi F (eds): Imaging in Endocrine Disorders.
Front Horm Res. Basel, Karger, 2016, vol 45, pp 55–69 (DOI: 10.1159/000442313)

Adrenal Imaging: Magnetic Resonance Imaging and Computed Tomography

Colin J. McCarthy[a] · Shaunagh McDermott[b] · Michael A. Blake[c]

Divisions of [a]Interventional Radiology, [b]Thoracic Imaging and Intervention and [c]Abdominal Imaging, Department of Radiology, Massachusetts General Hospital, Harvard Medical School, Boston, Mass., USA

Abstract

The adrenal glands are located superior to the kidneys and play an important role in the endocrine system. Each adrenal gland contains an outer cortex, responsible mainly for the secretion of androgens and corticosteroids, and an inner medulla, which secretes epinephrine and norepinephrine. Here, we review the anatomy of the adrenal glands and explain the current imaging modalities that are most useful for the assessment of the various conditions – both benign and malignant – that can affect these glands. As adrenal lesions are often identified incidentally on cross-sectional imaging performed for other reasons, the management of such adrenal 'incidentalomas' is also discussed. In many cases, adrenal lesions have distinctive imaging features that allow for a full characterization with noninvasive techniques. In some cases, invasive studies such as adrenal vein sampling or adrenal biopsy become necessary. This review should give the reader a wide overview of how various imaging techniques can be useful in the assessment of adrenal pathology.

© 2016 S. Karger AG, Basel

Introduction

The Normal Adrenal Gland

The adrenal cortex is derived from the mesoderm and is responsible for secreting androgens and corticosteroids. The adrenal medulla is derived from neural crest tissue and secretes catecholamines as part of the sympathetic nervous system. The adrenal glands are located within the renal fascia [1] (fig. 1). The glands weigh approximately 5 g each, with the majority of the weight accounted for by the adrenal cortex. On computed tomography (CT), the maximum width of the normal right and left adrenal gland has been estimated at 6.1 and 7.9 mm, respectively. The maximum width of an individual adrenal limb should be at most 6.5 mm in the transverse section [2]. The glands are typically supplied by three adrenal arteries and a single adrenal vein.

Adrenal Lesions

Adrenal lesions are frequently encountered as incidental findings during imaging studies performed for a variety of reasons. It is estimated that approximately 4–5% of patients with no history of endocrine disorder or malignancy have adrenal abnormalities on abdominal CT studies [3]. Furthermore, the incidence of adrenal 'incidentalomas' increases with age [4]. There is also a cohort of patients in whom adrenal pathology may represent the major finding, and explain the patients' signs and symptoms. This is particularly the case in the field of endocrinology, where imaging assessment of the adrenal glands is often critical during the workup of patients with adrenal disorders. Modern imaging techniques allow for the accurate characterization of adrenal lesions into benign and malignant categories in the majority

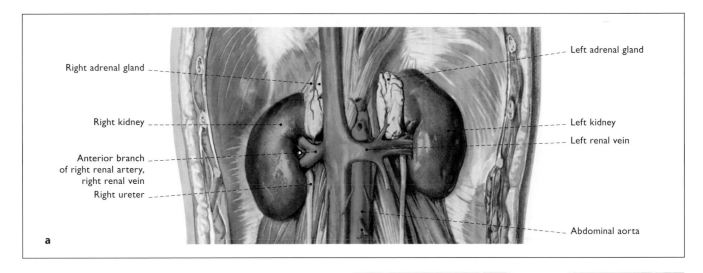

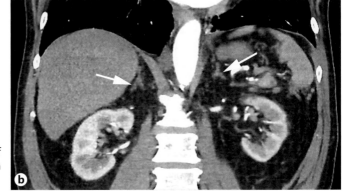

Fig. 1. a, b Coronal-reformatted CT reveals the normal appearance of the adrenal glands (arrows). **a** Reproduced with permission from Köpf-Maier [54].

of cases, with additional investigation (including the use of biopsy) now required only in a minority of cases [5]. In addition to lesion size and morphology, adrenal lesions can be further characterized by the confident identification of its lipid content, its intravenous contrast washout characteristics, as well as by its metabolic activity. In this review, we discuss the role of CT and magnetic resonance imaging (MRI) – now established modalities in the evaluation of adrenal pathology – and briefly present the role of other modalities and developments, including position emission tomography (PET)-CT and MR spectroscopy.

Lesion Morphology

Some lesions can be immediately identified based on their morphological features alone. For example, lesions that are large in size with irregular margins are often suspicious findings, and may represent metastatic disease from a remote primary tumor, or represent a malignancy of the adrenal gland itself (i.e. adrenal cortical carcinoma; ACC). An-

other useful feature is the change in size observed over time with serial imaging. Stability of a lesion over time is relatively reassuring, whereas increasing size may prompt additional investigation, making comparison with any prior imaging covering the adrenal glands helpful at the time of adrenal imaging interpretation. It is important to note, however, that not all enlarging lesions represent malignancy. For example, benign adrenal lesions will increase in response to elevated levels of adrenocorticotropic hormone, and spontaneous or traumatic hemorrhage involving the adrenal gland will cause a more abrupt enlargement in size [6]. Indeed, the typical abundant adrenal arterial supply – via three arteries with drainage only by a single adrenal vein which can be vasoconstricted by medullary catecholamines – is considered to represent a form of vascular dam which predisposes to adrenal hemorrhage [7]. It has also been noted that adrenal lesions >4 cm in size are more likely to represent malignancy, although benign adrenal lesions can also be this size and larger [8].

McCarthy · McDermott · Blake

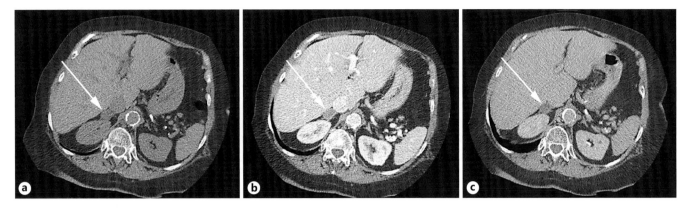

Fig. 2. A 63-year-old woman with a right adrenal lesion discovered on imaging performed for another reason. Selected images from a noncontrast (**a**), portal venous (**b**) and 10-min delayed CT (**c**) are shown. This lesion demonstrated absolute washout of 63% and relative washout of 52%, in keeping with a benign adrenal adenoma.

Computed Tomography

The resolution of modern CT scanners is such that small adrenal lesions can now be identified with relative ease. In addition to the overall morphological features described above, CT can be used to evaluate for the presence of lipid and measure the perfusion characteristics of an adrenal lesion.

Lipid Content

As it is known that the majority of adrenal adenomas contain a high amount of intracellular lipid, the identification of such lipid is very useful during evaluation of an adrenal lesion. This is best performed using noncontrast CT, where Hounsfield measurements of the lesion can be taken, giving an indication of the amount of lipid within the lesion. The value of CT densitometry [9] in differentiating lipid-rich adenomas from nonadenomatous lesions is now well established. In clinical practice, a Hounsfield measurement <10 Hounsfield units (HU) is generally accepted to be a reliable indicator of a lipid-rich adrenal adenoma, with a sensitivity of 71% and specificity of 98% [10].

Although useful when present, the absence of intracytoplasmic lipid on unenhanced CT does not exclude the diagnosis of an adrenal adenoma. It does, however, require the use of additional techniques to further evaluate the lesion. In practical terms, when an adrenal lesion has a mean attenuation value >10 HU on noncontrast CT, such lesions are indeterminate and require additional evaluation.

In those cases where a lesion cannot be confidently labeled as a lipid-rich adenoma based on the 10 HU threshold, some authors have found the use of histogram analysis useful. Rather than focusing on the mean Hounsfield measurement, this technique involves the identification of negative-attenuation (<0 HU) pixels after placing a region of interest around the examined lesion. The authors who originally described this technique for adrenal lesion characterization found that its use increased sensitivity for the detection of adrenal adenomas [11]. However, other studies have found this technique to be of relatively low sensitivity [12]. In particular, some metastases and pheochromocytomas have also exhibited negative pixel values, thereby somewhat limiting the usefulness of this technique that currently is not part of routine clinical practice.

Tissue composition analysis can also be performed with dual-energy CT. This involves the acquisition of two image sets at different tube voltages (kVp), usually at the same time or after a short delay. This method takes advantage of the fact that lipid-containing tissue is known to exhibit a reduction in attenuation with reducing tube voltages [13]. In one study, the authors found that a reduction in attenuation between the 140 and 80 kVp levels was a highly specific feature of an adrenal adenoma. Using this technique, the researchers reported 50% sensitivity and 100% specificity in the diagnosis of adrenal adenoma [14].

Dual-energy CT may also have a role in further characterizing indeterminate adrenal lesions. For example, it is capable of generating virtual unenhanced imaging from post-IV contrast studies, which may be particularly useful when a postcontrast study is performed for another reason. If an adrenal lesion is seen, the dataset can be reconstructed to produce virtual unenhanced imaging. Similarly, the tissue composition information gleaned from dual-energy CT

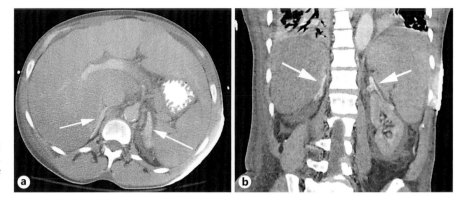

Fig. 3. A 63-year-old man in hypovolemic shock. Axial (**a**) and coronal (**b**) CT with characteristic symmetric hyperenhancement of the adrenal glands (arrows).

may also assist in the differentiation of adrenal adenoma from metastasis [15]. It has also been shown that the increased radiation dose associated with performing a dual-energy CT scan is still less than the dose when a dedicated multiphasic CT is performed [16]. The theory behind the technique involves using CT data to identify the composition of various tissues, which have different characteristics based on the atomic number of the constituent elements at different CT energies (i.e. 80 and 140 kVp). The image sets can be acquired using two different tubes, or using the same tube that can alternate voltages rapidly. Technical factors that must be considered include the presence of motion artifact between the two acquisitions (although this is less of a problem with modern CT scanners), and the fact that the second tube often utilizes a smaller field of view, which in theory may limit dual-energy coverage, particularly in obese patients. Nonetheless, advances in the clinical application of dual-energy CT mean that this may become a valuable tool for adrenal imaging in the near future.

Dynamic Computed Tomography Imaging
In general, adrenal adenomas are known to rapidly accumulate and excrete intravenous iodinated contrast. Such 'contrast washout' can be used to further evaluate adrenal lesions that are indeterminate on the basis of unenhanced CT. Studies have shown that adenomas washout at a faster rate than other lesions, such as metastases [17]. The time after contrast administration in which to obtain delayed imaging is the matter of some debate, although delays of 5–15 min are the most common [18]; a 15-min delay is used at our institution.

The technique involves acquiring noncontrast imaging followed by dynamic contrast-enhanced images (60–75 s), and a final delayed acquisition after 15 min. This allows both the relative and absolute washout values to be calculated (fig. 2).

The washout is calculated as follows:
– absolute percentage washout (APW) = (E – D)/(E – U) × 100,
– relative percentage washout (RPW) = (E – D)/E × 100,

where E = enhanced, D = delayed and U = unenhanced. In cases where unenhanced imaging is not obtained, as is often the case in oncology, an additional delayed acquisition in follow-up studies can provide enough information to calculate the RPW, and may be sufficient to accurately characterize an adrenal lesion as adenoma or non-adenoma. It has been shown that after 15 min, absolute and relative washout values of 60 and 40%, respectively, identify adrenal adenomas with a high degree of accuracy [19, 20]. With a 10-min delayed acquisition, an APW value of 52% or higher appears to be 100% sensitive and 98% specific in the identification of an adrenal adenoma. In the same study, an RPW value of 38–40% or higher had a reported sensitivity of 98% and specificity of 100%, respectively, for the detection of adrenal adenoma [17]. However, it should be borne in mind that these studies excluded pheochromocytomas, which typically show intense enhancement and may demonstrate marked washout. Of further note, a study by Northcutt et al. [21] found that lesions exhibiting higher enhancement during the arterial phase, absolute arterial enhancement measurements of greater than 110 HU and overall lesion heterogeneity were more likely to represent pheochromocytomas than adrenal adenomas.

Perfusion Imaging
Efforts have also been made to identify adrenal lesions based on their early, perfusional characteristics. Information such as blood flow, mean transit time and blood volume can be ascertained using this technique. At least some of these perfu-

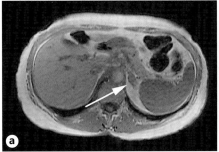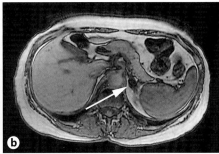

Fig. 4. A 58-year-old man with a left adrenal lesion identified on abdominal CT at an outside facility. T1-weighted axial chemical shift MRI with in-phase (**a**) and out-of-phase (**b**) imaging shows a small lesion in the left adrenal gland. Note the characteristic drop in signal on the out-of-phase image (**b**), typical of a lipid-rich adrenal adenoma.

sion parameters can be explained by the expression of vascular endothelial growth factor and microvessel density within the adrenal tumors; however, this technique is not yet in widespread use [22]. Of note, the importance the body places on adrenal functioning is highlighted by the adrenals' striking relative hyperenhancement in patients in hemodynamic shock, particularly relative to other abdominal organs (fig. 3).

Position Emission Tomography-Computed Tomography
Providing a combination of structural and functional information, PET-CT has been used in the evaluation of the adrenal glands. On PET alone the adrenals are rarely visible, with improved visualization when combined with CT anatomical data [23]. In one study, 41 adrenal lesions in 38 patients were evaluated with PET-CT. Of these, 32 were considered to be benign based on either stability on imaging (n = 31) or biopsy confirmation (n = 1). Thirty out of 32 benign lesions showed ^{18}F-FDG (fluorodeoxyglucose) activity that was less than that of the liver. In addition, all malignant adrenal lesions were detected using PET-CT, with no false negative results [17].

In another study, Boland et al. [24] reviewed 150 consecutive patients undergoing PET-CT with a documented malignancy and known adrenal lesions. The authors found that combined PET-CT identified malignant lesions with a sensitivity of 100% and specificity of 99%. When it came to detecting benign lesions, combined PET-CT had a sensitivity and specificity of 99 and 100%, respectively.

Metser et al. [25] showed that the combination of PET and CT was superior to PET alone in differentiating benign from malignant adrenal lesions in those patients with a known malignancy. Additionally, they noted that using an SUV threshold of 3.1 could identify malignant lesions with a sensitivity and specificity of 98.5 and 92%, respectively. Importantly, a number of studies have noted caution when it comes to false negatives, as adrenal metastases from tu-

mors such as neuroendocrine tumors and lung tumors previously categorized as bronchoalveolar lung cancer may be non-FDG avid [26, 27].

Magnetic Resonance Imaging
MRI offers excellent soft tissue information without the use of ionizing radiation. In brief, MRI involves placing the patient in a strong magnetic field, which causes the axes of all protons in the body to line up and spin, or more accurately, precess around the axis of the external magnetic field. The frequency of precession is directly related to the strength of the magnetic field, as defined by the Larmor equation. When a radiofrequency (RF) wave is applied at the same frequency as the precessing protons (resonance), the protons can absorb that energy. When the RF wave is turned off, the energy is released and can be measured by coils on the surface of the body; this is analyzed and used to produce images. As tissues have different chemical properties (i.e. fat and water content), the return of the protons to their original state after removal of the RF pulse varies depending on the chemical structure of the tissue, producing T1 and T2 times which can lead to the production of clinically useful diagnostic images.

A fundamental imaging technique with MRI is the ability to identify fat using chemical shift imaging. This takes advantage of the slightly different resonant frequencies of lipid and water protons. At a 1.5-tesla field strength, the difference in resonant frequencies of fat and water protons is approximately 224 Hz [28].

An important parameter during MRI acquisition is the time between the RF pulse and the echo (signal returning from the tissue), known as the echo time (TE). Fat protons precess more slowly than water protons, causing the protons to cycle between 'in' and 'out-of-phase'. After 4.4 ms in a 1.5-tesla magnet, the protons of water and lipid are briefly in sync or 'in-phase'. By selecting a TE of 2.2 ms (exactly half of 4.4 ms), the protons in water and fat will be maximally

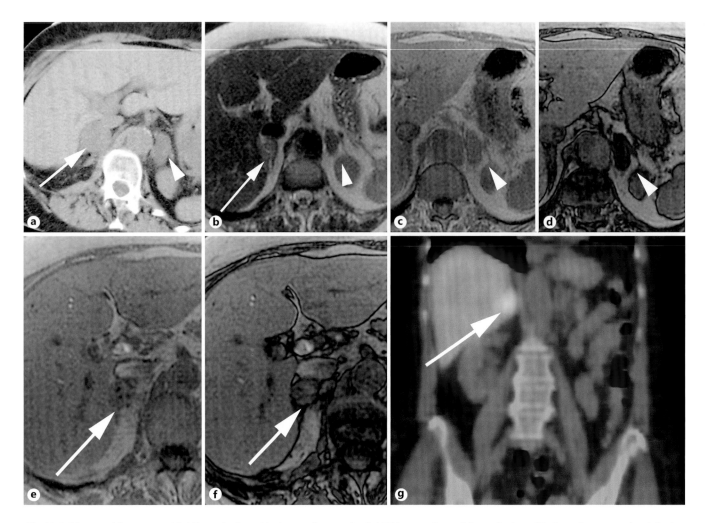

Fig. 5. A 62-year-old woman with bilateral adrenal lesions. **a** A curved axial CT image shows bilateral adrenal lesions, larger on the right (arrow) than the left (arrowhead). **b** The right adrenal lesion exhibits mildly increased T2 signal (arrow). **c, d** T1-weighted chemical shift imaging shows dramatic loss in signal of the left adrenal lesion (arrowhead), compatible with an adrenal adenoma. The right adrenal lesion (**e, f**, arrow) does not drop in signal, and also the coronal fused MIBG/CT image (**g**) shows increased uptake in the right adrenal lesion, and this lesion represented a right adrenal pheochromocytoma.

'out-of-phase', a phenomenon which can be used to identify the presence of lipid and water in the same area of tissue or voxel. Again, because many adrenal adenomas contain lipid [29] unlike most metastases, imaging can be optimized to highlight the presence of fat, thereby allowing the noninvasive diagnosis of adrenal adenoma (fig. 4–6).

The identification of lipid in adenomas can be performed using MRI or CT, as described above. The sensitivity for identification is similar for both CT densitometry and MR chemical shift imaging, although there is evidence that MRI may be superior in the case of lipid-poor adrenal adenomas measuring between 10 and 20 HU on noncontrast CT [30].

Nonadenomatous exceptions to the general rule regarding lesions containing lipid include tumors such as myelolipomas (which contain macroscopic foci of fat), rarely pheochromcotytomas (atypical) and adrenocortical carcinomas, and some metastases from clear-cell renal cancer, liposarcoma and some hepatocellular cancers.

Postcontrast (gadolinium) imaging may be performed in addition to chemical shift imaging. Similar to CT, benign adrenal adenomas typically exhibit prompt mild enhancement and rapid washout on dynamic imaging, whereas malignant lesions tend to enhance more avidly and are slower to washout.

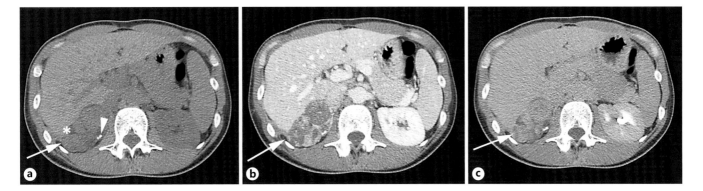

Fig. 6. A 49-year-old woman with an incidental right adrenal mass. Axial noncontrast (**a**), postcontrast (**b**) and delayed (**c**) CT images revealed a large, right, 6.1 × 3.9 × 3.9 cm lobulated soft tissue mass (arrow) arising from the right adrenal gland, containing foci of possible lipomatous elements (*) and punctate calcifications (arrowhead). The mass was excised, revealing adrenocortical adenoma composed of two cell components with lipomatous and cystic degenerative changes. Although ultimately benign, this mass may be difficult to categorically define as such on imaging alone, and given the relative increased risk of malignancy in large adrenal masses, masses such as this are often resected.

The third MR technique is conventional spin-echo MRI, where standard T1- and T2-weighted imaging can be performed. The T2-weighted sequence is of particular importance as pheochromocytomas are known to exhibit a high T2 signal in a relatively large percentage of cases, although the intense T2 bright 'light bulb' sign is less common than once thought and a non-T2 bright lesion does not exclude a pheochromocytoma [31].

Adrenal Lesions – General Approach to Imaging Evaluation
Most adrenal lesions are identified incidentally during abdominal imaging [4]. These so-called 'adrenal incidentalomas' are generally defined as a focal adrenal lesion measuring ≥1 cm. In 2002, an NIH conference was held which heard presentations from 21 experts in adrenal incidentalomas, with one of the most important recommendations being the need for the multidisciplinary management of such lesions [32].

As noted previously, the prevalence of adrenal incidentalomas is relatively high and was estimated at 4.4% in a large population [3], with an increasing prevalence with older patient age [33]. Such lesions are bilateral in approximately 10–15% of cases, in which case metastatic disease, congenital adrenal hyperplasia, bilateral cortical adenomas and infiltrative diseases of the adrenal glands are the most common underlying etiologies [34]. Upon discovery, the main issues are determining whether the mass is functioning and whether it represents a benign or malignant process. Although imaging can provide useful information, the input of an endocrinologist is invaluable, particularly when it

comes to biochemical investigation and the coordination of patient follow-up.

It is important to note that the incidence of malignancy in incidentally discovered adrenal lesions is very low. A meta-analysis performed by Cawood et al. [35] found that the incidence of primary adrenal carcinoma and metastases from a nonadrenal tumor in such patients was of approximately 1.9–4.7 and 0.7–2.3%, respectively. Most studies have also shown that increasing lesion size also confers an increased risk of malignancy, either primary or metastatic [36]. In view of this, standard first steps for the radiologist are to compare the lesion with any priors to assess for any change in size and to also evaluate the lesion for the presence of lipid, often allowing the lesion to be characterized as an adrenal adenoma.

Benign Lesions

Adrenal Adenoma
Adrenal adenomas are commonly small (<4 cm) and exhibit evidence of intravoxel lipid as evidenced by low attenuation on CT (<10 HU) or drop in signal on chemical shift MRI. Postcontrast imaging should show an absolute washout of at least 60% at 15 min. The imaging characteristics were described in detail above.

Adrenal Myelolipoma
Another fat-containing lesion is the adrenal myelolipoma, a relatively uncommon tumor containing mainly fat and he-

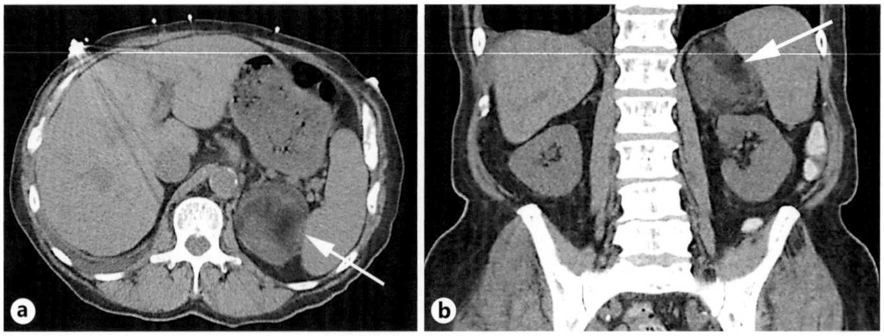

Fig. 7. A 56-year-old man with a 5.5-cm left adrenal mass. Axial (**a**) and coronal (**b**) CT images revealed that the lesion contains gross fat (low attenuation), in keeping with an adrenal myelolipoma.

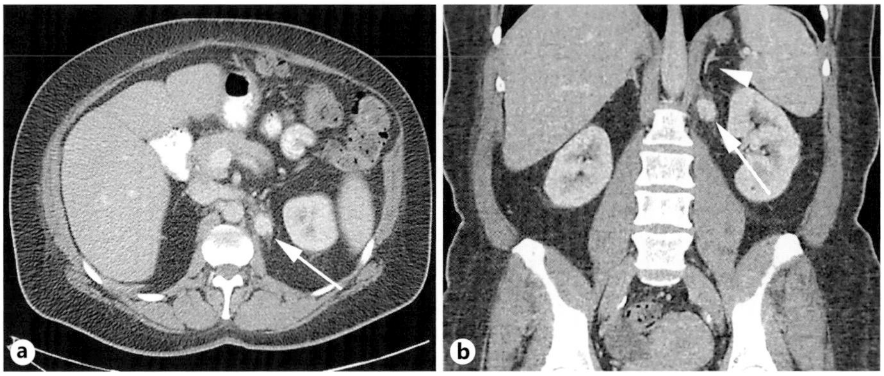

Fig. 8. A 42-year-old woman with hypertension. Serial CT examinations had shown a slow interval increase in size of a left para-aortic mass. Axial (**a**) and coronal (**b**) CT images showed a 2.6-cm hyperenhancing lesion in the left para-aortic region (arrow). Note the normal-appearing left adrenal gland (arrowhead). Surgical excision of the mass revealed a paraganglioma.

matopoietic elements resembling bone marrow. Myelolipomas are usually unilateral and nonfunctioning, but can be quite large in size. They are easily distinguished from adrenal adenomas by the presence of usually well-defined macroscopic fat on imaging (fig. 7), and sometimes contain small areas of calcification. Spontaneous intralesion hemorrhage has been described, particularly associated with increasing tumor size, although not very frequently [37]. Given the usual large amount of fat within these tumors, they exhibit characteristic T1 hyperintensity on MRI, with a drop in signal on fat-suppression imaging. If the noninvasive diagnosis is certain, further evaluation and follow-up is not typically required.

Pheochromocytoma
Pheochromocytomas are catecholamine-secreting tumors that typically (90%) arise from the adrenal medulla (pheochromocytoma), with extra-adrenal pheochromocytomas (more correctly referred to as paraganglioma) occurring anywhere along the sympathetic chain from the neck to the urinary bladder. The organ of Zuckerkandl, a ganglion at the level of the aortic bifurcation, is a common location of paraganglionoma (of note, pathologists still call lesions at this lo-

cation extra-adrenal pheochromocytomas). These tumors are characteristically solid masses, classically described as T2 hyperintense on MRI with avid contrast enhancement (fig. 8). They are often well circumscribed, and may be multiple in the case of a familial syndrome, including multiple endocrine neoplasia type II, von Recklinghausen's disease, Carney's syndrome and von Hippel-Lindau disease. Importantly, the typical imaging features may be absent, requiring the radiologist to be aware of the various appearances of these tumors [38]. Indeed, they can mimic many other pathologies, including adrenal adenomas. Correlation with biochemical markers and patient symptomatology (i.e. palpitations, sweating and hypertension) is often useful. The presence of disease at remote sites is currently the only reliable determinant of malignant behavior in these tumors. A relatively large study performed by Goldstein et al. [39] showed the incidence of malignancy to be in the order of 13%.

The incidence of malignancy is known to be higher in extra-adrenal paragangliomas when compared to adrenal pheochromocytoma, by a ratio of about 2:1. Workup assessing for local and metastatic disease may include the use of CT. Although there have been concerns in the past of iodinated contrast media exacerbating hypertension in pa-

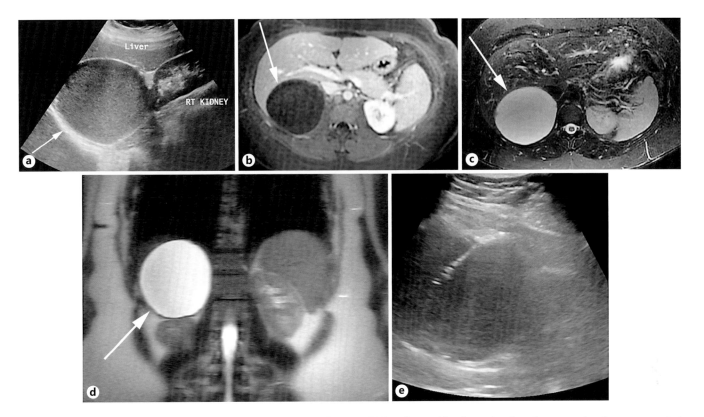

Fig. 9. A 55-year-old female with right upper quadrant pain. An ultrasound (**a**) performed for the evaluation of suspected gallstones revealed a large, well-defined fluid collection closely related to the upper pole of the right kidney. Axial T1 postcontrast (**b**) and T2-weighted (**c**) MRI revealed a 10-cm cyst arising from the right adrenal gland, with no solid components and no abnormal enhancement. Coronal T2-weighted MRI (**d**) showed the mass to be separate from the right kidney. Given its size and the patient's symptomatology, she elected to undergo ultrasound-guided aspiration (**e**), with analysis revealing benign cyst contents.

tients with pheochromocytoma, this is not felt to be of significant concern with modern low-osmolar contrast agents. In one small study, the authors found there to be a clinical and statistically significant increase in diastolic blood pressure immediately after infusion, with no change in plasma catecholamine levels in their group of patients [40].

If CT and MRI remain negative for pheochromocytoma in the presence of suspicious clinical and biochemical findings, an alternative imaging method, such as MIBG (^{123}I-metaiodobenzylguanidine) scintigraphy, should be considered.

Adrenal Cyst

Adrenal cysts are relatively rare findings, both in imaging and autopsy studies, with a reported incidence <1%. They are generally unilateral and asymptomatic, although abdominal pain, mass, hypertension and spontaneous hemor-

rhage have been reported [41]. A number of histological subtypes have been described, although for the most part it is not possible to discriminate these subtypes on imaging. The majority of adrenal cysts are histologically classified as endothelial (45%) or pseudocysts (39%), with epithelial and parasitic subtypes accounting for 9 and 7%, respectively [42]. Adrenal cysts are more common in females (fig. 9). Adrenal pseudocysts are considered to represent the sequelae of prior hemorrhage or trauma.

For all intents and purposes, adrenal cysts have very similar imaging appearances to simple renal cysts: they are generally of uniformly low attenuation on CT, exhibit high T2 signal on MRI and do not enhance. Their walls are usually thin and may contain calcification. Such lesions can somewhat mimic or be associated with other adrenal pathology, including cystic pheochromocytoma, ACC or adrenal metastases; however, all are rare and usually have at least a perceptible cuff of soft tissue. The management of adrenal cysts

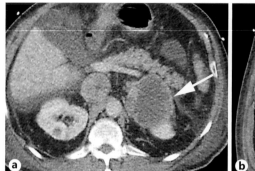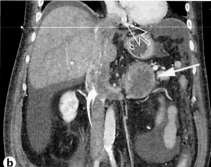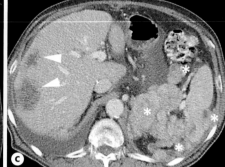

Fig. 10. A 75-year-old man undergoing investigation for weight loss. Axial (**a**) and coronal (**b**) CT revealed a 6-cm low-attenuation mass in the left adrenal (arrow). Note the filling defect in the left renal vein as it joins the inferior vena cava (curved arrow), with propagation of the thrombus to the inferior vena cava/right atrium junction (hollow arrow). The overall picture is that of an aggressive process, with biopsy confirming ACC. **c** Follow-up CT at 1 year showed progressive disease with multiple peritoneal (*) and liver (arrowhead) metastases.

is somewhat controversial; some authors suggest that the lesions can be followed on imaging, regardless of size [42], whereas others suggest that lesions larger than 5–6 cm require surgical evaluation [43].

Malignant Lesions

Adrenal Cortical Carcinoma

ACCs are rare and may be either functional or nonfunctional. They have an estimated incidence of 1–2/million people/year, and are more common in females [44]. Often large at presentation, they are commonly aggressive (fig. 10). Most cases are sporadic, although cases have been described in some of the hereditary syndromes, including Li-Fraumeni syndrome [45].

The incidence of malignancy in the adrenal glands is directly related to the increasing size of the tumor: over 90% of ACC are >4 cm when discovered [46]. The tumors exhibit a bimodal age distribution, with a peak in early childhood and between 40 and 50 years of age. Up to 60% of tumors are secretory and present with clinical signs and symptoms of hormone excess [44]. The tumors may overproduce glucocorticoids or androgens, resulting in Cushing's syndrome and virilization, respectively, although a combination of hormone hypersecretion may also be seen.

When compared to adrenal adenomas, ACC are generally larger when seen on both CT and MRI. ACCs may have irregular borders, internal heterogeneity, areas of calcification or evidence of invasion into adjacent structures or locoregional lymphadenopathy. Local invasion is often better

assessed with MRI, where improved soft-tissue contrast allows for more confident assessment of fat planes. Such lesions are often heterogeneous on both T1- and T2-weighted imaging, with areas of hemorrhage causing a high T1 signal and areas of tumor necrosis resulting in a high signal on T2-weighted sequences [5]. In contradistinction to adrenal adenomas, adrenocortical carcinomas demonstrate low-contrast washout similar to other malignancies [47]. These tumors also have a propensity to spread by tumor thrombus along the draining veins of the adrenal (fig. 10).

With PET-CT, ACC is known to exhibit increased FDG uptake. It has also been shown that this technique can be a useful tool for evaluating the presence of extra-adrenal disease, and may alter the management and prognosis [48]. However, the degree of increased uptake does not correlate with prognosis [49].

Adrenal Metastases

After lung, bone and liver, the adrenal glands are the fourth most common site of metastatic disease, despite their small size. Although frequently noted on autopsy series, very small adrenal metastases may not always be readily apparent on imaging, and may manifest with only a mildly nodular appearance of the adrenal gland. In other cases, discrete masses may be evident and sometimes large. Tumors that commonly metastasize to the adrenals include lung, breast and renal tumors, in addition to melanoma (fig. 11–13).

Adrenal metastases tend to be irregular in contour, may be bilateral and can exhibit increased FDG uptake on PET-CT. Given that the presence of an adrenal mass may be unrelated to the primary malignancy, many cen-

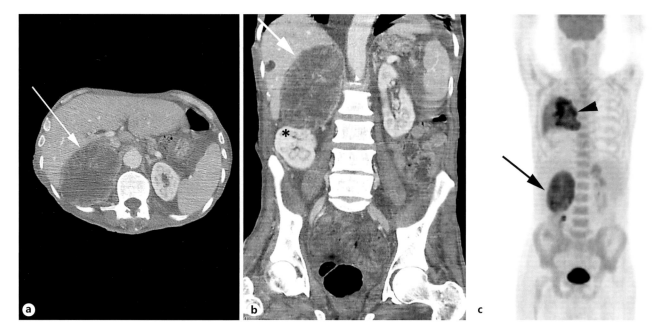

Fig. 11. A 75-year-old woman with a history of melanoma. Axial (**a**) and coronal (**b**) CT showed a large heterogeneous mass in the right adrenal gland (arrow), which most likely represented an adrenal metastasis. **c** Coronal MIP from a whole-body PET showed increased FDG uptake in the right adrenal lesion (arrow), together with a large mass in the right lung (arrowhead), which represented a biopsy-proven melanoma metastasis.

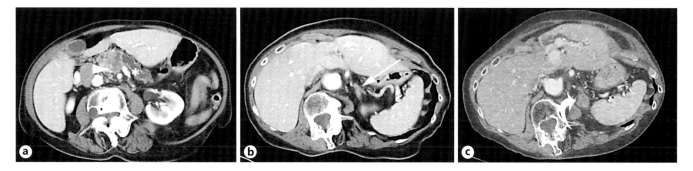

Fig. 12. A 79-year-old man with weight loss. **a, b** Initial axial CT revealed a pancreatic head mass (arrowhead) with pancreatic duct dilatation (*) and a mildly prominent left adrenal (arrow) without a discrete mass. **c** Follow-up CT performed 8 months later showed a new 2.5-cm left adrenal mass (curved arrow), suspicious for a metastatic deposit from the patient's biopsy-proven pancreatic adenocarcinoma.

ters will consider percutaneous biopsy when a definitive diagnosis is required. This is of particular importance when the exact nature of an adrenal lesion will dictate oncologic management of a primary tumor. However, it should be borne in mind that pathologists usually cannot reliably distinguish between an adrenal adenoma and an adrenocortical carcinoma on the basis of a fine-needle biopsy sample.

Adrenal Lymphoma

Lymphoma can sometimes involve the adrenal glands, usually as a manifestation of systemic disease rather than primary adrenal lymphoma, which is rare. In some cases, subtle lymphomatous infiltration of the adrenal glands may be difficult or impossible to identify on CT or MRI alone, whereas PET-CT provides additional functional information and may allow for the diagnosis of adrenal involvement. In general, the degree of increased FDG uptake tracks that of disease elsewhere [5].

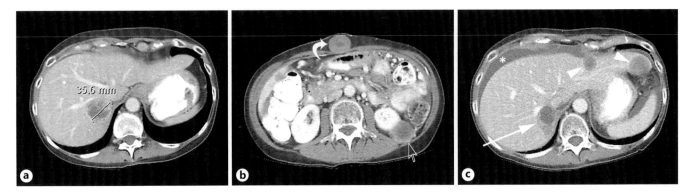

Fig. 13. A 66-year-old woman with a history of endometrial carcinoma. **a** Axial contrast-enhanced CT revealed a 3.6-cm right adrenal lesion. The patient underwent surgical excision, with the pathology confirming metastatic endometrial carcinoma. **b, c** Subsequent follow-up CT was performed. This revealed recurrence of the right adrenal metastasis (arrow), with new liver metastases (arrowheads), left renal metastasis (hollow arrow), ascites (*) and subcutaneous nodules, including a large deposit at the umbilicus (curved arrow), the so-called 'Sister Mary Joseph nodule'.

Fig. 14. a A 58-year-old man with a new diagnosis of lung cancer and an indeterminate left adrenal lesion measuring 2.5 cm. **b** He was referred for percutaneous biopsy, which was performed in the ipsilateral decubitus position, in an attempt to stabilize the left adrenal gland and reduce the risk of pneumothorax. Pathology revealed metastatic non-small-cell lung carcinoma.

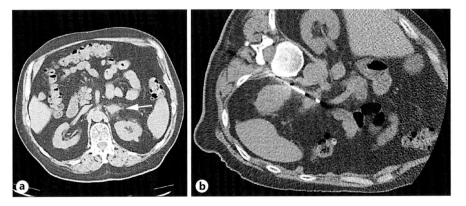

Image-Guided Intervention

Computed Tomography Biopsy

Radiologists are frequently asked to perform image-guided biopsy of the adrenal gland, usually when a focal lesion remains indeterminate by noninvasive studies and a definitive diagnosis is required. This is particularly important in oncologic imaging, where the presence of an adrenal metastasis from another site of malignancy may alter both the management and prognosis of a patient.

Percutaneous biopsy can be performed using ultrasound, CT or MRI. At our Institution the overwhelming majority of adrenal biopsies are performed using CT.

Our standard workup includes evaluation of the coagulation profile, complete blood count and basic metabolic panel. If there is any suspicion of a pheochromocytoma or extra-adrenal paraganglioma, it is imperative to perform a biochemical workup prior to any biopsy. Most adrenal biopsies are performed in the outpatient setting using monitored conscious sedation, or occasionally local anesthesia alone.

It is our preference to biopsy the adrenal gland in the ipsilateral decubitus position, using a direct posterior approach (fig. 14). For example, in the case of a right adrenal lesion, the patient lies on their right side. The reasoning for this approach is that the lung on the side nearest the table top expands less, therefore reducing the amount of lung between the adrenal gland and the skin. It is also theorized that the adrenal gland is more stable (and less likely to push away from the biopsy needle) in the lateral decubitus position. We generally adopt a paravertebral approach to biopsy of the adrenal gland. Occasionally, it may be necessary to traverse the pleura, liver or kidney to reach the adrenal gland.

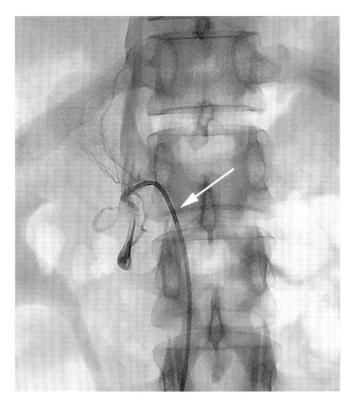

Fig. 15. A 36-year-old male with suspected primary hyperaldosteronism with bilateral adrenal nodules on CT (not shown). The image shows the catheter in the right adrenal vein.

Adrenal Vein Sampling

In cases where there is concern that an adrenal lesion is hormonally active, adrenal vein sampling can be performed. This can be a technically challenging procedure, particularly on the right side where the relatively short right adrenal vein enters directly to the inferior vena cava. On the left side, the adrenal vein enters the left renal vein, which is often more readily accessed. Venous samples will typically be obtained from both sides, in addition to obtaining peripheral blood at the same time. In cases of hyperaldosteronism, adrenal vein sampling can be used to differentiate aldosterone-secreting adrenal tumors from bilateral adrenal hyperplasia (fig. 15; online suppl. video clips; for all online suppl. material, see www.karger.com/doi/10.1159/000442313).

Monitoring of Adrenal Lesions

The American College of Radiology developed a white paper [50] that provides an outline for the image monitoring of adrenal lesions in those cases where such lesions cannot be immediately dismissed as benign on imaging. Three of the most useful determinants of benignity are the presence of lipid (adrenal adenoma), macroscopic fat (myelolipoma) or fluid (adrenal cyst). Lesions that are stable in size and appearance over a 1-year period can usually be dismissed as benign [50].

If lesions remain indeterminate or have not been monitored for 1 year, adrenal washout CT or chemical shift MRI may be useful investigations to identify those lesions representing adrenal adenomas. In order to confirm the stability of an indeterminate adrenal lesion, follow-up CT or MRI after 1 year is recommended. There is some concern associated with CT surveillance of adrenal lesions given the potential for high cumulative radiation doses, while MRI can provide the necessary change in size information without conferring any additional radiation in many cases [35].

Enlarging lesions, or those lesions larger than 4 cm, will require additional evaluation with either PET-CT, biopsy or resection [51]. A number of endocrine organizations and authors have released guidelines regarding the endocrine assessment and management of incidental adrenal lesions.

The American Association of Endocrinologists produced guidelines in 2009 concerning the management of such incidental lesions [52]. Their recommendations include the need for the clinical, biochemical and radiographic evaluation of adrenal incidentalomas, highlighting the importance of evaluating all patients for cortisol excess. In addition, when surgical resection is not required, follow-up imaging at 3–6 months and then annually for 1–2 years was recommended [52]. The Italian Association of Clinical Endocrinologists notes again the importance of the evaluation for cortisol excess, and also the need to exclude pheochromocytoma in all patients with an adrenal incidentaloma [33]. A 2002 NIH consensus panel recommended multidisciplinary management and, where necessary, follow-up imaging at 6–12 months. The panel also noted that long-term radiologic surveillance may not be indicated [32]. A clinical practice paper by Young [4] in 2007 recommended follow-up at 6, 12 and 24 months, and repeat hormonal evaluation on an annual basis for 4 years. On the other hand, Copeland [53] suggested that lesions that are not resected should be followed at 3, 6 and 18 months. Although there are minor variations in the recommendations and guidelines and they continue to evolve and be further refined, in general they provide a useful framework with helpful principles that can be applied to an individual patient in clinical practice.

References

1 Standring S: Suprarenal (adrenal) gland; in Standring S (ed): Gray's Anatomy. Amsterdam, Elsevier, 2008, pp 1197–1201.

2 Vincent JM, Morrison ID, Armstrong P, Reznek RH: The size of normal adrenal glands on computed tomography. Clin Radiol 1994;49:453–455.

3 Bovio S, Cataldi A, Reimondo G, Sperone P, Novello S, Berruti A, Borasio P, Fava C, Dogliotti L, Scagliotti GV, Angeli A, Terzolo M: Prevalence of adrenal incidentaloma in a contemporary computerized tomography series. J Endocrinol Invest 2006;29:298–302.

4 Young WF Jr: Clinical practice: the incidentally discovered adrenal mass. N Engl J Med 2007;356: 601–610.

5 Blake MA, Cronin CG, Boland GW: Adrenal imaging. AJR Am J Roentgenol 2010;194:1450–1460.

6 Russell C, Goodacre BW, van Sonnenberg E, Orihuela E: Spontaneous rupture of adrenal myelolipoma: spiral CT appearance. Abdom Imaging 2000;25:431–434.

7 Rao RH, Vagnucci, RH, Amico JA: Bilateral massive adrenal hemorrhage: early recognition and treatment. Ann Intern Med 1989;110:227–235.

8 McDermott S, O'Connor OJ, Cronin CG, Blake MA: Radiological evaluation of adrenal incidentalomas: current methods and future prospects. Best Pract Res Clin Endocrinol Metab 2012;26: 21–33.

9 Lee MJ, Hahn PF, Papanicolaou N, Egglin TK, Saini S, Mueller PR, Simeone JF: Benign and malignant adrenal masses: CT distinction with attenuation coefficients, size, and observer analysis. Radiology 1991;179:415–418.

10 Boland GW, Lee MJ, Gazelle GS, Halpern EF, McNicholas MM, Mueller PR: Characterization of adrenal masses using unenhanced CT: an analysis of the CT literature. AJR Am J Roentgenol 1998; 171:201–204.

11 Bae KT, Fuangtharnthip P, Prasad SR, Joe BN, Heiken JP: Adrenal masses: CT characterization with histogram analysis method. Radiology 2003; 228:735–742.

12 Remer EM, Motta-Ramirez GA, Shepardson LB, Hamrahian AH, Herts BR: CT histogram analysis in pathologically proven adrenal masses. AJR Am J Roentgenol 2006;187:191–196.

13 Raptopoulos V, Karellas A, Bernstein J, Reale FR, Constantinou C, Zawacki JK: Value of dual-energy CT in differentiating focal fatty infiltration of the liver from low-density masses. AJR Am J Roentgenol 1991;157:721–725.

14 Gupta RT, Ho LM, Marin D, Boll DT, Barnart HX, Nelson RC: Dual-energy CT for characterization of adrenal nodules: initial experience. AJR Am J Roentgenol 2010;194:1479–1483.

15 Shi JW, Dai HZ, Shen L, Xu DF: Dual-energy CT: clinical application in differentiating an adrenal adenoma from a metastasis. Acta Radiol 2014;55: 505–512.

16 Heye T, Nelson RC, Ho LM, Marin D, Boll DT: Dual-energy CT applications in the abdomen. AJR Am J Roentgenol 2012;199(5 suppl):S64–S70.

17 Blake MA, Kalra MK, Sweeney AT, Lucey BC, Maher MM, Sahani DV, Halpern EF, Mueller PR, Hahn PF, Boland GW: Distinguishing benign from malignant adrenal masses: multi-detector row CT protocol with 10-minute delay. Radiology 2006;238:578–585.

18 Kamiyama T, Fukukura Y, Yoneyama T, Takumi K, Nakajo M: Distinguishing adrenal adenomas from nonadenomas: combined use of diagnostic parameters of unenhanced and short 5-minute dynamic enhanced CT protocol. Radiology 2009; 250:474–481.

19 Caoili EM, Korobkin M, Francis JR, Cohan RH, Platt JF, Dunnick NR, Raghupathi KI: Adrenal masses: characterization with combined unenhanced and delayed enhanced CT. Radiology 2002;222:629–633.

20 Korobkin M, Brodeur FJ, Francis IR, Quint LE, Dunnick NR, Londy F: CT-time attenuation washout curves of adrenal adenomas and nonadenomas. AJR Am J Roentgenol 1998;170:747–752.

21 Northcutt BG, Raman SP, Long C, Oshmyansky AR, Siegelman SS, Fishman EK, Johnson PT: MDCT of adrenal masses: can dual-phase enhancement patterns be used to differentiate adenoma and pheochromocytoma? AJR Am J Roentgenol 2013;201:834–839.

22 Qin HY, Sun H, Wang X, Bai R, Li Y, Zhao J: Correlation between CT perfusion parameters and microvessel density and vascular endothelial growth factor in adrenal tumors. PLoS One 2013; 8:e79911.

23 Bagheri B, Maurer AH, Cone L, Doss M, Adler L: Characterization of the normal adrenal gland with 18F-FDG PET/CT. J Nucl Med 2004;45:1340–1343.

24 Boland GW, Blake MA, Holalkere NS, Hahn PF: PET/CT for the characterization of adrenal masses in patients with cancer: qualitative versus quantitative accuracy in 150 consecutive patients. AJR Am J Roentgenol 2009;192:956–962.

25 Metser U, Miller E, Lerman H, Lievshitz G, Avital S, Even-Sapir E: 18F-FDG PET-CT in the evaluation of adrenal masses. J Nucl Med 2006;47:32–37.

26 Yun M, Kim W, Alnafisi N, Lacorte L, Jang S, Alavi A: 18F-FDG PET in characterizing adrenal lesions detected on CT or MRI. J Nucl Med 2001;42: 1795–1799.

27 Erasmus JJ, Patz EF Jr, McAdams HP, Murray JG, Herndon J, Coleman RE, Goodman PC: Evaluation of adrenal masses in patients with bronchogenic carcinoma using 18F-fluorodeoxyglucose positron emission tomography. AJR Am J Roentgenol 1997;168:1357–1360.

28 Hood MN, Ho VB, Smirniotopoulos JG, Szumowski J: Chemical shift: the artifact and clinical tool revisited. Radiographics 1999;19:357–371.

29 Leroy-Willig A, Bittoun J, Luton JP, Louvel A, Lefevre JE, Bonnin A, Roucayrol JC: In vivo MR spectroscopic imaging of the adrenal glands: distinction between adenomas and carcinomas larger than 15 mm based on lipid content. AJR Am J Roentgenol 1989;153:771–773.

30 Israel GM, Korobkin M, Wang C, Hecht EN, Krinsky GA: Comparison of unenhanced CT and chemical shift MRI in evaluating lipid-rich adrenal adenomas. AJR Am J Roentgenol 2004;183: 215–219.

31 Reinig JW, Stutley JE, Leonhardt CM, Spicer KM, Margolis M, Caldwell CB: Differentiation of adrenal masses with MR imaging: comparison of techniques. Radiology 1994;192:41–46.

32 Grumbach MM, Biller BM, Braunstein GD, Campbell KK, Carney JA, Godley PA, Harris EL, Lee JK, Oertel YC, Posner MC, Schlechte JA, Wieand HS: Management of the clinically inapparent adrenal mass ('incidentaloma'). Ann Intern Med 2003;138:424–429.

33 Terzolo M, Stigliano A, Chiodini I, Loli P, Furlani L, Arnaldi G, Reimondo G, Pia A, Toscano V, Zini M, Borretta G, Papini E, Garofalo P, Allolio B, Dupas B, Mantero F, Tabarin A; Italian Association of Clinical Endocrinologists: AME position statement on adrenal incidentaloma. Eur J Endocrinol 2011;164:851–870.

34 Young WF Jr: Management approaches to adrenal incidentalomas: a view from Rochester, Minnesota. Endocrinol Metab Clin North Am 2000;29: 159–185.

35 Cawood TJ, Hunt PJ, O'Shea D, Cole D, Soule S: Recommended evaluation of adrenal incidentalomas is costly, has high false-positive rates and confers a risk of fatal cancer that is similar to the risk of the adrenal lesion becoming malignant; time for a rethink? Eur J Endocrinol 2009;161: 513–527.

36 Mantero F, Terzolo M, Arnaldi G, Osella G, Masini AM, Alì A, Giovagnetti M, Opocher G, Angeli A: A survey on adrenal incidentaloma in Italy: Study Group on Adrenal Tumors of the Italian Society of Endocrinology. J Clin Endocrinol Metab 2000;85:637–644.

37 Rao P, Kenney PJ, Wagner BJ, Davidson AJ: Imaging and pathologic features of myelolipoma. Radiographics 1997;17:1373–1385.

38 Blake MA, Kalra MK, Maher MM, Sahani DV, Sweeney AT, Mueller PR, Hahn PF, Boland GW: Pheochromocytoma: an imaging chameleon. Radiographics 2004;24(suppl 1):S87–S99.

39 Goldstein RE, O'Neill JA Jr, Holcomb GW 3rd, Morgan WM 3rd, Neblett WW 3rd, Oates JA, Brown N, Nadeau J, Smith B, Page DL, Abumrad NN, Scott HW Jr: Clinical experience over 48 years with pheochromocytoma. Ann Surg 1999;229: 755–764; discussion 764–766.

40 Baid SK, Lai EW, Wesley RA, Ling A, Timmers HJ, Adams KT, Kozupa A, Pacak K: Brief communication: radiographic contrast infusion and catecholamine release in patients with pheochromocytoma. Ann Intern Med 2009;150:27–32.

41 Neri LM, Nance FC: Management of adrenal cysts. Am Surg 1999;65:151–163.

42 Ricci Z, Cheryak V, Hsu K, Mazzariol FS, Flusberg M, Oh S, Stein M, Rozenblit A: Adrenal cysts: natural history by long-term imaging follow-up. AJR Am J Roentgenol 2013;201:1009–1016.

43 Rozenblit A, Morehouse HT, Amis ES Jr: Cystic adrenal lesions: CT features. Radiology 1996;201: 541–548.

44 Ng L, Libertino JM: Adrenocortical carcinoma: diagnosis, evaluation and treatment. J Urol 2003; 169:5–11.

45 Gonzalez KD, Noltner KA, Buzin CH, Gu D, Wen-Fong CY, Nguyen VQ, Han JH, Lowstuter K, Longmate J, Sommer SS, Weitzel JN: Beyond Li Fraumeni syndrome: clinical characteristics of families with p53 germline mutations. J Clin Oncol 2009;27:1250–1256.

46 Angeli A, Osella G, Alì A, Terzolo M: Adrenal incidentaloma: an overview of clinical and epidemiological data from the National Italian Study Group. Horm Res 1997;47:279–283.

47 Slattery JM, Blake MA, Kalra MK, Misdraji J, Sweeney AT, Copeland PM, Mueller PR, Boland GW: Adrenocortical carcinoma: contrast washout characteristics on CT. AJR Am J Roentgenol 2006; 187:W21–W24.

48 Becherer A, Viernhapper H, Potzi C, Karanikas G, Schmaljohann J, Staudenherz A, Dudczak R, Kletter K: FDG-PET in adrenocortical carcinoma. Cancer Biother Radiopharm 2001;16:289–295.

49 Tessonnier L, Ansquer C, Bournaud C, Sebag F, Mirallié E, Lifante JC, Palazzo FF, Morange I, Drui D, de la Foucardère C, Mancini J, Taieb D: ^{18}F-FDG uptake at initial staging of the adrenocortical cancers: a diagnostic tool but not of prognostic value. World J Surg 2013;37:107–112.

50 Boland GW, Blake MA, Hahn PF, Mayo-Smith WW: Incidental adrenal lesions: principles, techniques, and algorithms for imaging characterization. Radiology 2008;249:756–775.

51 Berland LL, Silverman SG, Gore RM, Mayo-Smith WW, Megibow AJ, Yee J, Brink JA, Baker ME, Federle MP, Foley WD, Francis IR, Herts BR, Israel GM, Krinsky G, Platt JF, Shuman WP, Taylor AJ: Managing incidental findings on abdominal CT: white paper of the ACR incidental findings committee. J Am Coll Radiol 2010;7: 754–773.

52 Zeiger MA, Thompson GB, Duh QY, Hamrahian AH, Angelos P, Elaraj D, Fishman E, Kharlip J; American Association of Clinical Endocrinologists; American Association of Endocrine Surgeons: American Association of Clinical Endocrinologists and American Association of Endocrine Surgeons Medical Guidelines for the Management of Adrenal Incidentalomas: executive summary of recommendations. Endocr Pract 2009;15:450–453.

53 Copeland PM: Approach to incidentally discovered adrenal masses. JCOM 2007;14:49–59.

54 Köpf-Maier P: Wolf-Heidegger's Atlas of Human Anatomy, ed 6. Basel, Karger, 2005.

Michael Blake, MD
Division of Abdominal Imaging, Department of Radiology
Massachusetts General Hospital, Harvard Medical School
55 Fruit Street, Boston, MA 02114 (USA)
E-Mail mblake2@partners.org

Buchfelder M, Guaraldi F (eds): Imaging in Endocrine Disorders.
Front Horm Res. Basel, Karger, 2016, vol 45, pp 70–79 (DOI: 10.1159/000442317)

Adrenal Molecular Imaging

Anders Sundin

Enheten för Radiologi, Institutionen för Kirurgiska Vetenskaper, Akademiska Sjukhuset, Uppsala Universitet, Uppsala, Sweden

Abstract

The major workload in the field of adrenal imaging comprises patients with adrenal tumors incidentally depicted by imaging performed for other reasons than adrenal disease. These so-called 'incidentalomas' are generally managed by CT and MRI, and molecular imaging techniques are required only for a few patients. PET/CT with ^{18}F-fluorodeoxyglucose (^{18}F-FDG) is useful for establishing whether an adrenal metastasis is the only lesion, and therefore is available for surgical resection, or if the disease is disseminated. ^{18}F-FDG PET/CT may be applied to differ benign from malignant incidentalomas and can be helpful in the imaging of pheochromocytoma and adrenocortical cancer (ACC). ^{11}C-metomidate PET/CT can differentiate adrenocortical from nonadrenocortical tumors and a suspected ACC may be characterized and staged before surgery. ^{11}C-metomidate PET/CT is currently also used to help diagnose Conn's adenomas in primary aldosteronism, but further development is needed. Scintigraphy with ^{123}I/^{131}I-metaiodobenzylguanidine (MIBG) remains the mainstay for molecular imaging of pheochromocytoma and is mandatory in patients for whom ^{131}I-MIBG therapy is considered. A PET tracer for the imaging of pheochromocytoma is the norepinephrine analogue ^{11}C-hydroxyephedrine that can be used to characterize equivocal lesions and for the follow-up and diagnosis of recurrent malignant disease. Other specialized PET tracers for the imaging of pheochromocytoma are ^{18}F-fluorodihydroxyphenylalanine (^{18}F-DOPA) and ^{18}F-fluorodopamine. © 2016 S. Karger AG, Basel

The vast majority of patients who are diagnosed with an adrenal tumor are those who undergo radiological imaging, usually CT (computed tomography) or MRI (magnetic resonance imaging), for reasons other than the suspicion of adrenal disease. Because of the escalating use of high-resolution MDCT (multidetector CT) and MRI, the number of these so-called adrenal 'incidentalomas' has increased considerably. Incidentalomas increase with age and are found in approximately 5% of CT examinations that include the adrenal region [1] and are also diagnosed by MRI and ultrasonography [2]. The finding of an incidentaloma warrants a biochemical workup, usually performed by an endocrinologist, to establish whether the incidentaloma is hormonally active or not. The radiological characterization of the tumor aims to differentiate benign from malignant lesions and was described in detail in the previous chapter. In patients without a cancer history, malignant incidentalomas are rare. This is opposed to cancer patients with the risk that the incidentaloma represents an adrenal metastasis. However, the reported incidence of adrenal metastases in incidentaloma patients varies greatly [3, 4]. Patients who present with clinical symptoms and/or with biochemistry indicating adrenal disease, and therefore undergo imaging, are rare in comparison with those with incidentalomas.

Molecular Imaging Techniques

Imaging with molecular imaging techniques (nuclear medicine imaging, functional imaging) mainly comprises scintigraphy using a gamma camera and PET (positron emission tomography) employing a PET camera. By molecular imaging methods, various aspects of biologic function may be imaged (e.g. metabolism, enzyme activity, receptor density, proliferation, blood flow, etc.) as opposed to radiological methods for imaging of anatomy and morphology.

Scintigraphy can be performed either by planar 2D imaging, producing anterior and posterior views, and/or by 3D transectional single-photon computed emission tomography (SPECT) utilizing gamma-emitting radionuclides, e.g. ^{99m}Tc, ^{123}I, ^{111}In. The radionuclide can be used alone (e.g. ^{123}I and ^{99m}Tc for thyroid scintigraphy) but more commonly the molecules, the biological function of which is imaged, are labelled with a gamma emitter to produce a so-called 'tracer'. Many tracers for scintigraphy are available as labeling kits to which the radionuclide is added. The tracer is usually administered intravenously and after a certain time period (depending on the tracer) allowing for distribution and tissue accumulation, the patient is positioned on the couch of the gamma camera. Planar image acquisition is accomplished by positioning the detectors in front of and/or behind the patient and stepwise, or by a slow continuous motion, moving the detectors to cover the anatomical area of interest. Transversal SPECT images are acquired by moving the detector heads stepwise around the patient in a circular fashion.

Positron-emitting radionuclides are generally produced in a low-energy cyclotron and their half-lives are usually short (^{18}F: 110 min, ^{11}C: 20 min, ^{15}O: 2 min). ^{18}F-tracers may be transported within approximately a 2-hour interval to PET units without a cyclotron. A PET camera resembles a CT scanner, with a patient couch and a short tunnel (gantry) in which thousands of detectors are arranged in several rings, typically with a 15- to 20-cm axial field of view. After tracer injection (and the distribution phase) the patient is positioned on the examination bed of the PET camera and is moved through the gantry during which an approximate 3-min acquisition is performed per 'bed position'. Most PET examinations are performed in oncological patients with ^{18}F-fluorodeoxyglucose (^{18}F-FDG) and typically as whole-body examinations, from the base of the scull to the proximal thighs. ^{18}F-FDG is usually administered 1 h before the examination, whereas with ^{11}C-labelled tracers, because of the shorter half-life, scanning is started earlier after injection

(10–20 min). In research studies, dynamical imaging may also be employed in which the image acquisition is started simultaneously with the tracer injection and the tracer pharmacokinetics may be registered over time for the tissues and organs included in this bed position. Unlike the gamma camera, the detectors in the PET camera indirectly register the positron emissions. The emitted positron collides with an electron upon which both are annihilated and converted into two high-energy (511 keV) photons. These travel in opposite directions and simultaneously (within a few nanoseconds) reach the detectors, allowing for registration of the line of decay. All lines of decay are reconstructed into transversal gray-scale or color-coded images representing the radioactivity concentration (Bq/ml).

Both SPECT and PET images are also regularly reformatted in the coronal and sagittal plane and as a 3D maximum intensity projection (MIP) that may be rotated and facilitates anatomical localization of the functional imaging findings. Also, to this end, SPECT and PET are currently performed on hybrid scanners together with CT (SPECT/CT, PET/CT). In some centers, a low radiation dose CT is used as a means for anatomical correlation; however, most current hybrid scanners allow the performance of a fully diagnostic CT, as regards radiation dose, including intravenous contrast-enhancement in order to fully take advantage of the potential of the hybrid imaging technique. In modern CT scanners a large number of detectors are arranged in parallel rows (multidetector CT, MDCT) and, by use of the rapidly rotating X-ray tube (0.5–1 s per rotation), typically more than one hundred high-resolution 0.5- to 1-mm sections are produced per second and both the abdomen and the thorax can usually be examined during one breath hold. These fast CT scanners also allow for better use of intravenous iodine-based contrast media, whereby the organs and tissues of interest may be examined in various contrast-enhancement phases for CT angiography, and hyper- and hypovascular lesions are displayed.

The CT examination is additionally used to correct the PET and SPECT images for attenuation. This is necessary because some of the photons are attenuated in the tissues and do not reach the detectors. The PET/CT and SPECT/CT examinations are evaluated on a computer workstation which is facilitated by the presentation of the three respective image volumes – (1) PET and SPECT, (2) CT (3) PET-CT fusion and SPECT-CT-fusion – in the transversal, coronal and sagittal planes. The attenuation-corrected PET images also allow for recalculation of the radioactivity concentrations to provide images of standardized uptake values (SUVs) whereby the radioactivity concentration data in the images (Bq/ml) are divided by the ratio between the injected dose (Bq) and the patient's body weight (g). The SUV recalculation is applied in order to normalize the tracer uptake in the patient's various tissues for differences in injected activity and distribution volume. This provides images for absolute quantification of the tracer accumulation in tissues of interest that may be compared between patients and between examinations in the same patient. This is, however, not yet a clinically established routine in SPECT/CT.

The high clinical impact of ^{18}F-FDG PET and PET/CT for many other tumor types has been reported in a large number of studies and reviews. ^{18}F-FDG PET/CT is mainly applied in oncology for tumor characterization, staging, detection of current disease and therapy monitoring, and is well established in lung cancer, lymphoma, colorectal cancer and melanoma. The use of ^{18}F-FDG for oncological PET/CT is based on its higher accumulation in malignant than in benign tumors and most normal tissues, except the brain. There is also a high accumulation in the kidney since ^{18}F-FDG is excreted into the urine and the high radioactivity concentrations in the urinary collective system and bladder makes the technique less useful for urological tumor imaging.

Recently, PET/MRI hybrid scanners have also become available and are currently being evaluated for various imaging applications. The radiation dose in PET/MRI is lower than that of PET/CT. PET/MRI is advantageous because of the better tissue contrast with MRI as compared to CT. Also, MRI can be applied in the patients who cannot receive intravenous iodine-based CT contrast media because of impaired kidney function or a previous severe adverse reaction. In PET/MRI, attenuation correction of the PET images needs to be performed using a segmented MRI sequence because no CT image volume is available for this purpose. This attenuation correction method has introduced image artifacts and also results in problems of quantifying the radioactivity concentrations that need to be solved.

Adrenal Incidentalomas

The radiological characterization and follow-up of the vast majority of adrenal incidentalomas may for the vast majority of patients be managed by CT and MRI, as described in the previous chapter, and the main emphasis of the present presentation will instead be put on patients for whom molecular imaging may be helpful. Due to the increasing risk of cancer with increasing size [2], patients with 'large' adrenal tumors,

unless obviously benign (adrenocortical adenoma, cyst and myelolipoma), are recommended to undergo surgical resection. The size cut-off varies depending on the local guidelines and expertise, but incidentalomas ≥4–6 cm are generally considered 'large'. The benign adrenocortical adenoma at CT appears morphologically benign – rounded to oval shape, well-delineated tumor borders, homogenous internal architecture, and clear separation of the tumor from surrounding organs and tissues. In contrast-enhancing lesions an attenuation ≤10 HU in the precontrast CT examination establishes the diagnosis with 65–71% sensitivity and 98–99% specificity [5, 6]. The abundance of microscopic cytoplasmic fat in adrenocortical adenomas may also be shown by MRI using signal sequences 'in-phase' and 'out-of-phase' [7, 8]. Myelolipomas are diagnosed because of their content of macroscopic fat (attenuation –100 HU), the variation of which may be considerable, with some tumors merely holding fatty islands of a few millimeters whereas other myelolipomas are almost completely made up of fat. The attenuation in cysts is typically below 20 HU and there is no contrast enhancement.

In patients who do not undergo surgical resection because of a large incidentaloma, nuclear medicine techniques may be helpful when the tumor remains uncharacterized by CT/MRI. However, in patients in whom radiology fails to characterize the lesion, it is mandatory to retrieve and review previous cross-sectional imaging examinations before referral to further imaging. These frequently provide important information, such as that the size and morphological characteristics of an incidentaloma may actually have been unchanged over a long (>6–12 months) observation time.

The results of biochemistry are of great importance for the clinical decision regarding surgical resection versus further imaging. Patients with biochemistry indicating functioning incidentalomas (Conn's adenoma, pheochromocytoma, paragangliomas and adrenocortical cancer, ACC) need to be managed according to the symptoms and signs at presentation and the results of the radiological, biochemical and clinical workup.

In oncological patients (current or previous cancer disease) the risk is much higher that the incidentaloma represents a metastasis than in those without a cancer history, which therefore needs to be considered. When an adrenal metastasis is suspected, core-needle biopsy or fine-needle aspiration cytology may be a more appropriate diagnostic procedure than further imaging. Before the biopsy is performed, pheochromocytoma must be ruled out biochemically because of the risk of inducing a hypertensive crisis by this intervention.

Molecular Imaging of Adrenal Tumors

^{18}F-FDG PET/CT for Characterization of Adrenal Tumors

Due to of the regularly higher accumulation of ^{18}F-FDG in malignant as compared to benign tumors, ^{18}F-FDG PET may be used to noninvasively characterize tumors, such as solitary pulmonary nodules [9]. Although unspecific, ^{18}F-FDG PET and PET/CT have in several studies also been applied to distinguish benign from malignant adrenal tumors. In a recently published systematic review and meta-analysis comprising 21 studies and including 1,391 lesions (824 benign and 567 malignant) in 1,217 patients, a mean 97% sensitivity and 91% specificity was found for differing malignant from benign adrenal tumors [10]. The results of ^{18}F-FDG PET and ^{18}F-FDG PET/CT were similar.

Another study instead applied the adrenal tumor-to-liver ratio at ^{18}F-FDG PET as a means of distinguishing benign from malignant adrenal tumors in 81 cancer patients. A cut-off value of 1.8 for the adrenal tumor-to-liver ratio corresponded to 87% sensitivity and 91% specificity, whereas a cut-off value of 1.7 corresponded to 90% sensitivity and 91% specificity [6]. An inherent problem with the use of uptake ratios, however, is that some benign adrenal lesions also demonstrate a moderate to high ^{18}F-FDG uptake, for example pheochromocytomas [11–13].

When an adrenal metastasis is suspected, ^{18}F-FDG PET/CT may be helpful to characterize the lesion, but the examination is perhaps even more important in order to establish if the adrenal tumor is the only metastatic lesion, and thereby available for surgical resection, or if it is a part of disseminated disease and therefore better suited for systemic oncological therapy (fig. 1).

^{18}F-FDG PET/CT in Adrenocortical Cancer

^{18}F-FDG PET/CT has also been applied for imaging of ACC. The results of ^{18}F-FDG PET/CT in 28 ACC patients were correlated to those at contrast-enhanced CT that was performed separately. The methods were concordant in 25 patients and showed a similar sensitivity (95%), whereas the specificity for ^{18}F-FDG PET/CT was lower (83%) than for CT (100%). In a lesion-based analysis, the sensitivity and specificity for ^{18}F-FDG PET/CT was 90 and 93%, respectively, and for CT was somewhat lower at 88 and 82%, respectively [14]. In a smaller study comprising 12 ACC patients, ^{18}F-FDG PET showed 83% sensitivity for the diagnosis of recurrent and/or metastatic ACC [15]. In 2 of these patients, ^{18}F-FDG PET failed to detect small lung metastases and a liver metastasis.

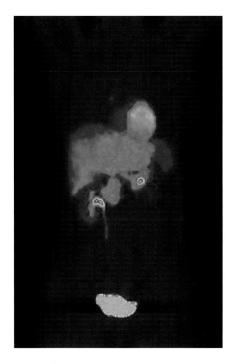

Fig. 1. ^{18}F-FDG PET image volume reconstructed as an MIP showing an intense focal FDG uptake corresponding to the left adrenal. This patient had previously undergone nephrectomy because of kidney cancer on the left side. Follow-up by CT showed a 3-cm incidentaloma in the left adrenal gland and needle biopsy showed metastasis from kidney cancer. Resection of the metastasis was then performed because FDG PET excluded other metastases than the single adrenal lesion.

^{11}C-Metomidate PET/CT for Characterization of Adrenal Tumors

The CYP11B enzymes 11β-hydroxylase (CYP11B1, P45011β) and aldosterone synthase (CYP11B2, P450aldo) are involved in the synthetic pathways of cortisol and aldosterone, respectively. Metomidate and etomidate are inhibitors of these enzymes and have been labelled with ^{11}C and ^{18}F for PET imaging of adrenocortical tumors. Due to its better radiochemical characteristics, ^{11}C-metomidate was chosen for the first clinical PET study in 15 patients with various adrenal tumors [16]. A high ^{11}C-metomidate uptake was found in all adrenocortical tumors (adenoma, hyperplasia, ACC) which were thereby unequivocally distinguished from the nonadrenocortical lesions (myelolipoma, pheochromocytoma, metastasis, cyst) without tracer uptake.

^{11}C-metomidate and ^{18}F-FDG were also compared in the same patients [17, 18] whereby PET with both tracers was performed in 19 and 16 patients, respectively, with various benign and malignant adrenal tumors. In the first study, all adrenocortical lesions were ^{11}C-metomidate positive and ^{18}F-FDG PET detected two thirds of the malignant tumors [17]. ^{11}C-metomidate PET distinguished the adrenocortical tumors from the nonadrenocortical lesions and ^{18}F-FDG PET identified the malignant from the benign tumors in the second trial [18].

In the largest study to date, comprising 73 patients with 75 adrenal tumors ranging from 1 to 20 cm in size (adrenocortical adenoma, hyperplasia, pheochromocytoma, ACC, metastasis, various tumors of nonadrenal origin), the results of ^{11}C-metomidate PET were correlated with the histopathological diagnosis [19]. ^{11}C-metomidate PET missed three small (≤1 cm) tumors and showed 89% sensitivity and 96% specificity in distinguishing adrenocortical from nonadrenocortical tumors. PET measurements of ^{11}C-metomidate uptake (SUV) failed to differ the benign from the malignant adrenocortical tumors.

The contribution of ^{11}C-metomidate PET in the imaging workup of adrenal incidentalomas was investigated in comparison with CT and MRI in 38 patients with 44 adrenal lesions [20]. Morphological imaging was found to be sufficient for the characterization of almost all incidentalomas whereas ^{11}C-metomidate PET could add information by defining the adrenocortical or nonadrenocortical origin of the lesions in the few patients in whom CT and MRI failed. It was concluded that ^{11}C-metomodate PET has a very marginal role in the management of patients with adrenal incidentalomas.

Primary Aldosteronism

In patients with a biochemical diagnosis of primary aldosteronism the diagnostic workup aims at identifying patients with a unilateral aldosterone-secreting adrenocortical tumor (Conn's adenoma), which may be surgically resected, from adrenal hyperplasia that, by contrast, is better suited for medical therapy. CT/MRI imaging of the adrenals is routinely included in this workup. However, the finding of a unilateral adrenal tumor is generally not sufficient for a surgical decision because the diagnosed tumor may be nonfunctioning and a small Conn's adenoma, escaping detection by CT/MRI, may instead be located in the contralateral adrenal. In order to avoid surgical resection of a nonsecreting adenoma, most patients additionally undergo selective venous sampling and subsequent hormonal analysis for lateralization of the Conn's adenoma before the surgical decision is taken. This is a technically challenging procedure and thorough training is required to achieve adequate bilateral sampling.

Previously, scintigraphy with ^{131}I-norcholesterol (NP-59) was used for preoperative localization of Conn's adenomas. However, the availability of the tracer is currently limited in most European countries since companies have generally stopped production. The technique requires considerable experience for adequate image interpretation and was therefore mainly used in specialized centers. Additional drawbacks were the high radiation dose to the patient and the need for thyroid blocking and repeated imaging at different time points.

[11]C-metomidate PET has also been evaluated for diagnosis and lateralization in primary aldosteronism [21, 22]. In a previous study [19] small adrenocortical adenomas were missed by ^{11}C-metomidate PET because of the similar tracer uptake in the ≤1-cm tumors and the normal adrenal. In order to increase the image contrast between the adenoma and the normal adrenal cortex a trial was conducted in 9 patients with small Conn's adenomas (average 1.7 cm, range 1.0–2.5 cm) who were examined by ^{11}C-metomidate PET and then reexamined after 3 days of per oral dexamethasone medication. It was hypothesized that corticoid treatment decreases ACTH secretion and thereby the 11-β-hydroxylase activity in normal adrenal parenchyma but not in Conn's adenomas. The tumor visibility was, however, similar in both examinations [21]. By premedication with a higher dose of per oral cortisone before ^{11}C-metomidate PET/CT it was, however, possible for another research group to increase the adenoma to normal adrenal ratio by a mean 25 ± 5%, and they also succeeded in visualizing subcentimeter adenomas [23]. The authors concluded that ^{11}C-metomidate PET/CT is a sensitive and specific noninvasive alternative to adrenal venous sampling in primary aldosteronism [23].

[11]C-Metomidate PET in Adrenocortical Cancer

In a report on ACC imaging, thirteen ^{11}C-metomidate examinations were performed in 11 patients and the results were correlated to findings at CT, surgery, autopsy and histopathology, together with clinical follow-up [24]. ^{11}C-metomidate PET visualized all viable tumors with high tracer uptake. ^{11}C-metomidate PET revealed two more lesions than CT and, interestingly, there were three necrotic tumors that were missed by PET but detected by CT. A suspected

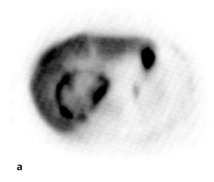 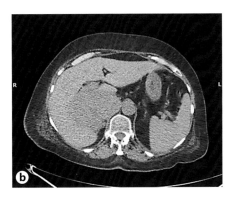 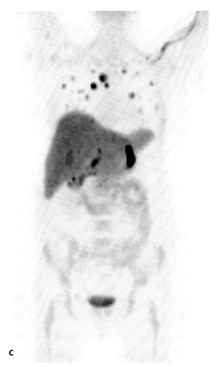

Fig. 2. ^{11}C-metomidate PET/CT of a patient with a large tumor in the right adrenal suspected to represent an ACC. **a** Transversal ^{11}C-metomidate PET image showing an intense uptake in the peripheral parts of the tumor whereas the central parts are devoid of tracer accumulation because of tumor necrosis, findings that support the ACC diagnosis. **b** Transversal CT image showing the large adrenal tumor in the right adrenal gland. **c** The ^{11}C-metomidate PET image volume reconstructed as an MIP showing the primary ACC and that there are multiple small focal ^{11}C-metomidate accumulations in the thorax confirming metastatic disease.

liver metastasis at CT was a true negative observation by ^{11}C-metomidate PET. In patients treated with adrenal steroid inhibitors (metapyrone, ketoconazole) and undergoing chemotherapy (streptozocin, p'-DDD, 5-FU), the ^{11}C-metomidate uptake was lower in tumors and normal tissues compared to examinations executed when the patients were without such treatment.

Currently, in the few centers where ^{11}C-metomidate PET/CT is available, it is used to verify the adrenocortical origin of tumors that CT/MRI fail to characterize, for example an ACC where biopsy should be avoided, and to detect regional and distant metastases (fig. 2). The method is also valuable for surveillance after surgery to detect recurrent disease.

^{123}I-Metomidate SPECT

SPECT systems are more generally available than PET/CT scanners and ^{123}I-iodometomidate has been developed [25]. The binding properties of ^{123}I-iodometomidate are comparable to those of metomidate and etomidate, and clinical evaluation has demonstrated a high and specific uptake of ^{123}I-iodometomidate in normal adrenals, adrenocortical tumors and distant ACC metastases. The long half-life of ^{123}I

makes it possible to distribute ^{123}I-iodometomidate to centers without their own tracer production. Another advantage of the long half-life of ^{123}I, as compared to ^{11}C, is that ^{123}I-iodometomidate allows for imaging at later time points. The spatial resolution of SPECT is, however, inferior to that of PET (1–1.5 vs. 0.5 cm).

Pheochromocytoma

In most patients with biochemically and/or symptomatically suspected or evident pheochromocytoma, a CT/MRI is usually sufficient to detect the pheochromocytoma before surgical resection. They are typically hypervascular and show a pronounced contrast-enhancement and a high signal in T2-weighted MR images. Further imaging with radionuclide techniques can be useful when an adrenal or extraadrenal tumor (in cases of extra-adrenal pheochromocytoma/paraganglioma) is not found by CT/MRI. Moreover, molecular imaging may be useful to diagnose recurrent malignant disease and for the staging of metastatic tumors.

Metaiodobenzylguanidine Scintigraphy
Metaiodobenzylguanidine (MIBG) is a norepinephrine analogue that is labelled with ^{123}I (and sometimes ^{131}I) for

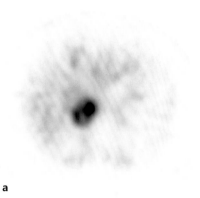
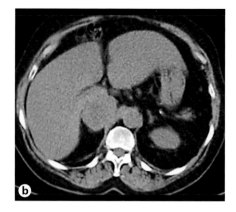

Fig. 3. a ^{123}I-MIBG scintigraphy SPECT image showing a high tracer uptake in a pheochromocytoma in the right adrenal gland. **b** Corresponding transversal CT image.

scintigraphy of pheochromocytomas and other sympatho-medullary tumors, such as neuroblastomas [26]. For diagnosis, ^{123}I-MIBG is preferred to ^{131}I-MIBG because of the lower radiation dose to the patient and better imaging characteristics [27, 28]. ^{131}I-MIBG in higher doses is used for therapy of disseminated disease and is beyond the scope of this review. Thyroid blockage with per oral iodine is needed before examination in order not to induce thyroiditis and thyroid dysfunction. Also, some antihypertensive drugs, tricyclic antidepressants and sympathomimetics may interact with MIBG uptake and need to be discontinued before examination and because of the risk for false negative results. ^{131}I-MIBG scintigraphy for the detection of pheochromocytomas shows 77–90% sensitivity and 95–100% specificity [28–30]. The corresponding sensitivity and specificity for ^{123}I-MIBG scintigraphy is 76–100% and 95–100%, respectively [13, 28, 29, 31] (fig. 3). In studies comprising many patients with extra-adrenal, multiple and hereditary pheochromocytomas, the sensitivity is lower (52–75%) [13]. In metastatic pheochromocytoma, ^{123}I-MIBG scintigraphy generally underestimates the disease [13]. When MIBG scintigraphy is negative, somatostatin receptor scintigraphy or ^{18}F-FDG PET/CT may detect the tumor. There are also specific PET tracers such as ^{18}F-fluorodopamine, ^{18}F-fluorodihydroxyphenilalanine (^{18}F-DOPA) or ^{11}C-hydroxyephedrine that can be tried when available (see below).

Somatostatin Receptor Imaging
Somatostatin receptor scintigraphy with ^{111}In-DTPA-pentetreotid (OctreoScan®) is the mainstay for radionuclide imaging of patients with neuroendocrine tumors [33]. Pheochromocytomas may also express somatostatin receptors and somatostatin receptor scintigraphy has shown 89% patient-based sensitivity and 69% region-based sensitivity in metastatic pheochromocytoma/paraganglioma [31]. However, the sensitivity for benign pheochromocytoma is low at 25–38% [31, 34]. The diagnostic yield of somatostatin receptor imaging has increased with the development of ^{68}Ga-labeled somatostatin analogues for PET. ^{68}Ga-labeled octreotide (^{68}Ga-DOTATOC and ^{68}Ga-DOTA-NOC) have increased the sensitivity and specificity in the detection of pheochromocytomas and paragangliomas to 100 and 86%, respectively [35], and in pheochromocytoma and neuroblastoma to 100 and 92%, respectively [36].

^{18}F-FDG PET/CT
As opposed to neuroendocrine tumors that generally do not accumulate ^{18}F-FDG, unless in high-grade tumors, pheochromocytomas can usually be visualized by ^{18}F-FDG PET/CT [11, 13, 32], although the sensitivity is higher for metastatic than benign pheochromocytoma/paraganglioma [11, 37]. ^{18}F-FDG PET/CT is therefore useful in cases when the tumors fail to concentrate MIBG. In patients with benign pheochromocytoma/paraganglioma, the performance of ^{18}F-FDG PET/CT was equal to that of ^{123}I-MIBG SPECT/CT, with a lesion-based sensitivity and specificity of 77 and 90% versus 75 and 92%, respectively [37]. In metastatic disease, the region-based sensitivity for ^{18}F-FDG PET/CT and ^{123}I-MIBG SPECT/CT was 83 and 50%, respectively [37]. In another study, MIBG scintigraphy showed 83% sensitivity and ^{18}F-FDG PET showed merely 58% in benign pheochromocytoma, but in malignant pheochromocytoma the corresponding sensitivities were 88 and 82% [11].

PET/CT with ^{18}F-DOPA and ^{18}F-Fluorodopamine
The amine precursor ^{18}F-DOPA PET can be used for the imaging of pheochromocytomas with high sensitivity for primary tumors and metastases [12, 38–41]. ^{18}F-DOPA PET

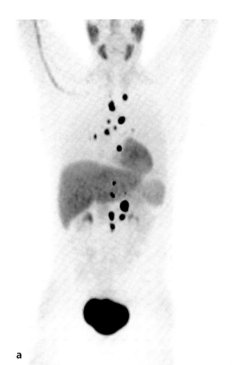

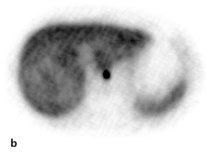

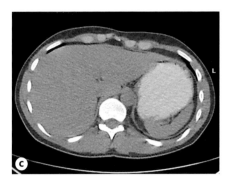

Fig. 4. ^{11}C-hydroxyephedrine PET/CT examination in a patient who previously underwent resection of an 8-cm pheochromocytoma. **a** MIP showing multiple small focal tracer accumulations confirming recurrent metastatic disease. **b** Transversal PET image showing a small retrocrural lymph node metastasis. **c** Corresponding transversal CT image.

was shown to be superior to ^{123}I-MIBG scintigraphy in localizing pheochromocytomas and paragangliomas with a lesion-based sensitivity and specificity 98 and 100% and 53 and 91%, respectively [40]. The use of ^{18}F-fluorodopamine PET/CT seems to be particularly advantageous for the localization of paragangliomas in the head and neck region [13].

The catecholamine precursor dopamine is formed by decarboxylation of DOPA. ^{18}F-fluorodopamine PET has been used for imaging of primary and metastatic pheochromocytoma/paraganglioma [12, 31, 37, 42–44]. In 99 patients ^{18}F-fluorodopamine PET ruled out pheochromocytoma in 39 patients and showed 78 and 77% lesion-based sensitivity and specificity for benign pheochromocytomas (n = 26) and 97% patient-based sensitivity for metastatic pheochromocytomas (n = 34). For ^{123}I-MIBG scintigraphy, the corresponding sensitivity/specificity was 78–92% and sensitivity was 85% [26]. Thus, the performance of ^{18}F-fluorodopamine PET and ^{123}I-MIBG scintigraphy was fairly similar in benign disease but the former was better in metastatic pheochromocytoma. This was further shown in comparison of ^{18}F-fluorodopamine PET and ^{131}I-MIBG scintigraphy in metastatic pheochromocytomas showing 100 and 56% patient-based sensitivity, respectively [43]. Moreover, in 53 patients with benign and metastatic pheochromocytoma, the patient-based sensitivity for ^{18}F-fluorodopamine PET

was 90%, for ^{123}I-MIGB scintigraphy was 76% and for somatostatin receptor scintigraphy was 22%, and the corresponding region-based sensitivities were 75, 63, and 64%, respectively [31]. In another comparative study, lesion-based sensitivity for benign pheochromocytoma/paraganglioma was 81% for ^{18}F-DOPA PET, 88% for ^{18}F-FDG PET/CT, 77% for ^{18}F-fluorodopamine PET/CT and 77% for ^{123}I-MIBG scintigraphy [12]. For metastatic pheochromocytoma/paraganglioma, the region-based sensitivity was 45% for ^{18}F-DOPA PET, 74% for ^{18}F-FDG PET/CT, 76% for ^{18}F-fluorodopamine PET/CT and 57% for ^{123}I-MIBG scintigraphy [12].

[11]C-Hydroxyephedrine PET/CT

[11]C-hydroxyephedrine is a synthetic norepinephrine analogue that enters the sympathetic neuron by the norepinephrine transporter [45]. ^{11}C-hydroxyephedrine is not metabolized in the sympathetic neurons and is therefore accumulated. Physiological ^{11}C-hydroxyephedrine uptake is found in organs with sympathetic innervation, for example the normal adrenal medulla, the heart and salivary glands [45]. In several studies, ^{11}C-hydroxyephedrine PET has been evaluated for the visualization of pheochromocytoma/ paraganglioma [46–50], and in occasional comparative reports has been shown to be superior to ^{123}I-MIBG SPECT/ CT, especially in detecting bilateral and extra-adrenal tu-

mors [46]. In 14 patients with a variety of tumors (neuroblastoma, pheochromocytoma/paraganglioma and ganglioneuroblastoma) ^{11}C-hydroxyephedrine PET detected 80/81 (99%) lesions compared to the 75/81 (93%) detected with ^{123}I-MIBG SPECT/CT [46]. A recent report included 134 patients with diagnosed or biochemically and/or symptomatically suspected pheochromocytoma who were examined by ^{11}C-hydroxyephedrine PET (n = 69) and PET/CT (n = 101). The patients were examined for detection of the primary tumor and for monitoring of malignant pheochromocytoma, and the results were compared to histopathology results and radiological and clinical follow-up. There were 6 false negative examinations but no false positive results (sensitivity 91%, specificity 100%) [50]. The sensitivity of ^{11}C-hydroxyephedrine PET in MEN2 patients was lower (73%) but still with maximum specificity. The tumor SUV_{max} was found to correlate with plasma normetanephrine and urinary norepinephrine. ^{11}C-hydroxyephedrine PET may be useful for follow-up and the early detection of recurrent malignant disease when malignant potential is suspected in the resected pheochromocytoma, for instance when the tumor is large (fig. 4).

References

1 Hammarstedt L, Muth A, Wängberg B, Björneld L, Sigurjónsdóttir HA, Götherström G, Almqvist E, Widell H, Carlsson S, Ander S, Hellström M: Adrenal lesion frequency: a prospective, cross-sectional CT study in a defined region, including systematic re-evaluation. Acta Radiol 2010;51: 1149–1156.

2 Mantero F, Terzolo M, Arnaldi G, Osella G, Masini AM, Alì A, Giovagnetti M, Opocher G, Angeli A: A survey on adrenal incidentaloma in Italy: Study Group on Adrenal Tumors of the Italian Society of Endocrinology. J Clin Endocrinol Metab 2000;85:637–644.

3 Hammarstedt L, Muth A, Sigurjónsdóttir HÁ, Almqvist E, Wängberg B, Hellström M: Adrenal lesions in patients with extra-adrenal malignancy – benign or malignant? Acta Oncol 2012;51: 215–221.

4 Boland GW, Blake MA, Hahn PF, Mayo-Smith WW: Incidental adrenal lesions: principles, techniques, and algorithms for imaging characterization. Radiology 2008;249:756–775.

5 Boland, GW, Lee MJ, Gazelle GS, Halpern EF, McNicholas MM, Mueller PR: Characterization of adrenal masses using unenhanced CT: an analysis of the CT literature. AJR Am J Roentgenol 1998; 171:201–204.

6 Ozcan Kara P, Kara T, Kara Gedik G, Kara F, Sahin O, Ceylan Gunay E, Sari O: The role of fluorodeoxyglucose-positron emission tomography/ computed tomography in differentiating between benign and malignant adrenal lesions. Nucl Med Commun 2011;32:106–112.

7 Korobkin M, Lombardi TJ, Aisen AM, Francis IR, Quint LE, Dunnick NR, Londy F, Shapiro B, Gross MD, Thompson NW: Characterization of adrenal masses with chemical shift and gadolinium-enhanced MR imaging. Radiology 1995;197:411–418.

8 Korobkin M, Giordano TJ, Brodeur FJ, Francis IR, Siegelman ES, Quint LE, Dunnick NR, Heiken JP, Wang HH: Adrenal adenomas: relationship between histologic lipid and CT and MR findings. Radiology 1996;200:743–747.

9 Nettelbladt OS, Sundin AE, Valind SO, Gustafsson GR, Lamberg K, Långström B, Björnsson EH: Combined fluorine-18-FDG and carbon-11-methionine PET for diagnosis of tumors in lung and mediastinum. J Nucl Med 1998;39:640–647.

10 Boland GW, Dwamena BA, Jagtiani Sangwaiya M, Goehler AG, Blake MA, Hahn PF, Scott JA, Kalra MK: Characterization of adrenal masses by using FDG PET: a systematic review and meta-analysis of diagnostic test performance. Radiology 2011; 259:117–126.

11 Shulkin BL, Thompson NW, Shapiro B, Francis IR, Sisson JC: Pheochromocytomas: imaging with 2-[fluorine-18]fluoro-2-deoxy-D-glucose PET. Radiology 1999;212:35–41.

12 Timmers HJ, Chen CC, Carrasquillo JA, Whatley M, Ling A, Havekes B, Eisenhofer G, Martiniova L, Adams KT, Pacak K: Comparison of ^{18}F-fluoro-L-DOPA, ^{18}F-fluoro-deoxyglucose, and ^{18}F-fluorodopamine PET and ^{123}I-MIBG scintigraphy in the localization of pheochromocytoma and paraganglioma. J Clin Endocrinol Metab 2009;94: 4757–4767.

13 Taïeb D, Timmers HJ, Hindié E, Guillet BA, Neumann HP, Walz MK, Opocher G, de Herder WW, Boedeker CC, de Krijger RR, Chiti A, Al-Nahhas A, Pacak K, Rubello D: EANM 2012 guidelines for radionuclide imaging of phaeochromocytoma and paraganglioma. Eur J Nucl Med Mol Imaging 2012;39:1977–1979.

14 Leboulleux S, Dromain C, Bonniaud G, Aupérin A, Caillou B, Lumbroso J, Sigal R, Baudin E, Schlumberger M: Diagnostic and prognostic value of 18-fluorodeoxyglucose positron emission tomography in adrenocortical carcinoma: a prospective comparison with computed tomography. J Clin Endocrinol Metab 2006;91:920–925.

15 Mackie GC, Shulkin BL, Ribeiro RC, Worden FP, Gauger PG, Mody RJ, Connolly LP, Kunter G, Rodriguez-Galindo C, Wallis JW, Hurwitz CA, Schteingart DE: Use of [^{18}F]fluorodeoxyglucose positron emission tomography in evaluating locally recurrent and metastatic adrenocortical carcinoma. J Clin Endocrinol Metab 2006;91:2665–2671.

16 Bergström M, Juhlin C, Bonasera TA, Sundin A, Rastad J, Akerström G, Långström B: PET imaging of adrenal cortical tumors with the 11β-hydroxylase tracer ^{11}C-metomidate. J Nucl Med 2000;41:275–282.

17 Minn H, Salonen A, Friberg J, Roivainen A, Viljanen T, Långsjö J, Salmi J, Välimäki M, Någren K, Nuutila P: Imaging of adrenal incidentalomas with PET using ^{11}C-metomidate and ^{18}F-FDG. J Nucl Med 2004;45:972–979.

18 Zettinig G, Mitterhauser M, Wadsak W, Becherer A, Pirich C, Vierhapper H, Niederle B, Dudczak R, Kletter K: Positron emission tomography imaging of adrenal masses: ^{18}F-fluorodeoxyglucose and the 11β-hydroxylase tracer ^{11}C-metomidate. Eur J Nucl Med Mol Imaging 2004;31:1224–1230.

19 Hennings J, Lindhe O, Bergström M, Långström B, Sundin A, Hellman P: [^{11}C]metomidate positron emission tomography of adrenocortical tumors in correlation with histopathological findings. J Clin Endocrinol Metab 2006;91:1410–1414.

20 Hennings J, Hellman P, Ahlström H, Sundin A: Computed tomography, magnetic resonance imaging and ^{11}C-metomidate positron emission tomography for evaluation of adrenal incidentalomas. Eur J Radiol 2009;69:314–323.

21 Hennings J, Sundin A, Hägg A, Hellman P: ^{11}C-metomidate positron emission tomography after dexamethasone suppression for detection of small adrenocortical adenomas in primary aldosteronism. Langenbecks Arch Surg 2010;395:963–967.

22 Razifar P, Hennings J, Monazzam A, Hellman P, Långström B, Sundin A: Masked volume wise principal component analysis of small adrenocortical tumours in dynamic [^{11}C]-metomidate positron emission tomography. BMC Med Imaging 2009; 9:16.

23 Burton TJ, Mackenzie IS, Balan K, Koo B, Bird N, Soloviev DV, Azizan EA, Aigbirhio F, Gurnell M, Brown MJ: Evaluation of the sensitivity and specificity of ^{11}C-metomidate positron emission tomography (PET)-CT for lateralizing aldosterone secretion by Conn's adenomas. J Clin Endocrinol Metab 2012;97:100–109.

24 Khan TS, Sundin A, Juhlin C, Långström B, Bergström M, Eriksson B: ^{11}C-metomidate PET imaging of adrenocortical cancer. Eur J Nucl Med Mol Imaging 2003;30:403–410.

25 Hahner S, Stuermer A, Kreissl M, Reiners C, Fassnacht M, Haenscheid H, Beuschlein F, Zink M, Lang K, Allolio B, Schirbel A: [123]Iodometomidate for molecular imaging of adrenocortical cytochrome P450 family 11B enzymes. J Clin Endocrinol Metab 2008;93:2358–2365.

26 Ilias I, Divgi C, Pacak K: Current role of metaiodobenzylguanidine in the diagnosis of pheochromocytoma and medullary thyroid cancer. Semin Nucl Med 2011;41:364–368.

27 Lynn MD, Shapiro B, Sisson JC, Beierwaltes WH, Meyers LJ, Ackerman R, Mangner TJ: Pheochromocytoma and the normal adrenal medulla: improved visualization with I-123 MIBG scintigraphy. Radiology 1985;155:789–792.

28 Furuta N, Kiyota H, Yoshigoe F, Hasegawa N, Ohishi Y: Diagnosis of pheochromocytoma using [123I]-compared with [131I]-metaiodobenzylguanidine scintigraphy. Int J Urol 1999;6:119–124.

29 Ilias I, Pacak K: Current approaches and recommended algorithm for the diagnostic localization of pheochromocytoma. J Clin Endocrinol Metab 2004;89:479–491.

30 Guller U, Turek J, Eubanks S, Delong ER, Oertli D, Feldman JM: Detecting pheochromocytoma: defining the most sensitive test. Ann Surg 2006;243: 102–107.

31 Ilias I, Chen CC, Carrasquillo JA, Whatley M, Ling A, Lazúrová I, Adams KT, Perera S, Pacak K: Comparison of 6-18F-fluorodopamine PET with 123I-metaiodobenzylguanidine and 111In-pentetreotide scintigraphy in localization of nonmetastatic and metastatic pheochromocytoma. J Nucl Med 2008;49:1613–1619.

32 Timmers HJ, Kozupa A, Chen CC, Carrasquillo JA, Ling A, Eisenhofer G, Adams KT, Solis D, Lenders JW, Pacak K: Superiority of fluorodeoxyglucose positron emission tomography to other functional imaging techniques in the evaluation of metastatic SDHB-associated pheochromocytoma and paraganglioma. J Clin Oncol 2007;25: 2262–2269.

33 Kwekkeboom DJ, Krenning EP, Scheidhauer K, Lewington V, Lebtahi R, Grossman A, Vitek P, Sundin A, Plöckinger U: ENETS Consensus Guidelines for the Standards of Care in Neuroendocrine Tumors: somatostatin receptor imaging with 111In-pentetreotide. Neuroendocrinology 2009;90:184–189.

34 van der Harst E, de Herder WW, Bruining HA, Bonjer HJ, de Krijger RR, Lamberts SW, van de Meiracker AH, Boomsma F, Stijnen T, Krenning EP, Bosman FT, Kwekkeboom DJ: [123I]metaiodobenzylguanidine and [111In]octreotide uptake in benign and malignant pheochromocytomas. J Clin Endocrinol Metab 2001;86:685–693.

35 Naswa N, Sharma P, Nazar AH, Agarwal KK, Kumar R, Ammini AC, Malhotra A, Bal C: Prospective evaluation of 68Ga-DOTA-NOC PET-CT in phaeochromocytoma and paraganglioma: preliminary results from a single centre study. Eur Radiol 2012;22:710–719.

36 Kroiss A, Putzer D, Uprimny C, Decristoforo C, Gabriel M, Santner W, Kranewitter C, Warwitz B, Waitz D, Kendler D, Virgolini IJ: Functional imaging in phaeochromocytoma and neuroblastoma with 68Ga-DOTA-Tyr 3-octreotide positron emission tomography and 123I-metaiodobenzylguanidine. Eur J Nucl Med Mol Imaging 2011;38:865–873.

37 Timmers HJ, Chen CC, Carrasquillo JA, Whatley M, Ling A, Eisenhofer G, King KS, Rao JU, Wesley RA, Adams KT, Pacak K: Staging and functional characterization of pheochromocytoma and paraganglioma by 18F-fluorodeoxyglucose (18F-FDG) positron emission tomography. J Natl Cancer Inst 2012;104:700–708.

38 Hoegerle S, Nitzsche E, Altehoefer C, Ghanem N, Manz T, Brink I, Reincke M, Moser E, Neumann HP: Pheochromocytomas: detection with 18F DOPA whole body PET – initial results. Radiology 2002;222:507–512.

39 Fiebrich HB, Brouwers AH, Kerstens MN, Pijl ME, Kema IP, de Jong JR, Jager PL, Elsinga PH, Dierckx RA, van der Wal JE, Sluiter WJ, de Vries EG, Links TP: 6-[F-18]Fluoro-L-dihydroxyphenylalanine positron emission tomography is superior to conventional imaging with 123I-metaiodobenzylguanidine scintigraphy, computer tomography, and magnetic resonance imaging in localizing tumors causing catecholamine excess. J Clin Endocrinol Metab 2009;94:3922–3930.

40 Fottner C, Helisch A, Anlauf M, Rossmann H, Musholt TJ, Kreft A, Schadmand-Fischer S, Bartenstein P, Lackner KJ, Klöppel G, Schreckenberger M, Weber MM: 6-18F-fluoro-L-dihydroxyphenylalanine positron emission tomography is superior to 123I-metaiodobenzyl-guanidine scintigraphy in the detection of extraadrenal and hereditary pheochromocytomas and paragangliomas: correlation with vesicular monoamine transporter expression. J Clin Endocrinol Metab 2010;95:2800–2810.

41 Luster M, Karges W, Zeich K, Pauls S, Verburg FA, Dralle H, Glatting G, Buck AK, Solbach C, Neumaier B, Reske SN, Mottaghy FM: Clinical value of 18F-fluorodihydroxyphenylalanine positron emission tomography/computed tomography (18F-DOPA PET/CT) for detecting pheochromocytoma. Eur J Nucl Med Mol Imaging 2010;37:484–493.

42 Timmers HJ, Eisenhofer G, Carrasquillo JA, Chen CC, Whatley M, Ling A, Adams KT, Pacak K: Use of 6-[18F]-fluorodopamine positron emission tomography (PET) as first-line investigation for the diagnosis and localization of non-metastatic and metastatic phaeochromocytoma (PHEO). Clin Endocrinol (Oxf) 2009;71:11–17.

43 Ilias I, Yu J, Carrasquillo JA, Chen CC, Eisenhofer G, Whatley M, McElroy B, Pacak K: Superiority of 6-[18F]-fluorodopamine positron emission tomography versus [131I]-metaiodobenzylguanidine scintigraphy in the localization of metastatic pheochromocytoma. J Clin Endocrinol Metab 2003;88:4083–4087.

44 Pacak K, Eisenhofer G, Carrasquillo JA, Chen CC, Li ST, Goldstein DS: 6-[18F]fluorodopamine positron emission tomographic (PET) scanning for diagnostic localization of pheochromocytoma. Hypertension 2001;38:6–8.

45 Rosenspire KC, Haka MS, van Dort ME, Jewett DM, Gildersleeve DL, Schwaiger M, Wieland DM: Synthesis and preliminary evaluation of carbon-11-meta-hydroxyephedrine: a false transmitter agent for heart neuronal imaging. J Nucl Med 1990;31:1328–1334.

46 Franzius C, Hermann K, Weckesser M, Kopka K, Juergens KU, Vormoor J, Schober O: Whole-body PET/CT with 11C-meta-hydroxyephedrine in tumors of the sympathetic nervous system: feasibility study and comparison with 123I-MIBG SPECT/CT. J Nucl Med 2006;47:1635–1642.

47 Shulkin BL, Wieland DM, Schwaiger M, Thompson NW, Francis IR, Haka MS, Rosenspire KC, Shapiro B, Sisson JC, Kuhl DE: PET scanning with hydroxyephedrine: an approach to the localization of pheochromocytoma. J Nucl Med 1992;33:1125–1131.

48 Trampal C, Engler H, Juhlin C, Bergström M, Långström B: Pheochromocytomas: detection with 11C hydroxyephedrine PET. Radiology 2004; 230:423–428.

49 Mann GN, Link JM, Pham P, Pickett CA, Byrd DR, Kinahan PE, Krohn KA, Mankoff DA: [11C]meta-hydroxyephedrine and [18F]fluorodeoxyglucose positron emission tomography improve clinical decision making in suspected pheochromocytoma. Ann Surg Oncol 2006;13:187–197.

50 Yamamoto S, Hellman P, Wassberg C, Sundin A: 11C-hydroxyephedrine positron emission tomography imaging of pheochromocytoma: a single center experience over 11 years. J Clin Endocrinol Metab 2012;97:2423–2432.

Prof. Anders Sundin, MD, PhD
Enheten för Radiologi, Institutionen för Kirurgiska Vetenskaper
Akademiska Sjukhuset, Uppsala Universitet
SE–751 85 Uppsala (Sweden)
E-Mail anders.sundin@radiol.uu.se

Buchfelder M, Guaraldi F (eds): Imaging in Endocrine Disorders.
Front Horm Res. Basel, Karger, 2016, vol 45, pp 80–96 (DOI: 10.1159/000442319)

Gonadal Imaging in Endocrine Disorders

Fabio Lanfranco • Giovanna Motta

Divisione di Endocrinologia, Diabetologia e Metabolismo, Dipartimento di Scienze Mediche, Università di Torino, Turin, Italy

Abstract

Ultrasound (US) is the most widely available method of diagnostic imaging for the evaluation and characterization of gonadal lesions and is usually the method of choice because of its high accuracy, low cost and wide availability. Today's high-resolution images allow for a confident diagnosis of many scrotal and adnexal lesions, with high sensitivity and specificity. Magnetic resonance imaging (MRI) is reliable in the detection of gonadal lesions in males, allowing the differentiation into testicular or nontesticular lesions, and their characterization. It is also an accurate and cost-effective diagnostic adjunct in those patients with solid scrotal lesions for whom the findings of clinical and US evaluations are inconclusive. In females, MRI is recommended as a second-line investigation for the characterization of complex adnexal masses that are indeterminate on US. In this review, gonadal pathologies related with the steroidogenic and gametogenic function of the testes and ovaries will be discussed. The main imaging features of benign and malignant lesions will also be presented.

Male Gonads

Introduction

Scrotal ultrasound (US) is the most widely available method of diagnostic imaging and is usually the method of choice for examining the scrotum because of its high accuracy, ex-cellent anatomic depiction, low cost and wide availability [1, 2]. Recent technical advances of US applications and post-processing developments have enabled new aspects in the structural and functional analysis of testicular tissue and can suggest a specific diagnosis for a wide variety of testicular diseases [3].

Magnetic resonance imaging (MRI) is reliable in the detection of scrotal lesions, allowing the differentiation into testicular or nontesticular lesions and their characterization, including cysts and fluid, solid masses, fat and fibrosis [4]. MRI is an accurate and cost-effective diagnostic adjunct in those patients with solid scrotal lesions for whom the findings from clinical and US evaluations are inconclusive [5].

CT (computed tomography) scan is not commonly used in testis imaging because it involves ionizing radiation and because it is expensive. However, it can play an important role in testis cancer staging and in cryptorchidism in order to localize undescended testes [6].

In this section, scrotal pathologies related with the steroidogenic and spermatogenic functions of the testes will be discussed. For a more comprehensive overview of other benign and malignant testicular or extratesticular scrotal lesions the reader is referred to recent reviews such as those by Appelbaum et al. [2], and Pearl and Hill [7].

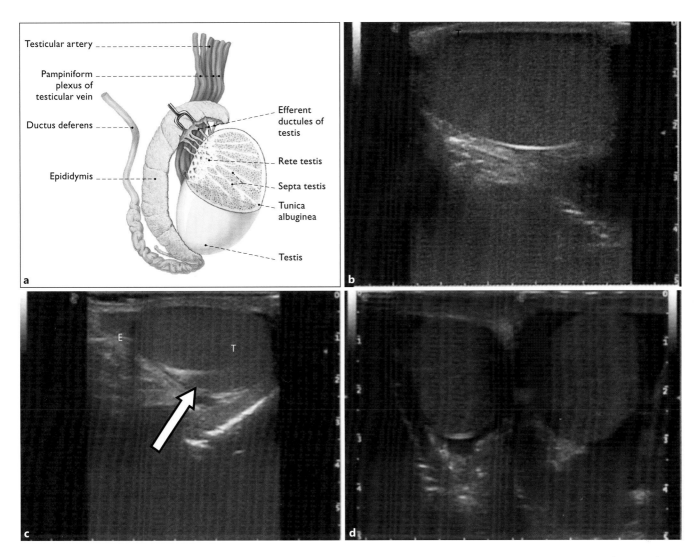

Fig. 1. a Sagittal view of the normal anatomy of the testicle, epididymis and mediastinum testis; reproduced with permission from Köpf-Maier [44]. Transverse (**b**) and longitudinal (**c**) US images showing a normal testis (T), epididymis (E) and mediastinum testis (arrow). **d** Transverse view of both testes for comparison of size, shape and echogenicity.

Normal Anatomy of the Scrotum

The normal postpubertal testes are symmetric and ovoid, and measure approximately 5 × 3 × 2 cm (fig. 1a). On US examination, the testis usually has medium level homogeneous echoes (fig. 1b–d), although normal variants have been described and include a unilateral striated pattern, thought to represent fibrosis (fig. 2), or hypoechoic intratesticular bands in the middle third of the testis which may contain arterial and venous components and represent a normal variant of intratesticular vessels. The fibrous tunica albuginea, which surrounds the testis, can be seen as a thin echogenic line [7].

The epididymis is a 6- to 7-cm tubular structure that normally courses inferiorly along the posterior aspect of the testis and is composed of a head, body and tail. The epididymal head measures 5–12 mm in diameter, is located at the superior pole of the testis and is round, triangular or pyramidal in shape [7, 8]. The body and tail are narrower, measuring 2–5 mm in diameter [8], and gradually taper as they course inferiorly along the testis to its lower pole (fig. 1a).

Testicular flow is supplied primarily by the testicular arteries, which arise from the aorta distal to the renal artery, course through the inguinal canal along the spermatic cord and reach the upper pole of the testes to divide into capsular

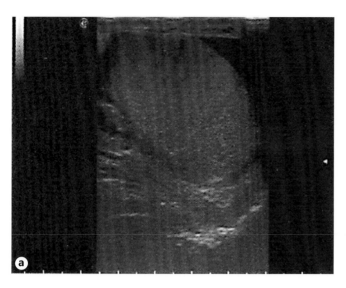 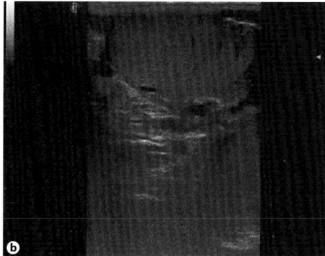

Fig. 2. Longitudinal (**a**) and transverse (**b**) US scans of a normal striated testis.

arteries [2] (fig. 1a). On color Doppler US (CDUS) normal testicular tissue shows a typical stellar vascular pattern [3].

The epididymis and the extratesticular tissues are supplied by the deferential and cremasteric arteries. Venous drainage is accomplished by the pampiniform plexus, which drains into the ipsilateral testicular vein and subsequently into the inferior vena cava on the right or the renal vein on the left testis (fig. 1a).

Scrotal Ultrasound: Technique of Examination
The patient lays supine with the scrotal sac supported by a draped towel over the thighs and the penis covered with a towel over the pubis. A large amount of gel is applied over the scrotal sac [2]. For structural analysis mainly grayscale or B-mode US with a high-resolution, near-focused, linear-array transducer with a frequency of 7.5–14 MHz or greater is used. Bilateral transverse and longitudinal slices of the scrotum and inguinal region are performed to allow side-to-side comparison of their sizes and echo texture [3]. Any intratesticular or extratesticular finding should be imaged and measured in different planes [2].

Grayscale US is mainly used for the measurement of testicular volume and for estimation of tissue texture based on alterations in echogenicity. This technique demonstrates the alteration of size and echogenicity in an atrophic testis as well as alteration of echogenicity in a testis with partial infarction or ischemia in comparison to normal testicular tissue. A slightly impaired echo texture indicates a decreased

testicular function. Testicular volume in infertile men is related to semen profiles. Up to 70–80% of the testicular volume consists of the seminiferous tubules and reflects spermatogenesis [3]. A strong correlation between testicular function and testicular volume measured by US or other techniques has been proven by Sakamoto et al. [9]. For further functional analysis the native or unenhanced CDUS, the contrast-enhanced CDUS and the advanced contrast agent detection techniques like MVI (microvessel imaging, Philips) and the calculation of TIC (time intensity curve) are implemented [3].

Unenhanced CDUS is well established to illustrate macrovascularity and therefore perfusion. Testicular perfusion can be evaluated with color Doppler, power Doppler and spectral Doppler US [3]. CDUS and power Doppler US represent a promising method for the assessment of patients affected by azoospermia by allowing the discrimination of obstructive azoospermia (normal vessel distribution) from nonobstructive azoospermia (reduced or absent testicular vessels) [3].

Contrast-enhanced US (CEUS) can be used for the illustration of macrovascularity and microvascularity. For this, micro bubbles with a lipid or galactose shell filled with an inert gas and a diameter of 7–10 μm are administered intravenously. These microbubbles can be used as an echo enhancer for CDUS leading to a visualization of blood flow also in the microvessels [3]. Thierman et al. [10] found out that CEUS is potentially applicable to the investigation of vascular disorders of the testis. The use of a pulse inversion technique, compared with conventional Doppler US methods, has been shown to provide superior assessment of perfusion in the setting of acute testicular ischemia [10].

CEUS appeared to be a useful adjuvant to CDUS in patients with epididymitis and a focal lesion in the testis [11]. Finally, hypervascularization is an important feature in the diagnosis of malignancy. In a recent publication, testicular lesion hyperenhancement had a positive predictive value of 97.4% for neoplasia [12].

Three-dimensional US (3D US) allows for imaging of the volume in many arbitrary planes, including the three classical axial, sagittal and coronal planes. 3D US can reduce imaging time and improve the demonstration of complex anatomy and vasculature [13]. 3D US offers a much more accurate assessment of volume of the testes and the tumor, and thus also more precise monitoring of the treatment [13]. The use of Doppler improves characterization of testicular lesions and confirms the lack of vascularity in benign abnormalities, such as epidermoid cysts, infarctions, abscesses and changes following trauma. Connection of the 3D and power Doppler mode offers the basis for a detailed study of the 3D vascular pattern of the lesion and the surrounding tissue. It can demonstrate the abnormal vasculature and calculate the vascularization index, which is a measure of the number of blood vessels in the tumor.

Another newly implemented technique is the real-time sonoelastography (RTE), which enables an illustration of the distribution of tissue elasticity in one US slice. This promising technique is calculated by postprocessing algorithms and needs no contrast media. RTE is therefore a real-time technique and shows different areas with different stiffness in a color-coded image simultaneously with the B-mode or grayscale image: 'stiff' or 'hard' lesions are suspicious for malignancy whereas benign lesions are in general 'soft', with normal or decreased tissue stiffness [2, 3]. RTE, due to its higher specificity, can provide additional information in cases with indeterminate sonographic findings [2].

Magnetic Resonance Imaging of the Scrotum

MRI is an accurate and cost-effective diagnostic adjunct in those patients with solid scrotal lesions for whom the findings from clinical and US evaluations are inconclusive [4]. Some tumor-like lesions, for instance, may appear mass-like on US images, but have a typical presentation at MRI.

MRI allows tissue characterization, with its signal intensity properties allowing the detection of fat, blood products, granulomatous tissue and fibrosis. MRI has a wider field of view than US and readily allows identification of an undescended testis. MRI imaging is less operator dependent than US and can help differentiate between a solid neoplasm and other entities, such as inflammatory or vascular abnormalities or scrotal hernia. Through the use of different sequence types and the administration of gadolinium, MRI can be used to characterize the pattern of scrotal disorders [5]. The correct classification of testicular lesions is crucial because the peak prevalence of testicular tumors occurs among 25- to 35-year-old men. Nonneoplastic lesions such as orchitis, hemorrhage and infarction can mimic a testicular mass because the US criteria for masses overlap those for neoplasms, which can lead to unnecessary orchiectomy.

Mohrs et al. [5] have recently analyzed the overall diagnostic value of MRI in the treatment of patients with suspected testicular and nontesticular scrotal lesions as encountered in routine clinical practice. They have shown a high diagnostic accuracy of MRI for differentiating intratesticular and extratesticular disorders. Moreover, MRI can be helpful in guiding surgical management because it allows precise localization of nonmalignant testicular lesions.

Male Infertility

The various causes of male infertility can be subcategorized as obstructive and nonobstructive azoo- or hypospermia. Nonobstructive disease includes varicocele, endocrinopathy, chromosomal abnormality, cryptorchidism, anabolic steroid abuse, gonadotoxin exposure, primary testicular failure and ejaculatory disorders. Obstructive disorders include congenital bilateral absence of the vas deferens, ejaculatory duct obstruction and prostatic cysts [14].

Varicocele

Varicocele, which is an abnormal dilatation of the pampiniform plexus, is present in approximately 15–20% of adult men and may be primary (idiopathic) or secondary [7]. US is the most frequently used method for varicocele diagnosis; a high-frequency transducer of at least 7 MHz should be used. Sonographically, varicoceles consist of multiple anechoic tubular structures around the epididymis that increase in size in the upright position and with a Valsalva manoeuver. The features on grayscale US include a prominence of at least two to three veins of the pampiniform plexus, of which one should have a diameter greater than 2–3 mm in a supine position [15]. The Valsalva manoeuver is an important component of the examination and should be performed routinely as it causes an increase in vessel size and conspicuousness [15].

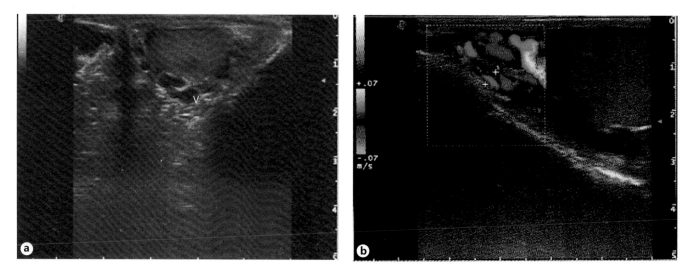

Fig. 3. Transverse (**a**) and CFD (**b**) images of a large left-sided varicocele (V).

Color Doppler can be used as part of the examination since it has been shown to improve diagnostic ability by the detection of reverse flow in the incompetent vein. The reflux is quantified as permanent, which is significant for a varicocele, intermittent or brief, which is physiological [15] (fig. 3). Varicocele may rarely be intratesticular, within the mediastinum testis or in a subcapsular location, and is usually associated with ipsilateral extratesticular varicocele [7].

In the past, thermography was a widely used technique but has largely been superseded by US [15]. Since a varicocele with venous stasis can cause an increased temperature of the affected testis and scrotal content, the temperature difference between both sides can provide information about the pathophysiological consequences of a varicocele. Thermography can be performed with thermosensitive films or continuously over 24 h by means of a portable gauge with thermal measuring devices (thermoport) [16].

Scrotal scintigraphy was met with enthusiasm in the early 1980s; however, the sensitivity was low and the technique was time consuming. More recent studies using dynamic varicocele scintigraphy have been more promising, especially in the group with a small or subclinical varicocele [17].

Although venography is still considered to be the gold standard, it is time consuming and invasive. If a varicocele is present, the internal spermatic vein is enlarged and there is reflux into the abdominal, inguinal, scrotal or pelvic portions of the spermatic vein. Venography is usually performed either in the assessment of difficult or uncertain cas-

es, or more commonly before definitive treatment by venous embolization [15].

Imaging with other techniques, such as MRI or CT, is only occasionally required, for example, to evaluate the presence of obstructing masses, particularly on the right side. When conventional venography is contraindicated (a history of anaphylaxis, etc.), magnetic resonance venography is a suitable alternative. Magnetic resonance angiography has been used for the assessment of recurrent varicocele [15].

Azoospermia

Azoospermia affects about 1% of the male population and may be present in up to 20% of infertility cases in men. RTE was evaluated for differentiating nonobstructive from obstructive azoospermia in a large patient cohort with promising results [18]. An average or low strain ratio (score 3–5) was seen in 81.7% of nonobstructive azoospermia. A significant difference in the strain ratio places the method as a promising imaging technique for the differential diagnosis of azoospermia types [2].

Chromosomal Abnormalities

Chromosomal abnormalities can lead to altered spermatogenesis, decreased sperm motility, impaired genital tract development and decreased fertilization capacity. When infertility is chromosomally mediated, it is more likely to be related to the sex chromosomes than to the autosomal chromosomes [19]. Klinefelter's syndrome is the most common sex chromosome disorder [20]. Less common abnormalities include mixed gonadal dysgenesis and XX male (46,XX) and XYY male (47,XYY) karyotypes. US reveals small and hypoechoic testes.

Cryptorchidism

Cryptorchidism, or undescended testes, is the most common genitourinary anomaly in male infants and leads to infertility [19, 21]. Moreover, the risk of malignancy is 20–46 times higher than males with normally descended testes and malignant degeneration usually occurs to seminoma [22].

When the testis fails to descend into the scrotum it is usually found in the inguinal canal, but it may be intra-abdominal. US is most commonly used for evaluation and may show a small and hypoechoic testis in comparison to the normal testis. Identification of the mediastinum testis confirms that the structure is the testis and not a lymph node or the pars infravaginalis gubernaculi, which is the inferior bulbous portion of the gubernaculum testis [7].

US is approximately 70% accurate in localizing the undescended testis; however, accurate detection of the intra-abdominal testis falls to less than 50% [22]. If US fails to identify the testis, MRI should be performed as the diagnostic accuracy in locating undescended abdominal testes has been reported as 90% [22]. Kanemoto et al. [23] reported that MRI had a sensitivity and specificity of 86 and 79%, respectively. Undescended testes have similar magnetic resonance signal characteristics to scrotal testes; there is low signal intensity on T1-weighted images and high intensity on T2-weighted images [6].

Congenital Bilateral Absence of the Vas Deferens

The most common abnormality of the extratesticular ductal system is congenital bilateral absence of the vas deferens [19, 21], which occurs in 1–2% of infertile men. At US evaluation, the epididymal heads are prominent and the rete testis is dilated. On MRI, low signal throughout the peripheral zone of the prostate gland is always seen. The seminal vesicles may be absent, as noted on transabdominal sonography or MRI [24].

Obstruction of the Ejaculatory Ducts

Obstruction of the ejaculatory ducts can be congenital and associated with midline cysts or acquired in relation to postinflammatory stenosis, typically from a prior sexually transmitted disease [24]. When an obstruction is suspected, MRI or transrectal US should be performed [14].

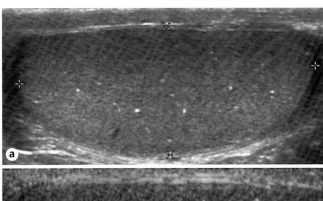
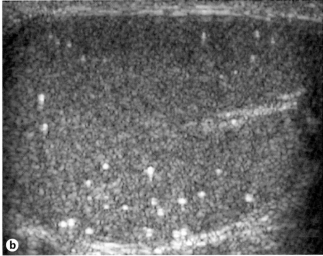

Fig. 4. a Longitudinal scan of the left testicle with TM. **b** Longitudinal scan of the right testicle with TM.

Testicular and Extratesticular Calcifications

Parenchymal testicular calcifications may be found in germ cell tumors, 'burned out' germ cell tumors and Sertoli cell tumors, or be secondary to prior trauma, infection (tuberculosis), infarction and inflammation (sarcoidosis) [7]. Testicular microlithiasis (TM) is identified as small 1- to 3-mm echogenic foci that may produce a comet tail artifact within the testicular parenchyma [25]. TM is defined as more than 5 echogenic foci in a single US image. It usually occurs bilaterally and may be diffuse (also referred to as classic) or limited (less than five hyperechoic foci per image) [25], which is associated with a lower rate of malignancy than classic microlithiasis [26] (fig. 4).

It is postulated that microlithiasis may be due to defective phagocytosis of degenerate tubular cells by the Sertoli cells, resulting in calcified cellular debris within the seminiferous tubules [7, 25]. TM is usually asymptomatic and may be found incidentally in patients presenting for a scrotal US

Table 1. Classification of intratesticular lesions

Nonneoplastic cystic lesions
Tunica albuginea cysts
Simple testicular cysts
Epidermoid cysts
Tubular ectasia of the rete testis
Intratesticular abscesses

Neoplastic lesions
Benign testicular lesions
    Segmental testicular infarction
    Fibrous pseudotumor of the testis
    Hamartomas in Cowden disease
    Granulomatous diseases
    Congenital testicular adrenal rests
    Focal orchitis
    Hematoma
    Focal changes after a testicular biopsy
Malignant testicular lesions
    Germ cell tumors
    Seminoma
    NSCGTs (embryonal carcinoma, yolk sac tumor,
    choriocarcinoma, teratoma, mixed germ cell)
    Stromal cell tumors
    Leydig cell tumors
    Sertoli cell tumors
    Lymphoma
    Leukemia
    Metastases

NSGCTs = Nonseminomatous germ cell tumors.

(1–2%) or be associated with cryptorchidism, Klinefelter's syndrome, Peutz-Jeghers syndrome and Down syndrome, and in patients with infertility [27].

TM has been associated with an increased risk of germ cell tumor (5–10%) and US follow-up has been recommended after the diagnosis. More recent literature, however, raises serious doubts regarding the association of TM to malignancy, and there is no consensus regarding the proper follow-up of patients with microlithiasis [28]. Annual sonographic surveillance, however, along with periodic self-examination, though not scientifically proven to be necessary, would probably be reasonable for the first years after the diagnosis [2, 7, 28].

Scrotal Lesions
Scrotal lesions, either symptomatic or asymptomatic, are one of the most common pathologies encountered in scrotal US. The aim of the US study in these cases is to identify the focal lesion, to determine its location (intratesticular or extratesticular), and to classify it according to the US charac-

teristics of the mass (solid vs. cystic, echogenicity, vascularity, etc.) [2].

Extratesticular lesions are more common and are usually benign, especially if the lesion is cystic. Intratesticular solid lesions are typically considered malignant; however, accurately diagnosing the rare benign intratesticular lesion is vital to avoid an unnecessary orchiectomy [27]. A classification of intratesticular lesions is reported in table 1.

Malignant testicular tumors account for less than 2% of all malignancies in men, but are the most frequent solid tumor in young male adults [7, 8]. Testicular tumors are divided into those derived from germ cells, gonadal stromal cells, along with lymphoma, leukemia and metastases (table 1). Germ cell tumors compose 95% of testicular cancers and are divided into seminoma and NSGCTs (nonseminomatous germ cell tumors), each with different treatments and prognosis [2].

Grayscale US is nearly 100% sensitive for the detection of testicular tumors [8]. Although a histologic diagnosis cannot be precisely established by US, patterns of sonographic findings permit a relatively accurate preoperative assessment as to whether a testicular mass is a seminoma or a nonseminoma testicular tumor. On US examination, in fact, seminomas are homogeneously hypoechoic and usually limited by the tunica albuginea [8] (fig. 5). Large seminomas can have a more heterogeneous appearance. Seminomas may be lobulated or multinodular, and can have cystic spaces (in 10% of them), which may be appreciated on a US image.

NSGCTs have multiple histologic patterns in 40–60% of cases [8], and the US features change according to the proportions of the different histologic components. They often have an inhomogeneous echotexture (71%), irregular or ill-defined margins (45%), echogenic foci (35%) and cystic components.

The majority of non-germ cell tumors are sex cord-stromal tumors, which represent 4% of testicular tumors. They are typically small and are usually discovered incidentally. They do not have any specific US appearance but show as well-defined hypoechoic lesions. These tumors are usually benign but malignancy can be encountered, mainly in older age [8].

Testicular lymphomas, almost exclusively diffuse non-Hodgkin B-cell lymphoma, constitute 5% of all testicular neoplasms [8]. Primary leukemia of the testes is rare but the testes are commonly the site of extramedullary relapse after chemotherapy-induced remission. Grayscale US of lymphoma and leukemia typically shows diffuse or focal regions of decreased echogenicity with maintenance of the normal ovoid testicular shape [8].

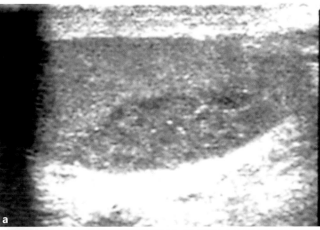

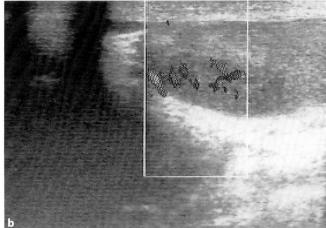

Fig. 5. Grayscale (**a**) and CFD (**b**) images of a seminoma. The tumor is solid and occupies a large portion of the testis.

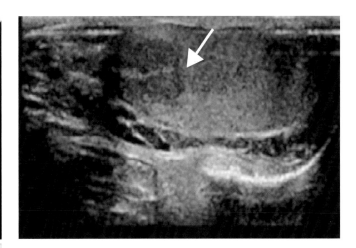

Fig. 6. TART of the right testis in B-mode (arrow).

Testicular metastases are uncommon, and usually occur in patients with a known malignancy in an advanced stage. The most common primary sources are the prostate (35%), the lung (19%), malignant melanoma (9%), the colon (9%) and the kidney (7%) [8]. Sonographically, they are generally hypoechoic but may be complex and even echogenic [7].

Rest Tumors

Testicular adrenal rest tumors (TART) are the nodular testicular lesions deriving from the adrenal remnant tissue in boys and men with congenital adrenal hyperplasia. TART are reported with great variability in 0–94% of congenital adrenal hyperplasia patients and often occur bilaterally. They may sometimes significantly enlarge, mimicking testicular malignant tumors, leading to damage to the structure of the testes, spermatogenesis disorders and infertility.

Until now, the diagnostics of TART have been based on a combination of clinical features (syndromes with hypercorticotropinemia), imaging methods (primarily 2D US), response of the foci to glucocorticosteroid therapy and the exclusion of the neoplastic process [1]. Routine application of 2D US provides a limited range of information about the size, volume, shape, demarcation, vascularization and elasticity of the lesion. Doppler studies have many limitations in quantitative vascular assessment [1]. Sonographic features of TART foci (fig. 6), such as hypoechogenicity and heterogeneity, clear delineation from the testicular parenchyma, encapsulation and poor vascular flow, are typical for other benign testicular lesions diagnosed in children, e.g. mature teratoma or epidermoid cyst. The latest advances in the field of US, such as sonoelastography and 3D US, may provide new opportunities for an early accurate diagnosis of TART and a much better understanding of the morphological pathology of scrotal mass lesions as well as the monitoring of treatment [1].

Hydrocele

A few milliliters of serous fluid are normally present in the potential space between the parietal and visceral layers of the tunica vaginalis. Hydrocele is an abnormal collection of fluid in this space and has a number of etiologies, which reflect the type of fluid accumulated. It may be idiopathic or secondary to trauma, prior inguinal hernia repair, testicular torsion, infection (acute epididymitis, acute epididymo-orchitis) or testicular neoplasm, and may contain serous fluid (simple hydrocele), pus (pyocele) or blood (hematocele) [7].

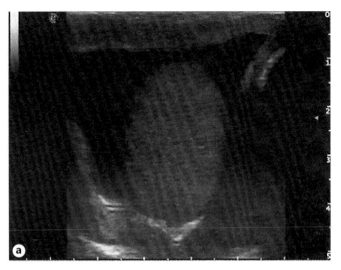 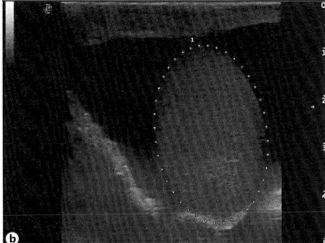

Fig. 7. Right (**a**) and left (**b**) hydrocele.

US evaluation is particularly useful in evaluating these patients as clinical evaluation of the underlying testis and epididymis is limited. Sonographically, the fluid surrounds the anterolateral margins of the testis as posteriorly the testis is adherent to the epididymis and scrotal wall. The fluid is usually anechoic with good sound transmission (fig. 7); however, it may contain low-level echoes due to fibrin bodies or cholesterol crystals. Complex hydroceles have internal septations and loculations, and may calcify if they become chronic [7].

Female Gonads

Introduction
US, specifically transvaginal US (TVUS), is the primary imaging modality for the evaluation and characterization of adnexal masses. Today's high-resolution images allow for the confident diagnosis of many adnexal lesions, with high sensitivity and specificity [29].

Color and duplex Doppler US have been proposed as further ways to distinguish between malignant and benign adnexal masses. Malignant masses are usually vascular (because of tumor-induced angiogenesis) with decreased peripheral blood flow resistance and increased blood flow velocity compared with benign tissue [30].

Studies have demonstrated that 3D US has a greater sensitivity compared with 2D US. The advantage of 3D US is that it visualizes the adnexal mass and associated vessels in all 3 planes, and a volume of US data is acquired and stored [30].

MRI is recommended as a second-line investigation for the characterization of complex adnexal masses that are indeterminate on US. Most studies have shown MRI to be superior to TVUS in the differentiation of benign from malignant adnexal lesions [29, 30]. Typical protocols include both T1- and T2-weighted sequences, with imaging performed in 3 planes. Fat-saturated T1-weighted imaging will help distinguish between fat or hemorrhage within an adnexal mass. Dynamic multiphase contrast-enhanced MRI after the administration of intravenous gadolinium is very useful for the characterization of adnexal masses. Solid components will demonstrate enhancement, enabling the distinction between fibrinous debris or retracting clot in the cyst wall from papillary projections. Gadolinium also improves the detection of peritoneal and omental implants in the case of ovarian carcinoma. Dynamic contrast-enhanced MRI (DCE-MRI; perfusion MRI) and diffusion-weighted imaging are not yet routinely performed for the evaluation of adnexal masses, although preliminary studies have demonstrated their value in the characterization of ovarian epithelial tumors, with early enhancement patterns enabling clinicians to distinguish between benign, borderline and invasive tumors [30].

CT is not routinely recommended for the evaluation of adnexal masses because it has poor contrast resolution and involves ionizing radiation. The advantages to CT are that it is widely available and it provides, with the use of intrave-

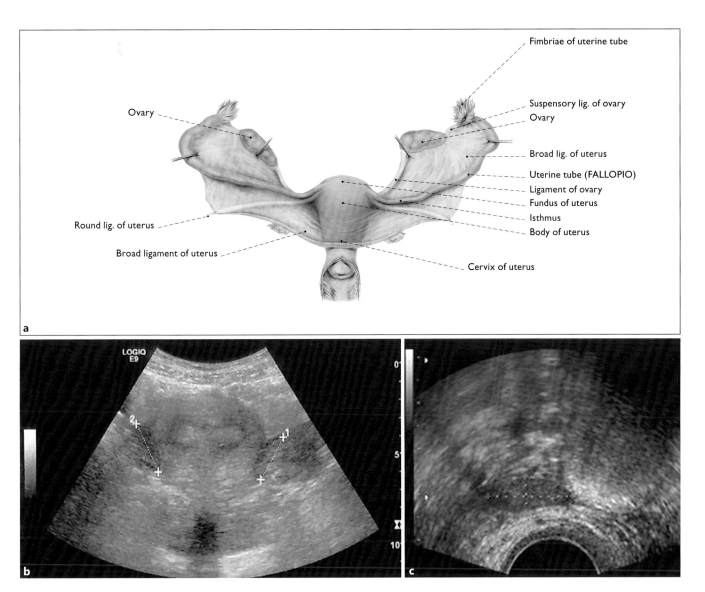

Fig. 8. a Coronal view of normal anatomy of the uterus and adnexa; reproduced with permission from Köpf-Maier [44]. **b** Grayscale transabdominal US demonstrating the uterus and adnexa. **c** Transvaginal US demonstrating a postmenopausal ovary.

nous and oral contrast medium, a comprehensive examination of the abdomen and pelvis, which is very useful in the case of ovarian carcinoma staging [30]. However, dynamic multiphase contrast-enhanced MRI has been shown to be more accurate than CT in staging ovarian carcinoma [31].

Normal Anatomy of the Adnexa

The adnexal region is the region lateral to the uterus that includes the ovary, the fallopian tube and the supporting ligaments (broad and round ligament). The normal ovary is an ovoid structure measuring approximately 3 × 2 × 2 cm,

with an average volume of 10 cm³; ovary size decreases after menopause [29] (fig. 8a).

The ovary is located in the posterior pelvic compartment because of its suspension by the mesovarium in the posterior and superior portion of the broad ligament. Additional support is provided by the fimbria of the fallopian tube draping over each ovary. The suspensory ligament inserts at the superior pole of the ovary orienting the long axis of the ovary in a craniocaudal direction (fig. 8a).

Despite the multiple mesenteric and ligamentous attachments, the ovarian position is highly variable and depends on the uterine size, ovarian size, bladder volume, distention of the rectosigmoid colon and the presence of other pelvic masses. In nulliparous women, the ovary is in close proximity to the lateral pelvic sidewall in the ovarian fossa [29] (fig. 8a).

The ovary is divided into outer cortical and inner medullary regions. The cortex consists primarily of follicles in different stages of maturation. The medulla consists of stromal cells, lymphatics, blood vessels and nerves. The appearance and structure of the ovary is highly variable owing to the cyclic influence of the hypothalamic-pituitary hormonal axis, which determines ovarian hormone production, follicular maturation and degeneration [29] (fig. 8b, c).

Although appreciated on US, the ovary zonal anatomy is better demonstrated on T2-weighted MR images. The cortex is characterized by a lower signal intensity and multiple small T2 bright follicles, whereas the central medulla is more intermediate in T2 signal [29].

Adnexal Ultrasound: Technique of Examination

Before a pelvic US examination is begun, relevant clinical information should be obtained, including the indication for the study, the date of the patient's last menstrual period and possible hormonal therapy, in the form of either birth control or hormonal replacement therapy (in postmenopausal patients) [32]. Unless the study is a follow-up examination, it is usually beneficial to begin with a quick transabdominal overview of the pelvis. In the interest of improving both patient throughput and patient comfort, distending the urinary bladder is no longer considered necessary and is not routinely done [32].

Transvaginal images should be obtained with the patient's urinary bladder empty, the transducer frequency should be at least 5 MHz and harmonic imaging should be used if deemed beneficial. To locate the ovary, the search can be started by imaging in the coronal plane at the level of the uterine fundus. The transducer is then gradually angled toward one of the adnexa. Often, there is visible thickening of soft tissues that are in continuity with the uterine fundus, likely representing a combination of the fallopian tube, mesosalpinx and ovarian ligament. This tissue serves as a useful anatomic landmark that can be followed as it leads toward the ovary. Once the ovary is identified, images should document its appearance in both the coronal and sagittal planes. If the ovary is not seen transvaginally, a second attempt should be made to locate it using a transabdominal approach [32].

A variety of US approaches have been used to evaluate and characterize ovarian masses. These range from sophis-

ticated analyses using statistically derived scoring systems, probability-based logistic regression analysis and mathematically derived neural networks [32], to a simpler subjective method that makes use of a pattern recognition approach [33]. Any mass with findings suggestive of malignancy must be identified and distinguished from masses with benign features.

Magnetic Resonance Imaging of Ovarian Masses

The entire pelvic anatomy is exquisitely depicted on pelvic MRI. On T1-weighted imaging the ovaries display a homogeneous low to intermediate signal intensity, whereas on T2-weighted imaging the follicles, if present, become hyperintense compared with the surrounding stroma [34]. Immature follicles are usually smaller than 1 cm in size, although normal ovaries may contain follicles up to 3 cm in size. With the advent of high-resolution imaging, the ovaries are now frequently identified in postmenopausal women. They appear as predominantly solid structures with a relative increase in stromal tissue, which is T2 hypointense, and may contain small T2 hyperintense follicles, although dysfunctional cysts up to several centimeters in size may also be encountered.

The greatest strength of MRI lies in its ability to characterize the physical and biochemical properties of different tissues (e.g. water, iron, fat and extravascular blood and its breakdown products) through the use of multiple imaging sequences. It is important to recognize that as there are no MRI signal intensity characteristics that are specific for malignant epithelial tumor, such tumors must be distinguished based on morphologic criteria [34]. The MRI features most predictive of malignancy are an enhancing solid component or vegetations within a cystic lesion and the presence of necrosis within a solid lesion, as well as the presence of ascites and peritoneal deposits [35]. Both TVUS and contrast-enhanced MRI have high sensitivity (97 and 100%, respectively) in the identification of solid components within an adnexal mass. MRI also shows high specificity (92%; fig. 9) [35].

Other MRI techniques also have a role in characterizing ovarian masses. Multiphase and DCE-MRI helps differentiate solid components or papillary projections from clots and debris [36]. In addition, DCE-MRI might play a role in the preoperative evaluation of borderline ovarian malignancies [36].

In the case of primary tumors, MRI enables local staging and detection of metastatic disease to help guide management options, such as complex surgery or the consideration of neoadjuvant chemotherapy. Functional MRI techniques,

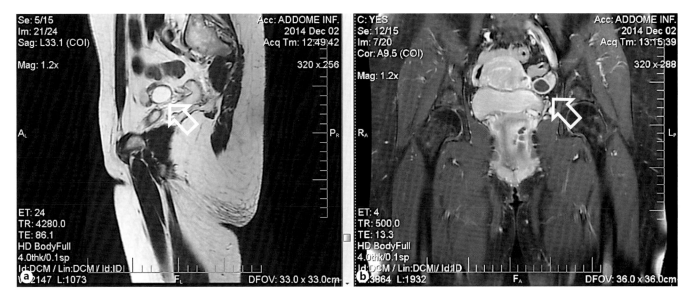

Fig. 9. Sagittal (**a**) and coronal (**b**) MR images of a left ovarian cyst (arrow).

such as diffusion-weighted MRI, DCE-MRI and tumor-selective molecular imaging, are currently being evaluated as possible predictive and prognostic biomarkers in the context of ovarian malignancy, and may play a larger role in routine clinical practice in the future [34].

Benign Ovarian Lesions
In most clinical practices, the great majority of ovarian masses are benign, easily recognizable and can be classified as one of six entities, known as the 'big six', including: physiological and functioning follicles, corpora lutea, hemorrhagic cysts, endometriomas, polycystic ovaries and benign cystic teratomas (dermoids) [32] (table 2).

Physiological and Functioning Follicles
In healthy premenopausal women monthly dynamic changes initially occur due to the preovulatory development of a dominant follicle. During this phase of the cycle (preovulatory phase), TVUS depicts a developing follicle as a thin-walled, round to oval, avascular simple-appearing cyst. At ovulation, its diameter ranges from 1.7 to 2.8 cm, but a diameter of up to and including 3.0 cm is considered normal [32]. Immediately before ovulation, a tiny peripheral curved line may be visible, which indicates that the ovum is surrounded by a cumulus oophorus within the mature follicle. A functional follicle develops when ovulation fails to occur, and the follicle continues to enlarge but remains simple in its US appearance.

Table 2. Classification of benign ovarian masses

Cystic lesions
    Physiological and functioning follicles
    Corpora lutea
    Hemorrhagic cysts
    Endometriomas
    Polycystic ovaries
    Benign cystic teratomas (dermoids)
Solid lesions
    Fibromas
    Thecomas
    Adenofibromas
    Brenner tumors

Corpora Lutea
A postovulatory corpus luteum can measure up to 3.0 cm, but its grayscale appearance is more varied and ranges from a thick-walled cyst with an irregular crenulated margin to a cyst that appears more collapsed, giving it a relatively solid appearance. In all cases, Doppler US demonstrates a prominent peripheral blood flow with a low-resistance waveform. Typically, physiological cysts resolve within a few weeks [32]. A functioning corpus luteum develops when the corpus luteum fails to resorb following ovulation. It too often enlarges and, given its inherent vascular wall, often evolves into a hemorrhagic cyst.

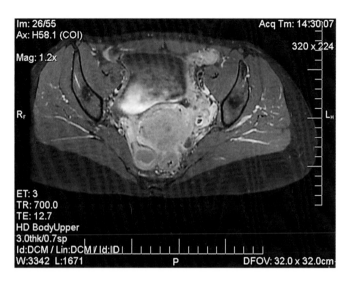

Fig. 10. MR image of a right ovary endometrioma.

high signal intensity on T1-weighted imaging (caused by methemoglobin) and low signal intensity on T2-weighted imaging because of a high iron concentration from the presence of blood (fig. 10) [30].

Polycystic Ovary Syndrome

Polycystic ovary syndrome is a clinical syndrome characterized by clinical or biochemical evidence of hyperandrogenism, chronic anovulation and polycystic ovaries on imaging. In 2003, a consensus report was published that included the following description of morphologic ovarian changes consistent with polycystic ovarian morphology: an involved ovary should demonstrate 12 or more follicles measuring 2–9 mm in diameter (fig. 11), an increased ovarian volume (>10 cm^3), or both [39]. A follow-up consensus statement was published that recommended the number of follicles used to suggest polycystic ovarian morphology should be increased from 12 to a threshold of 19, since smaller follicles can now be visualized with the improved US technology [32, 40].

The use of MRI for the assessment of polycystic ovaries has also been explored [41]. According to the American College of Radiology appropriateness criteria, pelvic MRI is recommended in cases in which US is inconclusive or nondiagnostic. The ovaries are typically enlarged (volume ≥10 ml) with a prominent central stroma of low to intermediate signal intensity on T2-weighted imaging and multiple small peripheral high T2 signal intensity follicles (≥12 follicles per ovary, each <10 mm in size) without a dominant follicle ≥10 mm in size or a corpus luteum cyst [34].

Mature Cystic Teratomas

Mature cystic teratomas (dermoids) are common benign avascular ovarian neoplasms with a variety of characteristic US features, which in most cases may be used to make a confident and accurate diagnosis [42]. Most dermoids contain a clump of hair, which both absorbs and reflects sound at US. The net effect is a focal hyperechogenic area that gradually attenuates sound and results in a characteristic gradual acoustic shadow [42].

On CT, dermoids are easily recognized due to the presence of macroscopic fat and calcifications. On MRI, the fat component will demonstrate high signal intensity on both T1- and T2-weighted imaging with the lipid-laden cyst fluid demonstrating a similar high signal intensity on T1-weighted imaging and intermediate signal intensity on T2-weighted imaging [30].

Hemorrhagic Cysts

Hemorrhagic cysts typically develop in premenopausal women due to hemorrhage within a corpus luteum. Acutely, a hemorrhagic ovarian cyst contains clotted blood which at US manifests as intensely echogenic, avascular, homogeneous or heterogeneous nonshadowing material. In its subacute state, the clot may retract, remain avascular and pull away from the cyst wall; its surface is often undulating and it has a characteristic concave contour. Another common feature is the presence of US findings that are consistent with fibrin strands. An ovarian cyst that demonstrates classic features consisting of fibrin strands, no septations and a smooth wall has been shown to be a hemorrhagic cyst with a likelihood ratio of 200, a sensitivity of 90% and a specificity of 100% [37].

On MRI, the presence of hemorrhage results in a high signal intensity on T1-weighted imaging and an intermediate to high signal intensity on T2-weighted imaging. The absence of papillary projections and nodular septa helps distinguish hemorrhagic cysts from ovarian tumors [30].

Endometriomas

The ovary is the most common site for extrauterine endometrial tissue deposition, and most endometriomas have a characteristic US 'signature' which consists of a well-defined, smooth-walled uni- or multiloculated cyst that contains homogeneous low-level echoes and imparts a characteristic 'ground-glass' appearance [38]. On MRI, endometriomas may appear as multicystic adnexal masses that show

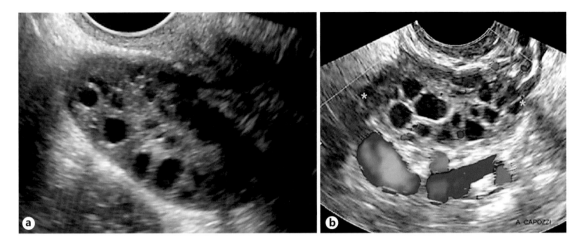

Fig. 11. Transverse (**a**) and CFD (**b**) images of the right ovary demonstrate the classic appearance of a polycystic ovary.

Cystic Lesions in Postmenopausal Women

Postmenopausal women may show simple cystic adnexal structures up to 5 cm (fig. 12). The American College of Radiology appropriateness criteria is used for ovarian cancer screening and follow-up [43]. A cystic structure that is less than 30 mm in size, unilateral, unilocular, and with no internal echoes, solid areas or nodules, which is avascular on color flow mapping, may be reevaluated 6 and 12 weeks later, and then annually if it does not increase or change in morphology. Any mass with abnormal vascularity and all masses greater than 50 mm in size warrant surgical evaluation. All masses associated with a rising CA 125 level warrant surgical exploration.

Benign Solid Ovarian Tumors

These tumors include ovarian fibromas, thecomas, adenofibromas and Brenner tumors. Fibrothecomas are the most common solid benign tumors of the ovary and are classified as sex cord-stromal tumors. Fibromas and fibrothecomas may mimic pedunculated myomas on US, appearing as well-circumscribed hypoechoic solid, round or oval tumors with sound attenuation. They are usually hypovascular on color Doppler [30]. On MRI, because of the extensive collagen content and hyalinized tissue, fibromas and the fibrotic component of fibrothecomas appear as intermediate signal intensity masses on T1-weighted imaging and low signal intensity masses on T2-weighted imaging. Calcification may occur, seen as foci of signal voids on T1- and T2-weighted imaging [30].

Adenofibromas are a subtype of benign epithelial tumor. They appear as a solid ovarian mass, being bilateral in 10–

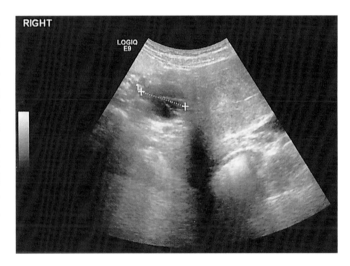

Fig. 12. Transabdominal image of a right ovarian cyst in a postmenopausal woman.

20% of cases. On color Doppler, there is increased vascularity demonstrated in 50% of tumors. On MRI, the fibrous component is of very low signal intensity on T2-weighted imaging, which is a very specific feature. Following intravenous gadolinium there is heterogeneous enhancement [30].

Brenner tumors are transitional cell tumors of the ovary. They are usually benign but borderline and malignant types can also arise. Benign tumors are usually unilateral, small (<5 cm) solid masses, appearing hypoechoic on US. Extensive calcification is characteristic, resulting in posterior acoustic shadowing on TVUS. On MRI the benign type appears solid and of low signal intensity on both T1- and T2-

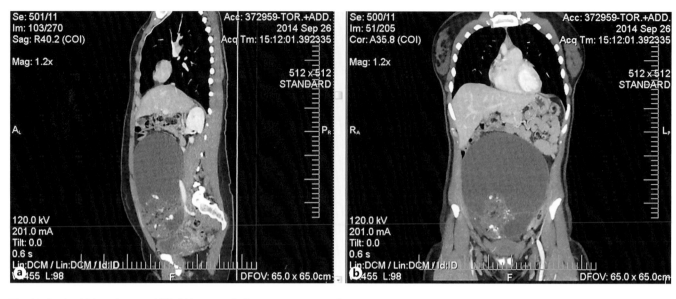

Fig.13. Sagittal (**a**) and coronal (**b**) CT images of a large ovarian cystadenocarcinoma.

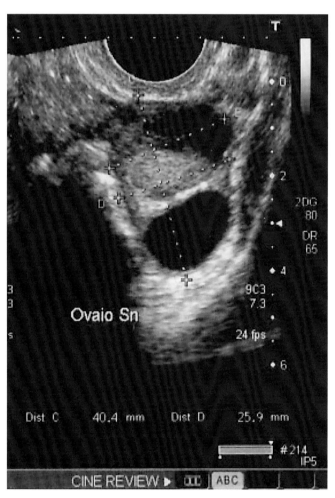

weighted imaging. There is homogeneous avid rapid enhancement after intravenous gadolinium. Borderline and malignant Brenner tumors may appear as multiloculated cystic masses with solid components or papillary projections [30].

Malignant Ovarian Tumors
Malignant ovarian tumors include surface epithelial stromal tumors [such as serous cystadenocarcinomas (fig. 13), mucinous cystadenocarcinomas, endometrioid and clear-cell carcinomas], sex cord-stromal tumors (granulosa cell and

Table 3. Classification of malignant ovarian tumors

Surface epithelial stromal tumors
    Serous cystadenocarcinomas
    Mucinous cystadenocarcinomas
    Endometrioid carcinomas
    Clear-cell carcinomas
Sex cord-stromal tumors
    Granulosa cell tumors
    Sertoli-Leydig cell tumors
Germ cell tumors

Fig. 14. Transvaginal US image of the left ovary demonstrates a multiseptated cystic lesion containing fluid and also solid areas (Sertoli cell tumor).

Sertoli-Leydig cell tumors) and germ cell tumors. Less common malignant tumors include mixed Müllerian tumors, undifferentiated carcinomas, carcinoids and lymphomas [30] (table 3).

Surface Epithelial Stromal Tumors

Borderline serous tumors account for 10–15% of all ovarian serous tumors and are bilateral in 30% of cases. There may be larger areas of necrosis and hemorrhage in malignant mucinous tumors compared with borderline tumors. On MRI solid components demonstrate marked enhancement [30].

Endometrioid carcinomas arise from the ovarian surface epithelium and can be associated with endometriosis, endometrial hyperplasia and cancer. On US and MRI they appear as mixed solid/cystic ovarian masses with vascularity and enhancement of solid components [30]. Clear-cell carcinomas are almost always malignant and present as unilateral large masses that can be either predominantly solid or cystic, containing one or more solid protrusions [30].

Sex Cord-Stromal Tumors (Granulosa Cell and Sertoli-Leydig Cell Tumors)

Granulosa cell tumors are rare sex cord ovarian tumors, accounting for 1–2% of all ovarian malignancies. The adult type is of low malignant potential and presents as a unilateral multiseptated cystic lesion containing fluid/blood products and also solid areas (fig. 14). On MRI it appears as a multilocular (sponge-like) cystic mass or as a solid mass with internal cysts. As these tumors produce estrogen, they are associated with endometrial hyperplasia and endometrial cancer in 5% of cases [30]. Sertoli-Leydig cell tumors are rare sex cord-stromal ovarian tumors with a variable appearance as solid, partially cystic or completely cystic.

Germ Cell Tumors

Germ cell tumors are derived from primordial germ cells and account for approximately 20% of all ovarian tumors. Only 5% are malignant. In general, malignant germ cell tumors tend to present as predominantly solid tumors with areas of hemorrhage and necrosis [30].

References

1 Jedrzejewski G, Ben-Skowronek I, Wozniak MM, Brodzisz A, Budzynska E, Wieczorek AP: Testicular adrenal rest tumors in boys with congenital adrenal hyperplasia: 3D US and elastography – do we get more information for diagnosis and monitoring? J Pediatr Urol 2013;9:1032–1037.

2 Appelbaum L, Gaitini D, Dogra VS: Scrotal ultrasound in adults. Semin Ultrasound CT MRI 2013; 34:257–273.

3 Schurich M, Aigner F, Frauscher F, Pallwein L: The role of ultrasound in assessment of male fertility. Eur J Obstet Gynecol Reprod Biol 2009; 144:S192–S198.

4 Hughes Cassidy F, Ishioka KM, McMahon CJ, Chu P, Sakamoto K, Lee KS, Aganovic L: MR imaging of scrotal tumors and pseudotumors. RadioGraphics 2010;30:665–683.

5 Mohrs OK, Thoms H, Egner T, Brunier A, Eiers M, Kauczor HU, Hallscheidt P: MRI of patients with suspected scrotal or testicular lesions: diagnostic value in daily practice. AJR Am J Roentgenol 2012;199:609–615.

6 Tasian GE, Copp HL, Baskin LS: Diagnostic imaging in cryptorchidism: utility, indications, and effectiveness. J Pediatr Surg 2011;46:2406–2413.

7 Pearl MS, Hill MC: Ultrasound of the scrotum. Semin Ultrasound CT MRI 2007;28:225–248.

8 Dogra VS, Gottlieb RH, Oka M, Rubens DJ: Sonography of the scrotum. Radiology 2003;227: 18–36.

9 Sakamoto H, Ogawa Y, Yoshida H: Relationship between testicular volume and testicular function: comparison of the Prader orchidometric and ultrasonographic measurements in patients with infertility. Asian J Androl 2008;10:319–324.

10 Thierman JS, Clement GT, Kalish LA, O'Kane PL, Frauscher F, Paltiel HJ: Automated sonographic evaluation of testicular perfusion. Phys Med Biol 2006;51:3419–3432.

11 Lung PF, Jaffer OS, Sellars ME, Sriprasad S, Kooiman GG, Sidhu PS: Contrast-enhanced ultrasound in the evaluation of focal testicular complications secondary to epididymitis. Am J Roentgenol 2012;100:345–354.

12 Lock G, Schmidt C, Helminch F, Stolle E, Dieckmann KP: Early experience with contrast-enhanced ultrasound in the diagnosis of testicular masses: a feasibility study. Urology 2011;77:1049–1053.

13 Riccabona M: Pediatric three-dimensional ultrasound: basics and potential clinical value. Clin Imaging 2005;29:1–5.

14 Simpson WL, Rausch DR: Imaging of male infertility: pictorial review. AJR Am J Roentgenol 2009; 192:S98–S107.

15 Beddy P, Geoghegan T, Browne RF, Torreggiani WC: Testicular varicoceles. Clin Radiol 2005;60: 1248–1255.

16 Jockenhövel F, Gräwe A, Nieschlag E: A portable digital data recorder for long-term monitoring of scrotal temperature. Fertil Steril 1990;54:694–700.

17 Prenen J, van Dis P, Feijen H: Varicocele scintigraphy: a simplified method for the detection of spermatic vein reflux. Clin Nucl Med 1996;21: 921–927.

18 Li M, Du J, Wang ZQ, Li FH: The value of sonoelastography scores and the strain ration in differential diagnosis of azoospermia. J Urol 2012;188: 1861–1866.

19 Brugh VM, Matschke HM, Lipshultz LI: Male factor infertility. Endocrinol Metab Clin N Am 2003; 32:689–707.

20 Lanfranco F, Kamischke A, Zitzmann M, Nieschlag E: Klinefelter's syndrome. Lancet 2004;364: 273–283.

21 Brugh VM, Lipshultz LI: Male factor infertility: evaluation and management. Med Clin N Am 2004;88:367–385.

22 Kolon TF, Patel RP, Huff DS: Cryptorchidism: diagnosis, treatment, and long-term prognosis. Urol Clin North Am 2004;31:469–480.

23 Kanemoto K, Hayashi Y, Kojima Y, Maruyama T, Ito M, Kohri K: Accuracy of ultrasonography and magnetic resonance imaging in the diagnosis of nonpalpable testis. Int J Urol 2005;12:668–672.

24 Cornud F, Amar E, Hamida K, Thiounn N, Hélénon O, Moreau JF: Imaging in male hypofertility and impotence. BJU Int 2000;86:153–163.

25 Cast JE, Nelson WM, Early AS, Biyani S, Cooksey G, Warnock NG, Breen DJ: Testicular microlithiasis: prevalence and tumor risk in a population referred for scrotal sonography. AJR Am J Roentgenol 2000;175:1703–1706.

26 Bennett HF, Middleton WD, Bullock AD, Teefey SA: Testicular microlithiasis: US follow-up. Radiology 2001;218:359–363.

27 Mirochnik B, Bhargava P, Dighe MK, Kanth N: Ultrasound evaluation of scrotal pathology. Radiol Clin North Am 2012;50:317–332.

28 Dutra RA, Perez-Boscollo AC, Melo EC, Cruvinel JC: Clinical importance and prevalence of testicular microlithiasis in pediatric patients. Acta Cir Bras 2011;26:387–390.

29 Heilbrun ME, Olpin J, Shaaban A: Imaging of benign adnexal masses: characteristic presentations on ultrasound, computed tomography, and magnetic resonance imaging. Clin Obstet Gynecol 2009;52:21–39.

30 Griffin N, Grant LA, Sala E: Adnexal masses: characterization and imaging strategies. Semin Ultrasound CT MRI 2010;31:330–346.

31 Forstner R, Hricak H, Occhipinti KA, Powell CB, Frankel SD, Stern JL: Ovarian cancer: staging with CT and MR imaging. Radiology 1995;197:619–626.

32 Laing FC, Allison SJ: US of the ovary and adnexa: to worry or not to worry? RadioGraphics 2012;32:1621–1639.

33 Patel MD: Practical approach to the adnexal mass. Radiol Clin North Am 2006;44:879–899.

34 Vargas HA, Barrett T, Sala E: MRI of ovarian masses. J Magn Reson Imaging 2013;37:265–281.

35 Hricak H, Chen M, Coakley FV, Kinkel K, Yu KK, Sica G, Bacchetti P, Powell CB: Complex adnexal masses: detection and characterization with MR imaging-multivariate analysis. Radiology 2000;214:39–46.

36 van Vierzen PB, Massuger LF, Ruys SH, Barentsz JO: Borderline ovarian malignancy: ultrasound and fast dynamic MR findings. Eur J Radiol 1998;28:136–142.

37 Patel MD, Feldstein VA, Filly RA: The likelihood ratio of sonographic findings for the diagnosis of hemorrhagic ovarian cysts. J Ultrasound Med 2005;24:607–614.

38 Patel MD, Feldstein VA, Chen DC, Lipson SD, Filly RA: Endometriomas: diagnostic performance of US. Radiology 1999;210:739–745.

39 Balen AH, Laven JS, Tan SL, Dewailly D: Ultrasound assessment of the polycystic ovary: international consensus definitions. Hum Reprod Update 2003;9:505–514.

40 Dewailly D, Gronier H, Poncelet E, Robin G, Leroy M, Pigny P, Duhamel A, Catteau-Jonard S: Diagnosis of polycystic ovary syndrome (PCOS): revisiting the threshold values of follicle count on ultrasound and of the serum AMH level for the definition of polycystic ovaries. Hum Reprod 2011;26:3123–3129.

41 Lee TT, Rausch ME: Polycystic ovarian syndrome: role of imaging in diagnosis. RadioGraphics 2012;32:1643–1657.

42 Patel MD, Feldstein VA, Lipson SD, Chen DC, Filly RA: Cystic teratomas of the ovary: diagnostic value of sonography. AJR Am J Roentgenol 1998;171:1061–1065.

43 Brown DL, Andreotti RF, Lee SI, Dejesus Allison SO, Bennett GL, Dubinsky T, Glanc P, Horrow MM, Lev-Toaff AS, Horowitz NS, Podrasky AE, Scoutt LM, Zelop CM: ACR Appropriateness Criteria© ovarian cancer screening. Ultrasound Q 2010;26:219–223.

44 Köpf-Maier P: Wolf-Heidegger's Atlas of Human Anatomy, ed 6. Basel, Karger, 2005.

Fabio Lanfranco, MD, PhD
Divisione di Endocrinologia, Diabetologia e Metabolismo
Dipartimento di Scienze Mediche
Università di Torino
Corso Dogliotti 14
IT–10126 Turin (Italy)
E-Mail fabio.lanfranco@unito.it

Buchfelder M, Guaraldi F (eds): Imaging in Endocrine Disorders.
Front Horm Res. Basel, Karger, 2016, vol 45, pp 97–120 (DOI: 10.1159/000442327)

Magnetic Resonance Imaging of Pituitary Tumors

Jean-François Bonneville

Service d'Endocrinologie, Centre Hospitalier Universitaire de Liège, Liège, Belgium

Abstract

Magnetic Resonance Imaging (MRI) is currently considered a major keystone of the diagnosis of diseases of the hypothalamic-hypophyseal region. However, the relatively small size of the pituitary gland, its location deep at the skull base and the numerous physiological variants present in this area impede the precise assessment of the anatomical structures and, particularly, of the pituitary gland itself. The diagnosis of the often tiny lesions of this region – such as pituitary microadenomas – is then difficult if the MRI technology is not optimized and if potential artifacts and traps are not recognized. Advanced MRI technology can not only depict small lesions with greater reliability, but also help in the differential diagnosis of large tumors. In these, defining the presence or absence of invasion is a particularly important task. This review describes and illustrates the radiological diagnosis of the different tumors of the sellar region, from the common prolactinomas, nonfunctioning adenomas and Rathke's cleft cysts, to the less frequent and more difficult to detect corticotroph pituitary adenomas in Cushing's disease, and other neoplastic and nonneoplastic entities. Finally, some hints are given to facilitate the differential diagnosis of sellar lesions.

© 2016 S. Karger AG, Basel

Pituitary adenomas represent the most common pathology of the sellar region. They become symptomatic if they exert a mass effect on the surrounding structures, or in cases of hormonal hypersecretion. Pituitary adenomas are frequently discovered by chance. The majority of this chapter will be devoted to the diagnosis of pituitary adenomas with magnetic resonance imaging (MRI). Most recent aspects will be particularly emphasized. Other tumors of the sellar region will be discussed more briefly at the end of the review.

MRI has totally supplanted CT (computed tomography) in the diagnosis of these lesions. The role of advanced techniques, such as high-field 3-tesla MRI, dynamic contrast-enhanced MRI, diffusion-weighted MRI and apparent diffusion coefficient (ADC) maps, spectroscopy or arterial spin-labeled perfusion imaging will be discussed. CT is still obtained in rare cases, including the search for tumor calcifications when a craniopharyngioma is suspected, or of bone erosion in the presurgical assessment of the clivus in aggressive pituitary adenomas.

The Normal Pituitary Gland

The pituitary gland is routinely examined in sagittal and coronal projections in every case, and in axial projections in some particular circumstances. In our practice, gadolinium

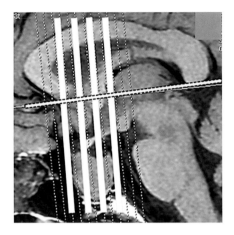

Fig. 1. Sagittal T1-weighted image obtained to determine coronal projections. Coronal sequences are obtained perpendicularly to the subcallosal plane.

injection is not always mandatory and depends on the results of nonenhanced sequences. Coronal T1- and T2-weighted sequences are always performed perpendicularly to a reference plan drawn on the sagittal view, e.g. a line tangential to the inferior surface of the corpus callosum [1] (fig. 1). This strategy permits a perfect comparison of images on serial MRIs. In normal subjects, the shape of the anterior pituitary is variable on coronal images, with a flat, concave or convex upper surface; its height can vary considerably from 1–2 to 7–8 mm. The T1-weighted signal of the normal anterior pituitary gland is strictly identical to that of the cerebral white matter, and this accurate relationship is very useful in clinical practice. The posterior lobe can be masked by the dorsum sellae in the T1-weighted sagittal view, so that its demonstration is best obtained on axial T1-weighted fat-saturated sequences. After intravenous gado-

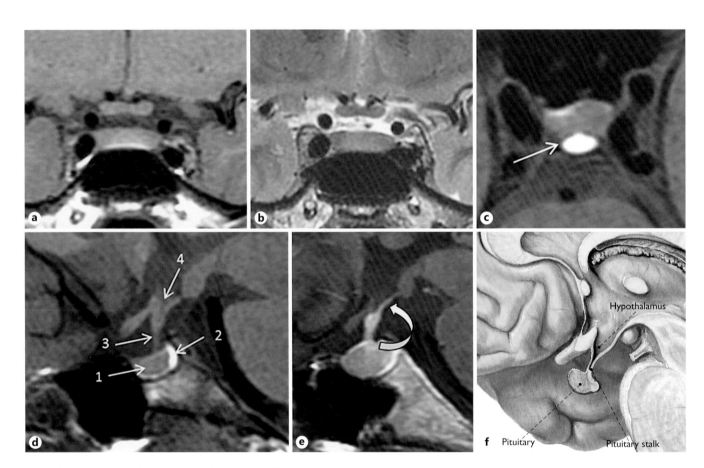

Fig. 2. MRI of the normal pituitary gland. **a, b** Coronal T1- and T2-weighted images. **c** Axial T1-weighted fat-saturated image (the arrow points to the posterior lobe). **d** Sagittal T1-weighted image: anterior pituitary (1); posterior pituitary (2); pituitary stalk (3); 3rd ventricle (4). **e** Contrast-enhanced sagittal T1-weighted MRI: enhancement of the anterior pituitary, the pituitary stalk and the tuber cinereum (arrow). **f** Anatomic representation of the normal sellar region; reproduced with permission from Köpf-Maier [41].

linium injection, enhancement of the anterior pituitary, pituitary stalk and tuber cinereum is normally observed [1] (fig. 2).

Pituitary Adenomas

The MRI aspect of pituitary adenomas is herein described according to their size and their hormonal secretion. Some particular conditions are separately mentioned.

Pituitary Microadenomas

Pituitary microadenomas are defined as tumors measuring less than 10 mm in diameter. They are typically represented by distinct small intrasellar lesions. We have proposed the term 'picoadenomas' for adenomas measuring less than 3 mm that frequently need specific technical options, such as the search for corticotropic adenomas. Traps and pitfalls are numerous [1].

Pituitary microadenomas have to be differentiated from:
– artifacts, in particular partial volume artifacts [2];
– normal anatomical structures, such as the posterior pituitary or the 'fossula hypophyseos' [2];
– variants from normal, such as unusual intrasellar arteries, an unusually well-developed inferior coronal sinus or a sellar spine [2];
– intrasellar cysts, such as Rathke's cleft cysts (RCC), that are encountered very frequently [2];
– a small sella turcica can also mimic a pituitary gland enlargement; indeed, such a small sella can be flat and frequently associated with an extensive sphenoidal sinus pneumatization, short (e.g. with a thick dorsum sellae) or narrow, when the sellar floor is <10 mm in width [2] (fig. 3).

Dynamic imaging has to be read with caution and can be the source of false positive diagnoses: early normal enhancement of a posterior pituitary, laterally located within the sella, could be interpreted erroneously as a controlateral defect in enhancement of the anterior pituitary [1, 2] (fig. 4).

Microprolactinomas

Microprolactinomas are by far the most frequent pituitary microadenomas. They are usually round or oval in shape, located off midline, hypointense on T1-weighted images, as compared to the normal anterior pituitary gland, and more or less hyperintense on T2-weighted images. Microprolactinomas generally have a T1-weighted signal similar to the cerebral gray matter, while the normal unaffected anterior pituitary gland has the same T1-weighted signal as the cerebral white matter [1] (fig. 5). High signal intensity on T1-weighted images can sometimes be observed, reflecting hemorrhagic transformation, not uncommon even in asymptomatic patients with prolactinomas [3]. Intratumoral calcifications are very rare, but do not rule out the diagnosis of pituitary adenomas, particularly in men. An additional CT scan can be helpful in these cases [1, 2].

There is probably some relationship between the tumor T2 signal and the serum prolactin levels; in our experience, the more hyperintense the tumor, the lower the prolactin levels are. T2 hypointense microprolactinomas are very unusual; they seem to be associated with higher prolactin levels and can possibly have a different evolution, e.g. arise during pregnancy [4] (fig. 6, 7).

There is generally a good correlation between the prolactin level and adenoma size, except for extremely T2-hyperintense and T1-hyperintense lesions as these situations usually correspond to tumors secreting low amounts of prolac-

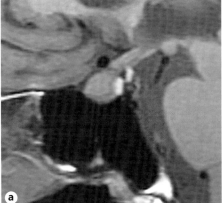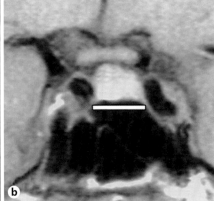

Fig. 3. a, b Small sella, short sellar floor and hyperpneumatization of the sphenoid bone (frontal view).

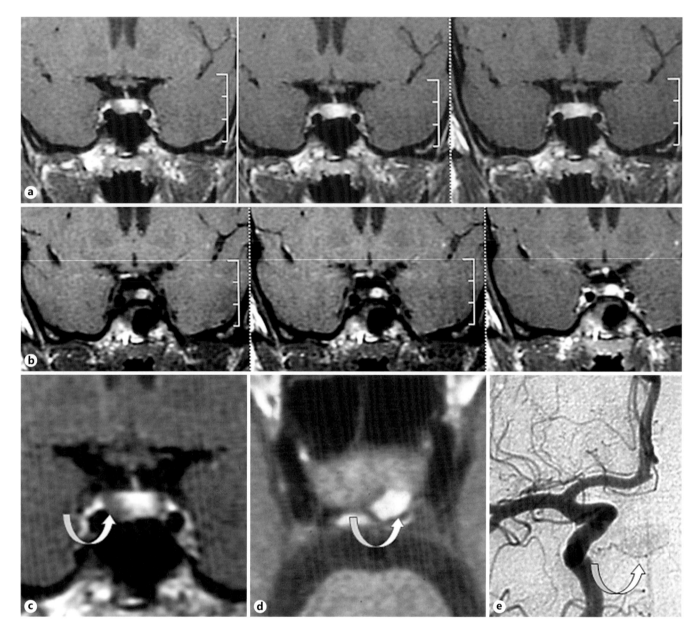

Fig. 4. a–e Hazard of dynamic MRI: normal delayed enhancement of the anterior pituitary gland wrongly interpreted as a microadenoma (arrow in **c**). The off-midline posterior lobe enhances earlier because of its direct blood supply.

tin [4]. We have almost never detected a microprolactinoma with a prolactin level <1,000 mIU/l (35 μg/l) on MRI.

Indirect radiological signs of a microadenoma are changes of the sellar floor and an upper convex surface. The pituitary stalk displacement is not always helpful for diagnosis. However, a localized subtle deformation of the sellar floor is a valuable indicator, even for small microadenomas [1].

When the radiological diagnosis is obvious after T2- and T1-weighted sequences in a context of infertility, amenorrhea-galactorrhea and hyperprolactinemia, we consider contrast-enhanced sequences unnecessary. On the contrary, contrast medium injection must be used in all uncertain situations, e.g. if an isointense or hypointense pituitary microadenoma is suspected [1].

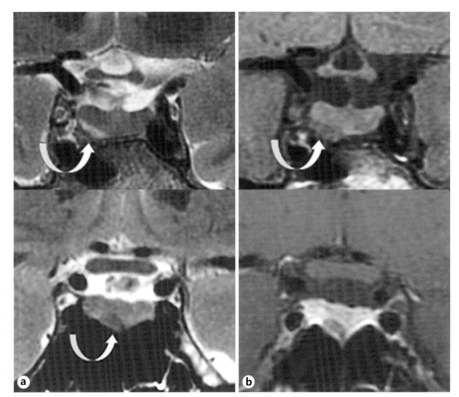

Fig. 5. Typical microprolactinoma MRI pattern: the adenoma is located in the top right side of the pituitary and appears hypointense on T1-weighted images and hyperintense on T2-weighted images (**a**); unusual hypointense microprolactinoma on a T2-weighted image, before and after gadolinium injection (**b**).

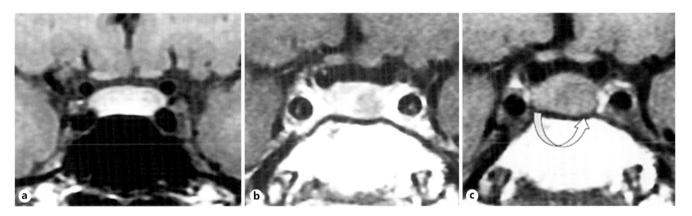

Fig. 6. Normal appearance of the pituitary in the 7th month of a normal pregnancy: the gland is enlarged and hyperintense on T1-weighted MRI images (**a**); microprolactinoma before cabergoline treatment (**b**), and moderate adenoma enlargement in the 7th month of pregnancy after cabergoline withdrawal (**c**).

Shrinkage of microprolactinomas is normally observed after a few weeks of treatment with dopamine agonists. Most of the time, an accentuation of high T2-intensity is also seen. A partial hemorrhagic transformation of the adenoma can mask its shrinkage [3].

Enlargement in size, usually a doubling, of the microadenoma occurs during pregnancy, principally during the third trimester, if dopamine agonists have been withdrawn [3–5]. In the same way, the volume of the normal anterior pituitary gland increases – on average by 0.08 mm per week – and its T1-weighted signal increases. Return to the prepregnancy size of the adenoma and of normal pituitary gland shape is usually observed a few weeks after delivery [5]. In some particular conditions, such as hemorrhagic

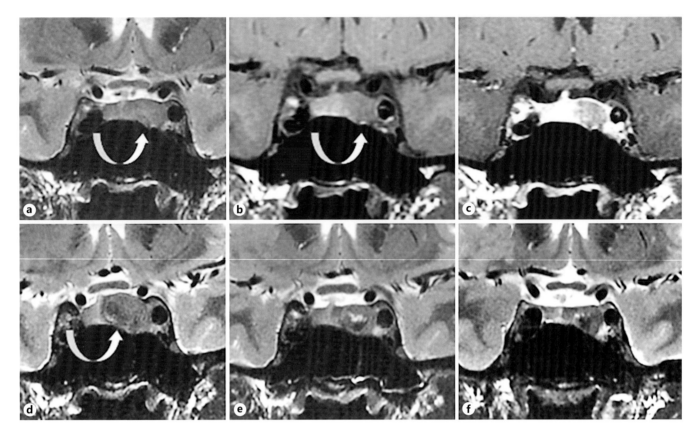

Fig. 7. A 27-year-old female with 'post-pill' amenorrhea; prolactin was 4,000 mIU/l. Left-sided prolactinoma with an unusual T2-hypointense signal (**a**); T1- (**b**) and post-contrast T1-weighted sequences (**c**). Pregnancy occurred quickly after dopamine agonist treatment and was stopped as soon as the pregnancy was determined (**d**). On the coronal T2-weighted image, a clear enlargement of the adenoma in the 8th month of pregnancy is seen, with tilting of the optic chiasm. Cabergoline was reintroduced and normal delivery occurred. At follow-up, 4 months after delivery, there was shrinkage of the mass and a slight hemorrhagic transformation of the adenoma (**e**). **f** Further reduction of the lesion 1 year after delivery.

transformation of the adenoma, a second pregnancy or prolonged medical treatment during pregnancy, a reduction of size or even the disappearance of the adenoma at MRI can sometimes be observed, paralleled by the normalization of prolactin levels [5, 6].

Growth Hormone-Secreting Microadenomas
Growth hormone (GH)-secreting microadenomas were previously underdiagnosed, while to date they represent one third of all somatotropinomas. Indeed, with high-resolution MRI, particularly in elderly subjects, it has become possible to reveal tiny pituitary adenomas – sometimes within an enlarged sella, erroneously called 'empty sella' – corresponding to involuted adenomas, either spontaneously or after hemorrhage, [1]. More than half of micro-somatotropinas as well as GH-secreting pituitary mac-

roadenomas present with hypointensity on T2-weighted images, if compared with the unaffected pituitary gland [1] (fig. 8).

Corticotroph Microadenomas
Corticotroph microadenomas represent a difficult challenge for the neuroradiologist, their size being sometimes at the limit or below the radiological visibility (fig. 9) [7]. In cases of negative MRI examination, it is recommended to resume MRI and to add alternative sequences, such as delayed imaging studies, dynamic MRI, 3D imaging and other variants [8]. Sun et al. [7] considers that the use of pituitary-specific technical parameters can improve the detection of adrenocorticotropic hormone (ACTH)-secreting pituitary tumors. Nevertheless, dynamic procedures improve the sensibility of MRI for the visualization of micro-

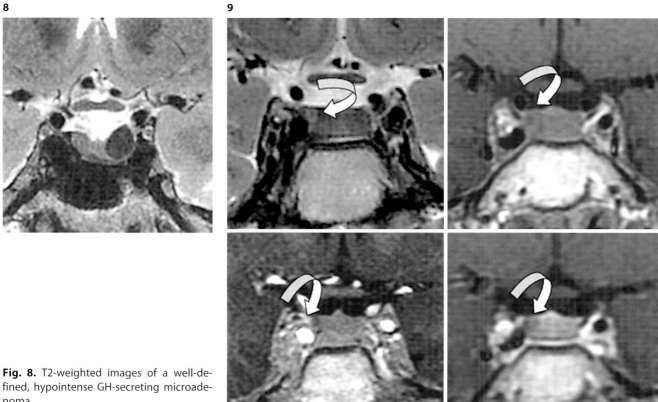

Fig. 8. T2-weighted images of a well-defined, hypointense GH-secreting microadenoma.
Fig. 9. Corticotroph 'picoadenoma' demonstrated with optimized MRI techniques.

adenomas, but unfortunately they also decrease its specificity as compared to conventional methods. Recently, Erickson et al. [9] have confirmed that 3-tesla MRI is significantly more sensitive than 1.5-tesla MRI and should become the gold standard for the evaluation of patients with ACTH-dependent Cushing's disease. Thanks to the application of 3-tesla MRI, the percentage of MRI-negative patients with Cushing's disease has fallen from 50% in the 1990s to 20%, as reported by several more recent surgical series. Erickson et al. [9] have demonstrated that the administration of corticotropin-releasing hormone during 3-tesla MRI does not improve the detection rate of microadenomas. Ikeda et al. [10] found a high accuracy of microadenoma localization at surgery using composite images from methionine positron emission tomography (MET-PET) and 3-tesla MRI, but this has not been introduced into clinical practice. Finally, it is important to recall that experienced neuroradiologists are probably more able to use optimizing-specific parameters, to recognize incidentalomas and artifacts, and to differentiate these from true ACTH-secreting microadenomas. Such a second opinion should be

obtained before requesting inferior petrosal sinus sampling in a patient with suspected ACTH-dependent Cushing's disease.

Nonfunctioning Pituitary Microadenomas
Nonfunctioning pituitary microadenomas are very rarely diagnosed. These lesions are usually not visible on thick-section CT or routine MRI examinations obtained for other reasons (e.g. head trauma, headache or sinusitis).

Pituitary Macroadenomas
Pituitary macroadenomas are reliably depicted by standard MRI investigations as space-occupying, predominantly intrasellar lesions. The issue here is not so much to demonstrate the presence of a pituitary lesion, but rather to assess the extension of the tumor and, if possible, its consistency and vascularization, and to characterize its nature. Analysis of their volume change over time – either by segmentation and contouring or by a rough approximation using geometric models – is a critical factor for treatment decisions [9]. In every case, a follow-up MRI should be precision engi-

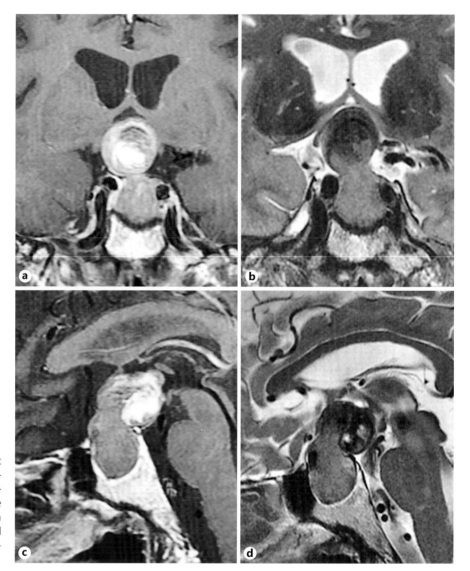

Fig. 10. So-called 'snowman' hemorrhagic pituitary macroadenoma with hyperintensity of the upper part of the tumor on the T1-weighted image and hypointensity on the T2-weighted image. **a, b** Postgadolinium coronal T1- and T2-weighted images. **c, d** Postgadolinium sagittal T1- and T2-weighted images.

neered, i.e. obtained strictly with the same acquisition parameters and the same anatomical landmarks as the previous studies.

Pituitary Nonfunctioning Macroadenomas
Pituitary nonfunctioning macroadenomas are predominantly localized within an enlarged sella turcica. They often also present with extrasellar extension, upwards into the suprasellar cistern, downwards into the sphenoid sinus or laterally into the cavernous sinus. The normal residual pituitary tissue is compressed and pushed laterally, towards one side, and superiorly, but never inferiorly.

Upwards extension is present in more than 70% of patients [11] with possible contact, or even compression, of the optic chiasm. The sellar diaphragm can function like a 'belt', thus giving the adenoma an hourglass shape (fig. 10). The suprasellar component of large macroadenomas is often multilobular. Hyperintensity of the optic chiasm on T2-weighted images can indicate a poor prognosis for the visual function even after quick removal of the pituitary adenoma responsible for optic pathway compression (fig. 11). After surgery, some degree of descent of the optic chiasm with a V-shaped appearance is usually observed [11, 12].

Downwards extension of pituitary nonfunctioning adenomas is more rare than in GH-secreting tumors. Special

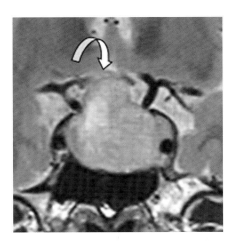

Fig. 11. Pituitary macroadenoma with suprasellar extension. T2 hyperintensity within the optic chiasm could indicate a nonrecovery of the visual field defect despite surgery.

attention has to be devoted to clival invasion, which is present in about 8% of macroadenomas, preferentially in female patients with large-volume adenomas [13]. MRI, or even better CT, demonstrates a focal or widespread defect of the more anterior, upper portion of the clivus and a decreased attenuation of the underlying trabecular bone (fig. 12). Surgical complications can be anticipated, especially if the clival invasion is not recognized preoperatively.

The signal intensity of nonfunctioning macroadenomas is usually inhomogeneous, particularly on the T2-weighted images, with disseminated areas of hyperintensities which reflect cystic or necrotic components. The posterior lobe is hyperintense in T1-weighted sequences. It is compressed, flattened and best identified in the axial noncontrast projection. Aberrant storage of antidiuretic hormone in the so-called 'ectopic posterior lobe' occurs when the pituitary stalk is severely compressed, i.e. in practice with pituitary adenomas >20 mm in height [14]. An ectopic posterior lobe may be present with smaller adenomas after hemorrhagic events or after surgery. Enlargement of an ectopic posterior lobe can occur with time, sometimes described as a 'nodule' in the opticochiasmatic cistern, particularly on CT examination.

Pierallini et al. [15] tried to evaluate preoperatively the consistency of pituitary macroadenomas using diffusion-weighted MRI and ADC maps. He found that the mean value of ADC was lower in soft macroadenomas than in firm ones. A similar study by Suzuki et al. [16] did not confirm these results. Thus, at present, a reliable prediction of the

adenoma consistency cannot be made on the basis of MRI characteristics. Magnetic resonance spectroscopy (MRS) of pituitary tumors is also globally disappointing. Insufficient representation of the tumoral tissue within the MRS voxel and poor spectral quality by contamination of the MRS voxel (e.g. by the bony structures of the sellar region) are considered the major limitations of the technique. However, in macroadenomas with large suprasellar extension, metabolic data can be obtained. Typical spectra are characterized by a significant reduction of NAA (N-acetylaspartate) peak. In functioning pituitary adenomas, MRS demonstrates an elevated choline peak which is a marker of cellular proliferation, compatible with hormonal hyperactivity [17].

Gadolinium injection enhances the normal pituitary tissue, which is located superiorly and/or laterally on one side, but never inferiorly (fig. 13). Visualization of the normal residual pituitary gland is of crucial importance for the neurosurgeon. Postgadolinium enhancement of the dura, the so-called 'dural tail', is not specific of meningiomas and has been described with large pituitary adenomas, particularly if they are hemorrhagic or soon after surgery, as well as with perisellar aneurysms [18].

Gadolinium injection offers a more clear-cut demonstration of tumoral contours by enhancing the solid portion of the adenoma, but the degree of enhancement does not reflect the vascular density. Gadolinium chelates rapidly equilibrate between the intravascular and extracellular matrix of the tumor. Sakai et al. [19] recently demonstrated that the arterial spin-labeled perfusion imaging – a noninvasive MRI technique that measures tumor blood flow using arterial water as a freely diffusing tracer – reflects the vascular density of nonfunctioning pituitary macroadenomas, which can be helpful in the prediction of perioperative hemorrhage.

Intratumoral Hemorrhage
Intratumoral hemorrhage typically occurs in pituitary adenomas and much less frequently in other types of pituitary tumors. Hemorrhage classically appears with high signal intensity on T1-weighted images, and either as an intratumoral dark mass or as a cyst with a dark rim on T2-weighted images, which indicates a hematoma or hemorrhagic cyst, respectively. Tosaka et al. [20] consider T2-weighted gradient-echo MRI the most sensitive technique for the detection of blood, in particular in hyperacute and chronic hemorrhages. They describe different patterns of dark lesions, i.e. rim, mass, spot and diffuse. The rim appearance is caused by perilesional hemosiderin. A fluid-fluid level can be apparent

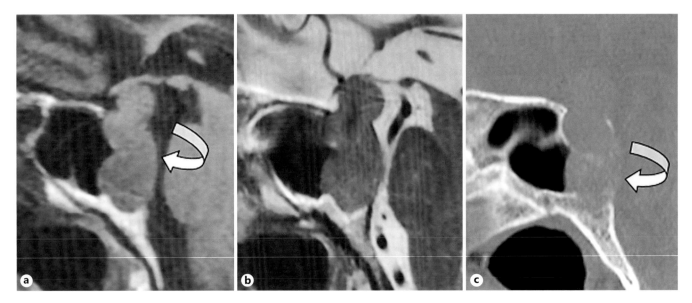

Fig. 12. Pituitary macroadenoma invading the sphenoid sinus and eroding the clivus. **a, b** Sagittal T1- and T2-weighted images. **c** Sagittal reformatted CT.

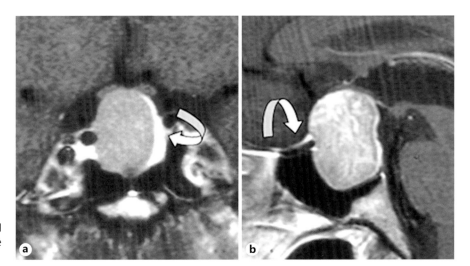

Fig. 13. Pituitary macroadenomas: lateral displacement of the normal pituitary tissue (**a**) and the dural tail (not specific; **b**).

in large chronic hematomas due to the sedimentation of de-oxyhemoglobin, methemoglobin and cellular debris (fig. 14).

Pituitary Apoplexy
The diagnosis of pituitary apoplexy is made clinically. It is usually caused by infarction or hemorrhage of a previously undiagnosed pituitary macroadenoma, typically a nonfunctioning adenoma. This clinical syndrome, characterized by sudden headache, oculomotor nerve palsy and asthenia, can mimic subarachnoid hemorrhage, stroke or meningitis. A

radiological diagnosis may be difficult in the early stage. The classical predominant hyperintensity on T1-weighted images is frequently absent because infarction or hemorrhage are still in the form of deoxyhemoglobin [21]. However, sequential MRI will demonstrate the progressive increase of T1-weighted hyperintensity, with the passage from deoxy-hemoglobin to methemoglobin. T2-weighted gradient-echo MRI can be helpful in this case, making pituitary hemorrhage appear as a 'dark mass'. Diffusion-weighted images can show increased signal intensity if compared to normal brain gray and white matter, and a low apparent diffusion

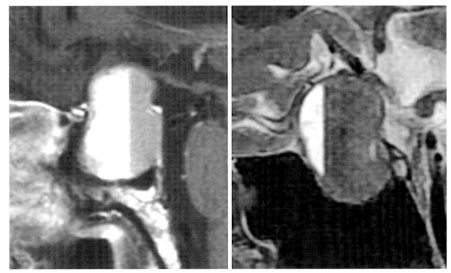

Fig. 14. Pituitary macroadenomas: the fluid-fluid level indicates an old hemorrhage.

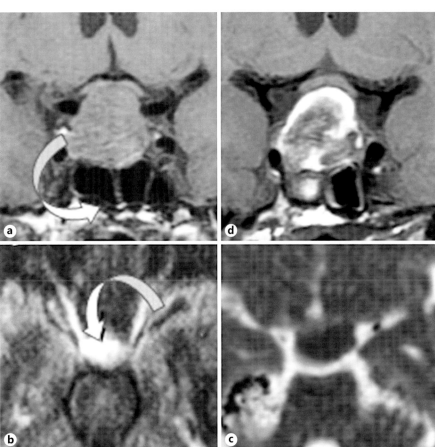

Fig. 15. Pituitary apoplexy with a sudden onset of headache 24 h before. **a** Coronal T1-weighted image: 'striated' pattern of a pituitary mass without evidence of hemorrhage. **b** Diffusion-weighted MRI: increased signal intensity (arrow) within the pituitary mass. **c** ADC map showing decreased signal intensity. **d** Coronal T1-weighted image 2 days later: peripheral T1-hyperintensity represents methemoglobin.

[21] (fig. 15). Finally, reactive thickening of the sphenoid sinus mucosa constitutes a reliable sign, present from the early stage [22]. It corresponds to a swelling of the subepithelial layer of the sphenoid sinus mucosa; it does not indicate infectious sinusitis, nor rule out the option of the transsphenoidal route for surgery. If surgery is postponed or not indicated, shrinkage of the mass usually occurs within several weeks.

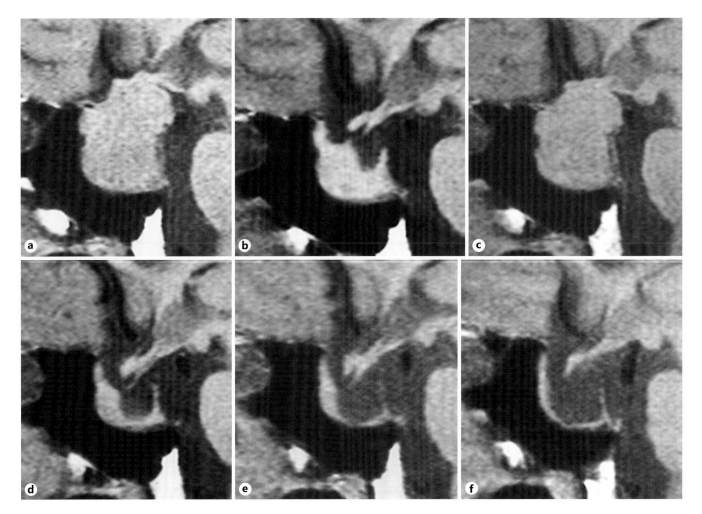

Fig. 16. a Macroprolactinoma with suprasellar extension. **b** Six weeks after dopamine agonist treatment. **c** After the patient stopped treatment. **d–f** Shrinkage of the adenoma after reinstitution of medical treatment on sequential MRIs, 2 months, 1 and 2 years later, respectively.

Prolactinomas in Men

Prolactinomas in men are most often large or very large and frequently invasive. Extension into the sphenoid sinus can be impressive and mimic a primitive sphenoid sinus tumor. Prolactin levels are usually much higher than in females and can reach hundreds of thousands mIU/l [23, 24]. Tumor shrinkage and T2-weighted hyperintensity occur very rapidly with dopamine agonist treatment (fig. 16). Shrinkage of large invasive macroprolactinomas can exceptionally lead to cerebrospinal fluid fistula [23, 24].

GH-Secreting Macroadenomas

GH-secreting pituitary macroadenomas present specific characteristics. According to personal data obtained from MRI performed in 300 acromegalic patients, two thirds of them were macroadenomas and 71% extended predominantly downwards into the sphenoid sinus (fig. 17a). Chiasmatic compression and resulting visual field defects were present in only 17% of the cases [25]. This explains in part the long delay frequently observed between the onset of symptoms and the diagnosis. An isolated inferior extension, i.e. without any extension above the sellar diaphragm level (fig. 17b), was found by Zada et al. [26] in 24% of somatotropinomas; 40% of them corresponded to atypical adenomas according to the most recent WHO classification (MIB >3%, increased p53, increased mitoses) [27]. The cause of the predominant inferior extension of GH-secreting pituitary adenomas is unknown. Several theories have been proposed:
- a change in the collagenous sellar diaphragm under the influence of GH makes an upwards extension of the

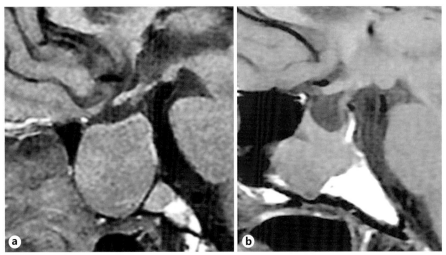

Fig. 17. GH-secreting macroadenomas: predominant inferior extension (**a**) and isolated inferior extension (**b**).

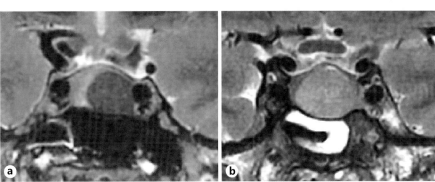

Fig. 18. Two different types of GH-secreting pituitary adenomas: T2-hypointense (**a**) and T2-hyperintense (**b**) to the normal pituitary gland.

pituitary adenoma impossible; this hypothesis is, however, unlikely, since an incompetence of the sellar diaphragm is very common;

– the posteroinferior location of GH-secreting cells within the sella could be a potential cause for microadenomas but not for large tumors;

– enlarged 'kissing internal carotid arteries' have also been suspected; however, in our MRI analysis of acromegalic patients [25], we have found only 64 out of 300 patients with dilated intracavernous carotid arteries, with no correlation to inferior extension;

– passive enlargement of the sella under the direct influence of GH; this hypothesis is also unlikely as, according to our data [25], a disproportionately large sella was only found in 42 out of 300 patients with GH-secreting adenoma, with a significant correlation to an older age at diagnosis. This suggests that this rather rare situation most likely results from a spontaneous involution of the adenoma. In our series we have found a positive correlation (p = 0.001) between the inferior extension of the adenoma and the pneumatization of the sphenoid

sinus [25]. Hyperpneumatization of the frontal sinuses, as well as of the sphenoid sinus, is believed to be related to a GH-induced bone turnover with apposition of bone along the outer surface of the sinus associated with internal resorption leading to an increased sinus cavity. We thus suspect that this phenomenon can lead to the fragilization of the sellar floor, thus enabling preferential inferior extension of GH-secreting pituitary adenomas.

The T2-weighted MRI signal appears hypointense in 52% of GH-secreting pituitary adenomas, as compared to the normal pituitary gland. Most of these T2-hypointense adenomas present a well-defined round or oval contour (fig. 18) and invade the cavernous sinus in only 29% of cases versus 58% of GH-secreting T2-hyperintense adenomas [24–26].

T2-weighted hypointense GH-secreting pituitary adenomas present are associated with significantly higher levels of IGF-I (insulin-like growth factor 1) and are suspected to be densely granulated [28]. The IRMA-2 study, aimed at assessing in a large sample of patients the association between T2-weighted MRI characteristics and response to treatment with somatostatin analogs, is ongoing.

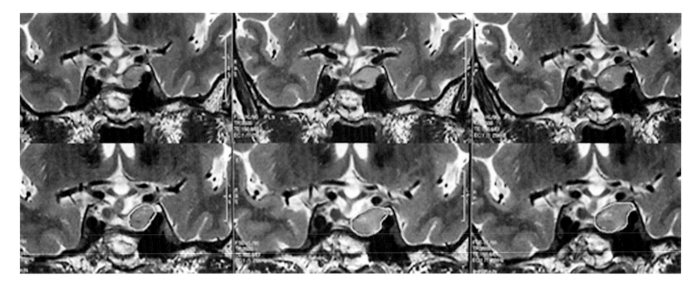

Fig. 19. Pituitary adenoma remnant. Progressive increase in size on sequential MRIs (top); note that coronal images can be strictly superimposed. Volumetric assessment (bottom).

Aggressive Pituitary Adenomas

The definition of 'aggressive' pituitary adenomas differs within medical specialties. From a radiological point of view, an aggressive pituitary adenoma presents with these characteristics [1]:

– a tumor with a rapid growth;
– a tumor extended beyond a natural barrier, or beyond the adenoma 'capsule';
– the presence of tumor metastases (pituitary carcinoma).

In the case of a pituitary adenoma with rapid growth it is strongly recommended to obtain reproducible MRI examinations in the follow-up using the same technical parameters and the same projections for coronal sequences, which can be easily obtained by tracing the subcallosal plane on the sagittal view and then orienting the coronal views perpendicularly to this plane of reference. In this way, diagnosis of recurrence of pituitary tumors can be made earlier and the speed of tumoral growth can be better assessed (fig. 19).

For pituitary adenomas with extrasellar extension, it could be difficult to differentiate true sphenoidal invasion from fair distortion of the sellar floor under the pressure of the macroadenoma. Abrupt/acute changes of the sellar floor, as well as focal tumoral extension outside the adenoma 'capsule', come out in favor of a true extrasellar invasion by the tumor [26].

Diagnosis of cavernous sinus invasion is of paramount importance, particularly with secreting pituitary adenomas. Cavernous sinus invasion, for instance, is found in more than half of T2-hyperintense GH-secreting macroadenomas hardly cured only by surgery. The diagnosis of subtle invasion remains difficult to define [29]. In our opinion, anatomical landmark assessments are of little help for the diagnosis of subtle invasion in an individual patient. Evaluation of the parasellar veins may be helpful [30]. Today, T2-weighted MRI allows, especially with thin coronal and axial T2-weighted sequences, the visualization of the thin medial dural wall of the cavernous sinus and of small tumoral herniations through the dural wall, usually located posteriorly, where the wall is thinner (fig. 20) [29]. T2-weighted images are of better quality with 3.0-tesla machines, but the dural wall of the cavernous sinus can also be seen with 1.5-tesla machines if the technical parameters are optimized. In the more aggressive lesions, tumoral tissue can extend into the temporal lobe (fig. 21).

Hyperintense T2-weighted tumors are more prone to invasion than hypointense ones. This is particularly true for GH-secreting pituitary adenomas, as previously mentioned (fig. 22). Thus, the chance of surgical or medical cure of acromegaly due to T2-weighted hyperintense GH-secreting pituitary adenomas is lower than for hypointense ones. Recently, a peculiar T2-weighted MRI pattern characterized by numerous small areas of hyperintensity has been described in silent corticotroph adenomas, the aggressiveness of which is well recognized (fig. 23) [31].

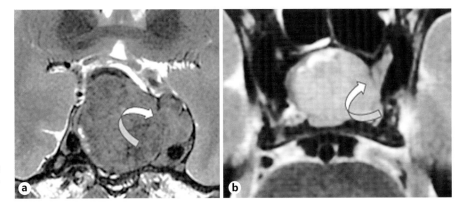

Fig. 20. Rupture of the internal wall of the cavernous sinus on T2 coronal (**a**) and T2 axial (**b**) images.

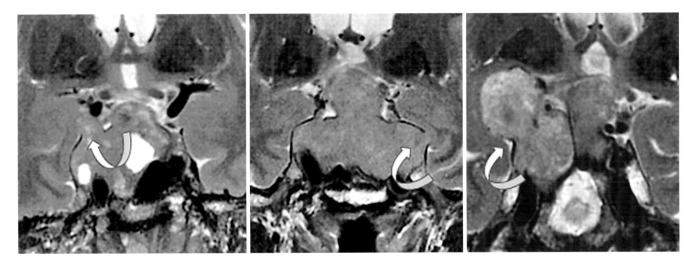

Fig. 21. Tumoral extension toward the subarachnoid space through the enlarged dural pocket of the third intracavernous nerve (arrows).

Finally, vascular density, as shown with spin-labeled perfusion MRI, could predict the possibility of tumoral hemorrhage in nonfunctioning pituitary adenomas. The imaging pattern of the rare pituitary carcinomas does not differ from that of aggressive pituitary adenomas except for the presence of metastases.

Collision Lesions of the Pituitary Region

The concomitant presence of a pituitary adenoma with a second sellar lesion is uncommon, but not exceptional. The diagnosis of an RCC combined with a pituitary adenoma can be very challenging [32]. It could be useful to remember that pituitary adenomas, even microadenomas, typically present with signs secondary to mass effect, particularly on the sellar floor, while intrasellar RCC do not.

The incidence of coexisting intracranial aneurysm and pituitary adenoma is higher than in other brain tumors (7.4 vs. 1.1%; fig. 24) [33], especially for GH-secreting adenomas, possibly because of the effect exerted by chronic excessive IGF-I levels on cerebral vascular walls. A useful recommendation could be to systematically add an MRI angiography of the circle of Willis in the check-up of acromegalic patients.

The Postoperative Sella

Secretions, blood or packing materials frequently keep the postsurgical tumor cavity from collapsing in the days or weeks following transsphenoidal adenomectomy. This situation can make early MRI quite similar to the preoperative pattern [34, 35]. For this reason, early postoperative MRI control is usually not obtained in the majority of pituitary

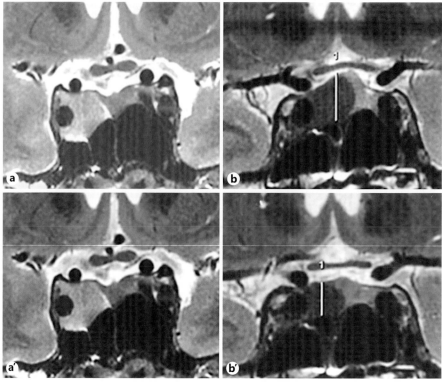

Fig. 22. GH-secreting pituitary adenomas before (**a**, **b**) and after somatostatin analogs (**a′**, **b′**). Only the T2-hypointense adenoma (**b**, **b′**) shrank.

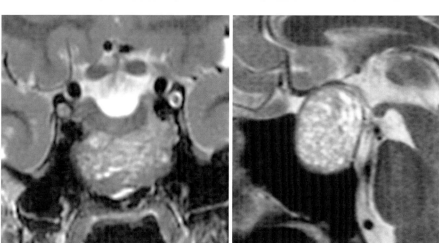

Fig. 23. Silent corticotroph adenomas: microcystic pattern in T2-weighted images in 2 cases.

centers. On the contrary, we strongly advocate MRI of the pituitary region before the discharge of the patient from hospital on day 3 or 4 postsurgery. This investigation checks for potential complications and may visualize a tumoral remnant, even if packing material has been placed into the sella (fig. 25). Blood, secretions and packing involute over the following months with the exception of fat grafts, which remain visible for years. The possibility of an increase in volume of such a fat graft in a patient together with a gain of weight has

recently been described [34, 35]. After involution of the postoperative sellar content, a tumoral remnant can be seen, particularly with large nonsecreting macroadenomas or with those invading the cavernous sinus. Remodeling of the residual anterior pituitary is observed on one side, with its T1-weighted signal remaining identical to that of cerebral white matter. The pituitary stalk is tilted towards the normal gland. The adenoma remnant signal is the same as before surgery, most of the time hyperintense on the T2-weighted MRI. Af-

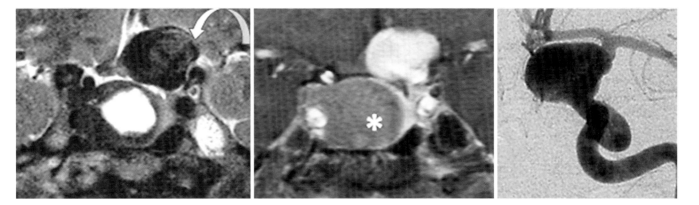

Fig. 24. Collision lesions: intrasellar degenerated GH-secreting adenoma (*) and supraclinoid internal carotid artery aneurysm (arrow).

Fig. 25. Surgical packing. **a** Typical pattern of Gelfoam occupying the surgical bed 3 days after adenomectomy; intrasellar remnant (arrow). **b** Fat fragment with chemical shift artifact on the right side of the sella.

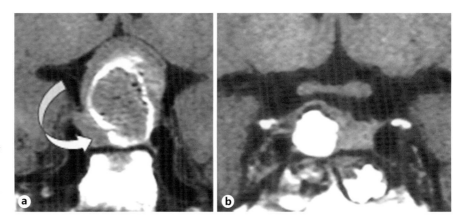

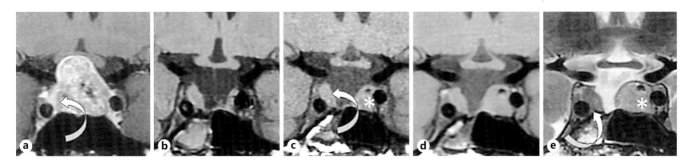

Fig. 26. Pituitary adenoma recurrence. **a** Initial presentation after gadolinium injection; the normal pituitary gland is compressed laterally (arrow). **b–d** Sequential T1-weighted MRI: remodeling of the normal pituitary, the volume of which is unchanged with time (arrow). A pituitary remnant (*) increases in size regularly. **e** T2-weighted image: clear signal differentiation of the normal pituitary and adenoma remnant.

ter gadolinium injection, enhancement of the normal pituitary tissue is more pronounced than that of the adenoma remnant. Pituitary adenoma recurrence – in fact increase in the volume of an adenoma remnant – is demonstrated much earlier when MRI follow-up examinations are obtained strictly with the same anatomical projections (fig. 26).

If the neurosurgeon has removed the sphenoid sinus mucosa before transsphenoidal adenomectomy – to avoid the

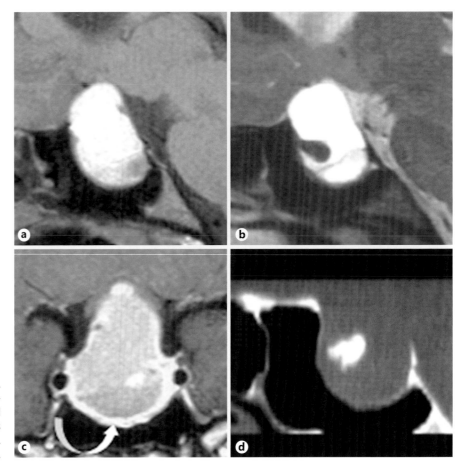

Fig. 27. Adamantinous craniopharyngioma. The cystic component is hyperintense on T1-weighted images (**a**) and on T2-weighted images (**b**). **c** The pituitary gland (arrow) is displaced inferiorly against the sellar floor. **d** Calcification is better demonstrated on CT.

formation of a sphenoidal mucocele – fatty changes of cortical bone occur, as demonstrated by the T1-weighted hyperintensity of the wall of the sphenoid sinus [34, 35].

Differential Diagnosis of Sellar Space-Occupying Lesions

Craniopharyngiomas
Diagnosis of the classic adamantinous type of craniopharyngiomas, usually occurring in childhood or adolescence, is easy when the tumor presents with three components: solid, cystic and calcified portions which occupy the suprasellar cistern. The cystic component is usually, but not always, hyperintense on T1- and T2-weighted images (fig. 27). The demonstration of calcifications can be difficult with MRI; if any doubt exists, CT is indicated [36].

The papillary type of craniopharyngiomas is found in adult patients. These lesions often occupy the third ventri-

cle, are solid, noncalcified and enhance uniformly after gadolinium injection.

Peritumoral edema spreading along the optic tracts was first described as specific on T2-weighted MRI and useful for distinguishing craniopharyngiomas from other tumors of the sellar region (fig. 28). More recently, Saeki et al. [37] observed such edema changes in pituitary region tumors other than craniopharyngiomas. He postulated that optic tract edema is related to the distension of Virchow-Robin spaces, which represent a drainage route of interstitial fluid into the subarachnoid space, their outlet into the subarachnoid spaces being blocked by a pituitary region tumor.

Rathke's Cleft Cysts
RCC represent the most frequent lesion of the sellar region and are probably the source of the greatest number of radiological misreadings. The number of papers dealing with them has exploded since the advent of MRI, while these cysts were underdiagnosed previously, probably because most of

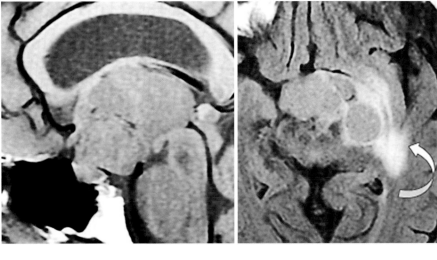

Fig. 28. Papillary craniopharyngioma: the lesion occupies the third ventricle with peritumoral edema along the optic tract on axial view (arrow).

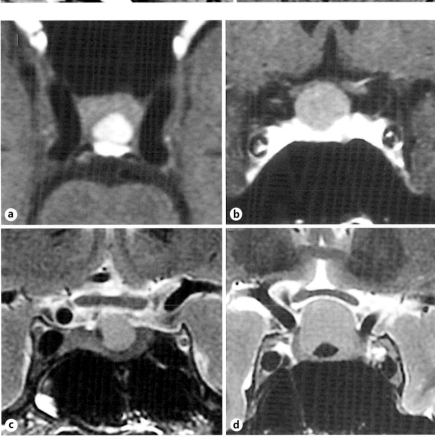

Fig. 29. RCC. **a** An axial T1-weighted image ideally separates the RCC from the posterior pituitary. **b** RCC appears as an egg in an egg cup without enhancement after gadolinium injection. **c, d** RCC on coronal T2-weighted images with hyperproteinic T2 hypointense nodules.

them are small, isodense on CT and asymptomatic. In fact, two main types of RCC, primarily intrasellar or suprasellar, can be described. However, they both can have an intra- as well as suprasellar location, and appear in duplicate or can even be ectopic (i.e. located within the pituitary stalk). The coexistence with a pituitary adenoma is not exceptional [38].

Most intrasellar RCC are small, asymptomatic and hyperintense on T1-weighted MRI images, so they are often mistaken with hemorrhagic microadenomas or the posterior pituitary. Diagnosis is very easy with a nonenhanced axial T1 fat-saturated sequence – the RCC, quite often hyperintense on T1-weighted images, is located on the mid-

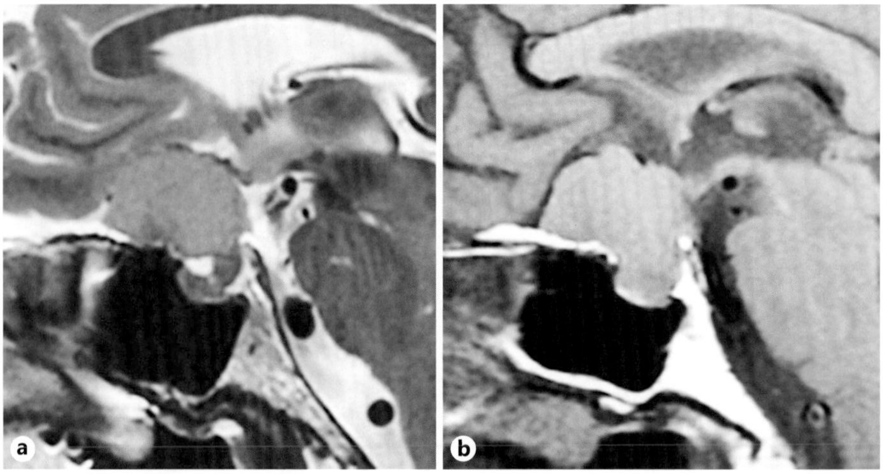

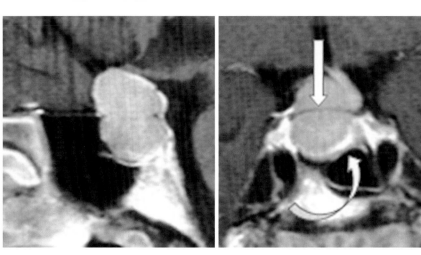

Fig. 30. Meningioma of the planum sphenoidale. **a** Visualization of a CSF cleft between the pituitary gland and meningioma on a T2-weighted image. **b** Osteoma of the planum on a T1-weighted image. The sella is not enlarged.

Fig. 31. Meningioma of the sellar diaphragm (arrow). Sagittal and coronal T1-weighted images after contrast. The pituitary gland is pushed inferiorly against the sellar floor (curved arrow).

line, between the anterior and posterior pituitary lobes. Its anterior surface is regularly convex, while its posterior surface is straight and clearly separated from the hyperintense posterior lobe by a thin T1-hypointense interface (fig. 29) [38].

Suprasellar RCC may become symptomatic if large enough to compress the optic chiasm, the pituitary stalk or the anterior pituitary gland, or be complicated. They can have a mucoid content, appearing hyperintense in T1-weighted images, or a serous content, harboring an MRI signal identical to that of the cerebrospinal fluid. Their signal can change spontaneously according to the protein concentration [38].

Their evolution is unpredictable. T2 hyperproteinic intracystic nodules floating in a T1-hyperintense intra- or suprasellar lesion are pathognomonic. The thin wall of RCC is made of a single layer of ciliated and mucus-secreting cells and typi-

cally does not enhance after gadolinium injection [38]. RCC may also become symptomatic through a complication such as hemorrhage, infection or rupture. Clinical symptoms are frequently severe with a brutal onset of headaches evoking aseptic meningitis associated with hypopituitarism symptoms. In these circumstances, postgadolinium enhancement of the thickened cyst wall may indicate local inflammation and simulate a craniopharyngioma. Diagnosis is here frequently delayed. Some so-called 'autoimmune hypophysitis' could be related to the rupture of RCC. Rapid changes in the volume or MRI signal of the cyst have to be considered as they can be observed after a cyst's puncture [38].

Meningiomas
Most meningiomas of the perisellar region arise from an osteoma, such as the meningiomas of the planum sphenoidale or of the anterior clinoid process. They are then easily diag-

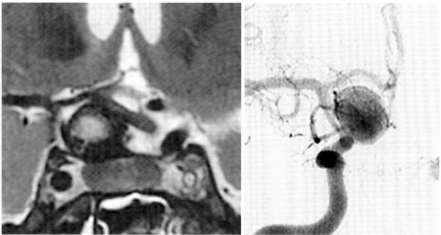

Fig. 32. Internal carotid artery aneurysm lying on the pituitary gland and threatening the optic chiasm.

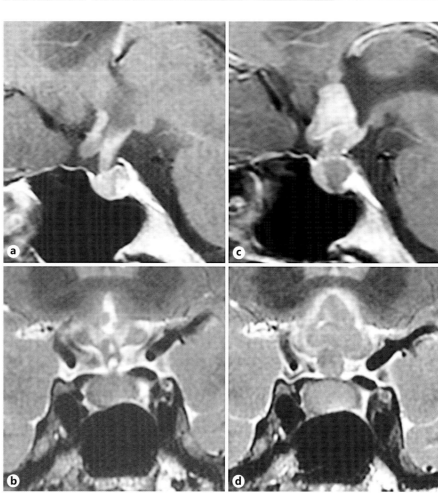

Fig. 33. Germinoma: isolated diabetes insipidus. **a**, **b** Initial MRI: thickened pituitary stalk and optic chiasm. **c**, **d** MRI follow-up 6 months later: presence of a hypothalamic mass; enlarged and heterogeneous pituitary content.

nosed although they are frequently isointense or, in T2-weighted images, slightly hyperintense to the pituitary gland. They are sometimes separated from the pituitary gland by a cerebrospinal fluid cleft (fig. 30). Homogeneous enhancement is observed after contrast medium injection. The so-called 'dural tail' is not completely specific. Meningiomas of the cavernous sinus can sometimes be misread as pituitary adenomas invading the cavernous sinus. Encase-

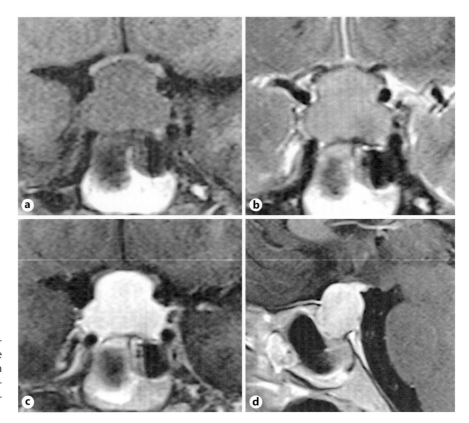

Fig. 34. Lymphocytic hypophysitis: intra- and suprasellar mass lesions. **a** Hypointense on T1-weighted imaging. **b** Hyperintense on T2-weighted imaging. **c, d** Strong enhancement after gadolinium injection with thickening of the surrounding dura mater.

ment of the internal carotid artery and narrowing of its lumen are in favor of the diagnosis of meningioma. Meningiomas of the sellar diaphragm lack a bone attachment and can be mistaken for a pituitary macroadenoma with a poor-quality examination. Dynamic MRI usually demonstrates an earlier enhancement of the meningioma if compared with the inferiorly displaced pituitary gland (fig. 31) [39].

Perisellar Aneurysms
Aneurysms of the sellar region arise mainly from the intracavernous or supraclinoid internal carotid artery (fig. 32). When nonthrombosed, they exhibit a hypointense signal on T1 and T2 related to the 'signal void' created by the rapidly flowing blood. Diagnosis of perisellar aneurysms can be less obvious in cases of complete or partial thrombosis [39].

Germinomas
Germinomas are suprasellar in location. They develop from the pituitary stalk and the hypothalamus towards the third ventricle, rarely from the optic chiasm (fig. 33). Extension to the sella can be observed. In some cases, the presence of a second localization of the tumor in the pineal region

makes the diagnosis easier. Diabetes insipidus is common: the absence of vasopressin storage is best evaluated on axial T1-weighted fat-saturated images. Germinomas appear iso- or hypointense on T1-weighted images and hyperintense on T2-weighted images. Contrast enhancement is usually intense after gadolinium injection. Evaluation of the complete craniospinal axis is mandatory to assess potential CSF (craniospinal fluid) tumor spread. Shrinkage of the mass is classically observed quickly after radiotherapy [39].

Hypophysitis
Adenohypophysitis
Lymphocytic hypophysitis is the most common type of hypophysitis. The characteristic imaging patterns are symmetric enlargement of the pituitary gland, an iso- or slightly hypointense signal on T1-weighted images, an iso- or slightly hyperintense signal on T2-weighted images, and a very pronounced enhancement after gadolinium injection (fig. 34). A 'tongue-like' enhancement along the pituitary stalk is frequently observed. Enhancement of the pituitary content is delayed on dynamic imaging as compared to the enhance-

ment pattern of a normal anterior pituitary gland. A peripheral dark rim, hypointense on T2-weighted images, consistent with fibrosis, can be noted as a sequel of the inflammatory tissue changes [40].

Infundibuloneurohypophysitis

Findings usually associated with central diabetes insipidus are encountered in neurohypophysis, i.e. a lack of T1 hyperintensity of the posterior lobe. Axial T1-weighted fat-saturated sequences are much more reliable than sagittal sequences to ascertain the absence of vasopressin storage. Thickening of the infundibulum is constant in the early phase of the disease. Measurement of the pituitary stalk does not help, but loss of its normal shape (i.e. the superior third being larger than the rest) has to be considered with suspicion. A somewhat tubular shape of the pituitary stalk is seen. In the majority of cases, after some months, the infundibulum becomes thin or even thread-like with a concomitant decrease in size of the anterior lobe [40].

References

1 Bonneville JF, Bonneville F, Cattin F: Magnetic resonance imaging of pituitary adenomas. Eur Radiol 2005;15:543–548.
2 Dietemann JL, Bonneville JF, Cattin F, Poulignot D: Computed tomography of the sellar spine. Neuroradiology 1983;24:173–174.
3 Sarwar KN, Huda MS, van de Velde V, Hopkins L, Luck S, Preston R, Powrie JK: The prevalence and natural history of pituitary hemorrhage in prolactinoma. J Clin Endocrinol Metab 2013;98:2362–2367.
4 Raverot G, Wierinckx A, Dantony E, Auger C, Chapas G, Villeneouve L, Brue T, Figarella-Branger D, Roy P, Jouanneau E, Jan M, Lachuer J, Trouillas HJ; Members of HYPOPRONOS: Prognostic factors in prolactin pituitary tumors: clinica, histological, and molecular data from a series of 94 patients with a long post-operative follow-up. J Clin Endocrinol Metab 2010;95:1708–1716.
5 Bonneville JF: When the pituitary swells up a little. J Radiol 2002;83:319–320.
6 Domingue ME, Devuyst F, Alexopoulou O, Corvilain B, Maiter D: Outcome of prolactinoma after pregnancy and lactation: a study on 73 patients. Clin Endocrinol 2014;80:642–648.
7 Sun Y, Sun Q, Fan C, Shen J, Zhao W, Su T, Ning G, Bian L: Diagnosis and therapy for Cushing's disease with negative dynamic MRI finding. Clin Endocrinol 2012;76:868–876.
8 Bonneville JF, Cattin F, Bonneville F, Schillo F, Jacquet G: Pituitary gland imaging in Cushing's disease. Neurochirurgie 2002;48:173–185.
9 Erickson D, Erickson B, Watson R: 3 Tesla MRI with and without corticotropin realeasing hormone stimulation for the detection of microadenomas in Cushing's syndrome. Clin Endocrinol 2010;72:793–799.
10 Ikeda H, Abe T, Watanabe K: Usefulness of composite methionine-positron emission tomography/3.0-tesla magnetic resonance imaging to detect the localization and extent of early-stage Cushing adenoma. J Neurosurg 2010;112:750–755.

11 Egger J, Kapur T, Nimsky C, Kikinis R: Pituitary adenoma volumetry with 3D slicer. PLoS One 2012;7:e51788.
12 Hagiwara A, Inoue Y, Wakasa K, Haba T, Tashiro T, Myamoto T: Comparison of GH-producing and non-GH producing pituitary adenomas: imaging characteristics and pathologic correlation. Radiology 2003;228:523–528.
13 Chen X, Dai J, Ai L, Ru X, Wang J, Li S, Young GS: Clival invasion on multidetector CT in 390 pituitary macroadenomas: correlation with sex, subtype and rates of operative complications and recurrence. AJNR Am J Neuroradiol 2011;32:785–789.
14 Bonneville F, Narboux Y, Cattin F, Rodiere E, Jacquet G, Bonneville JF: Preoperative location of the pituitary bright spot in patients with pituitary adenomas. AJNR Am J Neuroradiol 2002;23:528–532.
15 Pierallini A, Caramia F, Falcone C, Tinelli E, Ciddio AB, Bianco F, Ferrante L, Bozzao L: Pituitary macroadenomas preoperative evaluation of consistency with diffusion-weighted MR imaging. Radiology 2006;239:223–231.
16 Suzuki C, Maeda M, Hori K, Kozuka Y, Sakuma H, Taki W, Takeda K: Apparent diffusion coefficient of pituitary macroadenoma evaluated with line-scan diffusion-weighted imaging. J Neuroradiol 2007;34:228–235.
17 Stadlbauer A, Buchfelder M, Nimsky C, Saeger W, Salomonowitz, E, Pinker K, Richter G, Akutsu H, Ganslandt O: Proton magnetic resonance spectroscopy in pituitary macroadenomas: preliminary results. J. Neurosurg 2008;109:306–312.
18 Cattin F, Bonneville F, Andrea I, Barrali E, Bonneville JF: Dural enhancement in pituitary macroadenomas. AJNR Am J Neuroradiol 2002;23:528–532.
19 Sakai N, Koizumi S, Yamashita S, Takehara Y, Sakahara H, Baba S, Oki Y, Hiramatsu H, Namba H: Arterial spin-labeled perfusion imaging reflects vascular density in nonfunctioning pituitary macroadenomas. AJNR Am J Neuroradiol 2013;24:2139–2143.

20 Tosaka M, Sato N, Hirato J, Fujimaki H, Yamaguchi R, Kohga H, Hashimoto K, Yamada M, Mori M, Saito M, Yoshimoto Y: Assessment of hemorrhage in pituitary macroadenomas by T2*- weighted gradient-echo MR imaging. AJNR Am J Neuroradiol 2007;28:2023–2029.
21 Rogg JM, Tung GA, Anderson G, Cortez S: Pituitary apoplexia: early detection with diffusion-weighted MR imaging. AJNR Am J Neuroradiol 2002;23:1240–1245.
22 Liu JK, Couldwell WT: Pituitary apoplexia in the magnetic resonance imaging era: clinical significance of sphenoid mucosa thickening: J Neurosurg 2006;104:892–898.
23 Kreutz J, Vroonen L, Cattin F, Petrossians P, Thiry A, Rostomyan L, Tshibanda L, Beckers A, Bonneville JF: Intensity of prolactinoma on T2-weighted magnetic resonance imaging: toward another gender difference. Neuroradiology 2015;57:679–684.
24 Kurosaki M, Kambe A, Watanabe T, Fujii S, Ogawa T: Serial 3 T magnetic resonance imaging during cabergoline treatment of macroprolactinomas. Neurol Res 2015;37:341–346.
25 Potorac I, Petrossians P, Schillo F, Ben slama C, Nagi S, Sahnoun M, Brue T, Chanson P, Nasser G, Caron P, Bonneville F, Raverot G, Lapras V, Coton F, Delemer B, Higel B, Boulin A, Gaillard S, Goichot B, Dietemann JL, Kreutz J, Tshibanda L, Beckers A, Bonneville JF: Correlations significatives de l'aspect en IRM haute resolution des adénomes hypophysaires à GH avant traitement. Ann Endocrinol 2013;74:259–260.
26 Zada G, Lin N, Laws ER: Patterns of extrasellar extension in growth hormone-secreting and nonfunctional pituitary macroadenomas. Neurosurg Focus 2010;29:E4.
27 Louis DN, Ohgaki H, Wiestler OD, Cavenee WK, Burger PC, Jouvet A, Scheithauer BW, Kleihues P: The 2007 WHO classification of tumours of the central nervous system. Acta Neuropathol 2007;114:97–109.

28 Fougner SL, Casar-Borota O, Heck A, Berg JP, Bollerslev J: Adenoma granulation pattern correlates with clinical variables and effect of somatostatin analogue treatment in a large series of patients with acromegaly. Clin Endocrinol 2012; 76:96–102.

29 Cao L, Chen H, Hong J, Ma M, Zhong Q, Wang S: Magnetic resonance imaging appearance of the medial wall of the cavernous sinus for the assessment of cavernous sinus invasion by pituitary adenomas. J Neuroradiol 2013;40:245–251.

30 Bonneville JF, Cattin F, Tang YS: Radioanatomy of the laterosellar veins: value of computerized tomography. J Neuroradiol 1991;18:240–249.

31 Cazabat L, Dupuy M, Boulin A, Bernier M, Baussart B, Foubert L, Raffin-Sanson ML, Caron P, Bertherat J, Gaillard S: Silent but not unseen: multicystic aspect on T2-weighted MRI in silent corticotroph adenomas. Clin Endocrinol 2014;81: 566–572.

32 Noh SJ, Ahn JY, Lee KS, Kim SH: Pituitary adenoma and concomitant Rathke's cleft cyst. Acta Neurochir 2007;149:1223–1228.

33 Weir B: Pituitary tumors and aneurysms: case report and review of literature. Neurosurgery 1992;30:585:591.

34 Parrott J, Mullins ME: Postoperative imaging of the pituitary gland. Top Magn Reson Imaging 2005;16:317–323.

35 Ciric I, Fahrat H: The early versus late magnetic resonance imaging debate. World Neurosurg 2015;83:471–472.

36 Zada G, Lin N, Ojerholm E, Ramkissoon S, Laws ER: Craniopharyngioma and other cystic epithelial lesions of the sellar region: a review of clinical, imaging and histopathological relationships. Neurosurg Focus 2010;28:E4.

37 Saeki N, Uchino Y, Murai H, Kubota M, Isobe K, Uno T, Sunami K, Yamamaura A: MR imaging study of edema-like change along the optic tract in patients with pituitary region tumors. AJNR Am J Neuroradiol 2003:24;336–342.

38 Bonneville F, Cattin F, Bonneville JF, Jacquet G, Viennet G, Dormont D, Chiras J: Rathke's cleft cyst (in French). J Neuroradiol 2003;30:238–248.

39 Abele TA, Yetkin ZF, Raisanen JM, Mickey BE, Mendelsohn DB: Non-pituitary origin sellar tumours mimicking pituitary macroadenomas. Clin Radiol 2012;67:821–827.

40 Gutenberg A, Larsen J, Lupi I, Rohde V, Caturegli P: A radiological score to distinguish autoimmune hypophysitis from nonsecreting pituitary adenoma preoperatively. AJNR Am J Neuroradiol 2009; 30:1766–1772.

41 Köpf-Maier P: Wolf-Heidegger's Atlas of Human Anatomy, ed 6. Basel, Karger, 2005.

Jean-François Bonneville, MD
Service d'Endocrinologie
Centre Hospitalier Universitaire de Liège
Sart Tilman, B.35, BE-4000 Liège 1 (Belgium)
E-Mail bonnevillejf@gmail.com

Buchfelder M, Guaraldi F (eds): Imaging in Endocrine Disorders.
Front Horm Res. Basel, Karger, 2016, vol 45, pp 121–132 (DOI: 10.1159/000442328)

Intraoperative Magnetic Resonance Imaging for Pituitary Adenomas

Michael Buchfelder · Sven-Martin Schlaffer

Department of Neurosurgery, University of Erlangen-Nürnberg, Erlangen, Germany

Abstract

Surgery for pituitary adenomas attempts the optimally possible amount of tumor resection, which ideally is total excision. However, there are limitations in the resectability and in the intraoperative assessment of the radicality of an adenomectomy. Postoperative imaging is usually performed with a few months delay after tumor resection. Intraoperative magnetic resonance imaging (MRI) is used to depict the extent of tumor removal already achieved in the operating theater during surgery. To date, there are different low- and high-field intraoperative MRI systems available. Decompression of optic pathways, preservation of the pituitary and residual tumor can be largely predicted from the intraoperative images. Several studies convincingly show that intraoperative depiction of residual tumor allows targeted attack of the remnant. Not only is the amount of tumor resected increased, but also the percentage of total tumor excisions. Intraoperative MRI provides an immediate feedback to the surgeon and is thus a valuable quality control for pituitary surgery. It also allows the acquisition of data sets for precise intraoperative navigation. However, the MRI scanners are heavy and expensive and some systems even require extensive modification of the operating theater. Imaging slightly prolongs the operation but is not associated with an increased complication rate. There are also potential artifacts which must be considered.   © 2016 S. Karger AG, Basel

The radicality of tumor resection during pituitary tumor operations is intraoperatively estimated by the surgeon and depends on his or her ability to differentiate normal and pathological tissues and the complexity of the individual anatomy. As a rough estimate from the normalization of hormone secretion in secreting adenomas which are acknowledged as sensitive parameters, to date some 50–70% of pituitary macroadenomas can be resected completely [1, 2]. Especially in large and irregular adenomas, it is sometimes very difficult to assess how much of the entire tumor mass has been removed. Moreover, many adenomas are not completely resectable, even in very experienced hands, due to their giant size, extremely asymmetrical shape or invasive growth. Transsphenoidal surgery became safer when Hardy introduced the operating microscope for better visualization and the X-ray for orientation [3]. Fluoroscopy is still the most frequently used intraoperative imaging tool worldwide. However, it allows only the depiction of nonradiolucent instruments against the skull base. Several other intraoperative visualization tools have been assessed for clinical usefulness, such as cisternography, computed tomography, ultrasonography and color Doppler systems [4]. For neuronavigation, preoperative data sets referenced to the patient's head via fiducials were traditionally used and over time, at least partially, replaced fluoroscopy [2, 5]. Soon after magnetic resonance imaging (MRI) was introduced it became the standard diagnostic tool for both, pre- and postoperative imaging of pituitary tumors for its superior soft tissue contrast, the free orientation of slices and avoidance of ionizing radiation [6]. The idea of intraoperative MRI to objectively document the amount of tissue resection already achieved during the surgery of brain tumors with a low-field-strength system arose in Boston in 1994 [7–9]. Since then an increasing number of neurosurgical departments all over the world have integrated MRI systems into their operating rooms. Some have more recently evolved by upgrading low intra- to high-field MRI systems [10–12] or a high-field into an ultra-high-field system [13, 14]. The authors have used a 1.5-tesla Magnetom Sonata Maestro Class scanner (Siemens AG Medical Solutions, Erlangen, Germany) in a single room concept with a rotating surgical table since 2002 [11, 15]. They had previously gained initial experience with a low-field system which was in operation between 1996 and 2001 [10, 12]. Presently, there are many different intraoperative MRI systems available. They not only differ in the strength of the magnetic field, which directly determines the image quality, but also in constructional setup. The magnet strength ranges from 0.2 to 3 T. Most intraoperative high-field MRI scanners to date are 1.5 T and magnetic fields of or below 0.5 T are usually referred to as low-field systems. Since the estimation of the amount of tumor tissue removed in pituitary macroadenomas by the surgeon is highly subjective, documentation of the reality is to date obtained by postoperative MRI. The interpretation of early images might be difficult due to several artifacts resulting from the surgery. There might be hematoma or packing material visible within the resection cavity for some days postoperatively. Doubts then arise as to how efficacious the surgery was [6, 16]. Although the literature is somewhat controversial, a delayed postoperative MRI a few months after the intervention is recommended by most experts [2, 4, 6]. In nonfunctioning tumors there are no reliable biochemical parameters which could indicate a persisting tumor. In contrast, in secreting adenomas a residual hormonal excess is generally accepted as evidence of incomplete tumor resection. It has been questioned whether MRI follow-up is at all required if the remission of oversecretion is achieved [1]. However, visible residual tumor is usually equated with persistence of the endocrine disorder. Direct intraoperative depiction of this residual tumor portion offers the chance to extend or even complete tumor resection. Most of the currently available data were obtained during transsphenoidal operations. In neurosurgery, patient positioning is considered crucial. Owing to the limited diameter of the bore of the MRI scanners, it is generally not possible to use the semi-sitting positioning in pituitary surgery with intraoperative imaging. One also has to take into account that a large or very obese patient might just fit into an MRI scanner for diagnostic imaging, but may not when positioned for surgery, being draped and equipped with the necessary aesthetic lines and tubes. For imaging during transsphenoidal surgery a flexible MR head coil may be placed so that the head can be moved during surgery. Alternatively, the head can be fixed in a head holder with an integrated coil, especially when neuronavigation is utilized.

Scanners and Setups

The first dedicated MRI scanner within an operating theater was used in 1994 by Black and his coworkers [7] in Boston. It was called the 'double doughnut' since the surgeon stood between the 2 vertical magnets (0.5 T; General Electric Medical Systems) and although real-time imaging was possible, a major limitation of the system was the narrow space available for the surgical procedure. The Magnetic Resonance Imaging System used in Toronto resembled the Boston machine, but had a sliding tray on which the patient was shifted between the large vertical magnets [17]. 'Twin-room' concepts were developed in 1996 at the University Hospitals in Erlangen and Heidelberg, respectively, with an open intraoperative low-field MRI scanner (0.2 T; Magnetom Open, Siemens AG Medical Solutions). The patients were transported on air-cushioned trays so that technically unrestricted surgery could be performed in a standard shielded operating theater. The mean scanning time was 15 min [12, 18]. The low-field images allowed the proper documentation of the decompression of the optic chiasm and correlated reasonably with delayed postoperative standard 1.5-tesla MR images. Long-term follow-up data are now available for several patients (fig. 1). The implementation of a navigation system-compatible microscope within the fringe field of this MRI scanner [10] allowed the acquisition and processing of planning MR in the anesthetized patient to guide the surgical procedure and even to update navigation utilizing intraoperative MRI data. A similar system with an identical 0.2-tesla magnet but including a tiltable surgical table was described by Lewin et al. [19]. They required a mean time of 15.4 min for

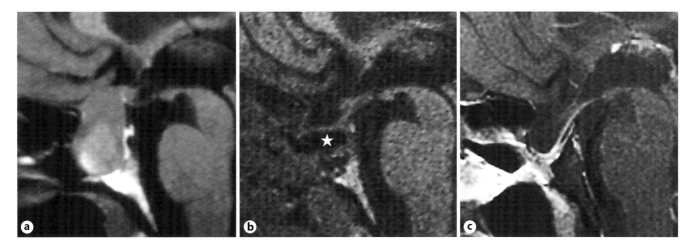

Fig. 1. Sagittal sections of preoperative 1.5-tesla (**a**) and intraoperative (**b**) low-field imaging (0.2 T) with some bone wax (☆) at the level of the sellar floor after tumor resection in a 34-year-old woman with a nonfunctioning pituitary adenoma. The most recent follow-up study with standard high-field (1.5 T) imaging (**c**) presents the long-term result 10 years after the operation, comparable to **b**.

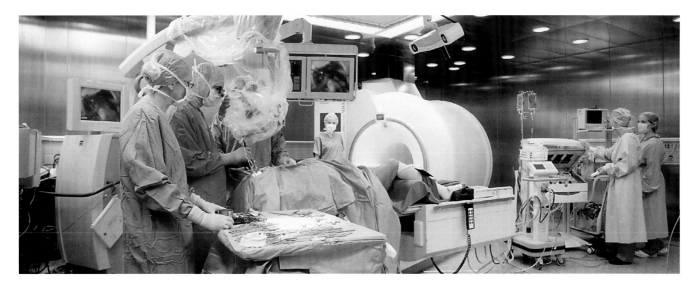

Fig. 2. The operating theater at the Neurosurgical Department in Erlangen with an integrated 1.5-tesla Siemens Magnetom MRI as it is used for transsphenoidal surgery with the head of the patient positioned outside the 5 Gauss line.

their intraoperative work and 11 min for postoperative imaging sessions. Darakchiev et al. [20] used a standard 0.3-tesla magnet and also a tilting table. There are several studies describing the use of the Pole Star N10 or N20 Medtronic systems in which the navigation tools are integrated (0.12 and 0.15 T, respectively) for assessing the extent of pituitary tumor operations [9, 18, 21–32]. A ceiling-mounted, mobile 1.5-tesla system was developed by IMRIS in 1997. It moves the magnet over the head of the patient,

who remains static [33]. One set of coronal and axial images added 20–30 min to the operative procedure. The system used in Erlangen was called the 'brain suite' [11]. It consists of a 1.5-tesla MRI scanner, is equipped with a rotating operating table and located in a radiofrequency-shielded operating theater (fig. 2). With a navigated microscope placed outside the 5 Gauss line and a ceiling-mounted navigation system, it allows for microscope-based neuronavigation in which the patient moves. Draping the patient and rotating the operating table for scanning takes some 2 min (see online suppl. video 1; for all online suppl. material, see www.karger.com/doi/10.1159/000442328). Principally, the MRI scanner can either be installed within the operation room or in a room adjacent to the theater ('twin room concept'). In the first option the use of normal surgical instruments is only possible when the surgical field is outside of the 5 Gauss line. Operations within a stronger magnetic field require nonmagnetic (e.g. titanium) instruments. The high-field system improved workflow, image quality and efficiency considerably in comparison to the low-field system in the same department [10]. More recently, even a few 3-tesla scanners have been installed in some operating theaters [13, 14, 34, 35]. However, the more heavy scanners and the even higher field strength of these magnets required new constructions or substantial modifications of existing operating rooms. The number of images acquired depends on the information needed for surgery. Both T1- and T2-weighted sequences can be used to determine tumor extension. Unfortunately, on T1-weighted images without contrast one cannot distinguish between blood and residual tumor. Thus, contrast medium is frequently used in patients when T1 images are acquired. T2 sequences, on the other hand, have proven to be the most accurate and quickly acquired images with which to identify not only all anatomical landmarks, critical structures and cystic components, but also to allow the distinguishing of residual adenoma from hematoma within the resection cavity. Prior to surgery, sagittal and coronal images are usually acquired, ideally in thin slices throughout the entire tumor. Intraoperatively, an identical data set is obtained when the surgeon believes that all the tumor tissue has been resected or the most radical resection possible has been achieved, if total resection is deemed impossible. To minimize the artifacts on the images, proper hemostasis must be secured and as little material as possible should be left in the resection cavity. Whenever a residual tumor is suspected, targeted dissection can be performed during the same operation. Visualization of residual tumor, unfortunately, cannot be equated with its resectability. This is a major limitation of the system.

Results of Low-Field Studies

In 1998, Steinmeier et al. [12] published a series of 18 transsphenoidal resections of 15 nonfunctioning pituitary adenomas and three craniopharyngiomas with intraoperative low-field (0.2 T) MRI scanning. They were able to extend the resection to complete in 3 out of 6 patients in whom residual tumor was identified. Moreover, Fahlbusch et al. [36] subsequently demonstrated that intraoperative low-field images compared favorably to delayed postoperative standard imaging. They stressed that the interpretation of intraoperative images requires experience. They resected additional tumor in 34% of their 44 patients, which increased the rate of total excision from 43 to 70% in these patients. In addition, they described the predilection sites for residual tumor. Likewise, Gerlach et al. [28] compared the intraoperative low-field images with standard postoperative 1.5-tesla images 3 months after surgery. An increase of the total resection rate of 38% resulted, as based on the assessment of intraoperative low-field images. A critical image analysis comparing the intraoperative images with delayed postoperative routine 1.5-tesla MRI, however, decreased the number of total resections to 12 out of 40, indicating that in low-field images small tumor residuals might not necessarily be ideally depicted. Ahn et al. [21] analyzed their 63 patients in two different groups. In 51 cases a complete transsphenoidal resection seemed to be possible, whereas 12 showed such an invasive growth that a complete resection was technically impossible. In the group of completely resectable tumors, the intraoperative MRI depicted residual tumor in 25%. They could thus increase the rate of complete resections from 75 to 94% and used gadolinium-coated paddies to better delineate the resection cavity [31]. Wu et al. [37] compared low-field intraoperative images to standard postoperative high-field 1.5-tesla MRI obtained within 72 h postoperatively. They revealed more residual tumor when the tumors had more pronounced parasellar extension. Also, intraoperative imaging led to an increase of the overall complete resection rate from 42 to 84%. Bellut et al. [24] not only compared intra- with standard postoperative images, but also with biochemical remission in acromegalic patients. Again, the complete resection rate dropped from 38 to 32 out of 39 when the postoperative images where critically analyzed. Baumann et al. [23] resected 3 of 5 giant adenomas. Whereas most of the available data derive from microsurgical practice, Anand et al. [22] used only the endoscope as a visualization tool. They described the low resolution and the limited field of view as disadvantages of the low-field system. Low-field intraoperative MRI is certainly able to reliably detect if a decompression of the visual pathways was performed. In several studies, recovery of vision was correlated to the amount of space created [25, 29, 38] between the upper tumor surface

Table 1. Results of intraoperative low-field imaging (0.12–0.3 T) on the extent of pituitary adenoma resection: an overview of the literature

First author (city) [Ref.]	Year	Scanner used	Patients and adenomas	Suspected residual tumor on intraoperative MRI	Eligible for further resection	Complete resection on further MRI	Complete resection at end of procedure	Intraoperative MRI leading to further tumor resection
Steinmeier (Erlangen) [12]	1998	Siemens Magnetom Open 0.2 T	n = 16; macroadenomas	6 of 16 (38%)	5 of 6	3 of 5	10 + 3 of 16 (81%)	5 of 16 (31%)
Martin (Boston) [49]	1999	General Electric Signa SP open configuration 0.5 T	n = 5; macroadenomas	MRI was performed at several stages of the procedure			3 of 5 (60%)	–
Bohinski (Cincinnati) [1]	2001	Hitachi AIRIS II vertical-field open magnet 0.3 T	n = 29; macroadenomas	19 of 29 (66%)	All 19	6 of 19	10 + 6 of 29 (55%)	19 of 29 (65%)
Fahlbusch (Erlangen) [36]	2001	Siemens Magnetom Open 0.2 T	n = 44; macroadenomas	25 of 44 (57%)	15 of 25	12 of 15	19 + 12 of 44 (70%)	25 of 44 (57%)
Walker (Boston) [50]	2002	General Electric Signa SP open configuration 0.5 T	n = 23; 4 micro- and 19 macroadenomas	13 of 19 macroadenomas (68%)	All 13	7 of 13 macroadenomas	4 microadenomas (100%); 6 + 7 of 19 macroade-nomas (68%)	13 of 23 (57%)
Schwartz (New York) [48]	2006	Polestar N-10 0.12 T	n = 15; macroadenomas	3 of 15 (20%)	All 3	3 of 3	12 + 3 of 15 (100%)	3 of 15 (20%)
Ahn (Seoul) [21]	2008	Polestar N-20 0.15 T	n = 63; macroadenomas; intended complete: n = 51 intended incomplete: n = 12	Intended complete: 13 of 51 (25%)	Intended complete: all 13; intended incomplete: 6 of 12	10 of 13	38 + 10 of 51 (94%)	19 of 63 (30%)
Gerlach (Frankfurt) [28]	2008	Polestar N-20 0.15 T	n = 40; macroadenomas	26 of 40 (65%)	7 of 26	1 of 7	14 + 1 of 40 (38%)	7 of 40 (18%)
Wu (Singapore) [37]	2009	Polestar N-20 0.15 T	n = 55; macroadenomas Hardy II: n = 26 Hardy III: n = 20 Hardy IV: n = 9	23 of 55 (42%) Hardy II: 5/26 (19%) Hardy III: 9/20 (45%) Hardy IV: 9/9 (100%)	23 of 55	14 of 23 Hardy II: 4/5 Hardy III: 6/9 Hardy IV: 4/9	32 + 14 of 55 (84%) Hardy II: 25/26 (96%) Hardy III: 17/20 (85%) Hardy IV: 4/9 (44%)	23 of 55 (42%)
Baumann (St. Gallen) [23]	2010	Polestar N-20 0.15 T	n = 6; giant adenomas	MRI was performed at several stages of the procedure			3 of 5 (60%)	
Bellut (Zurich) [24]	2010	Polestar N-20 0.15 T	n = 37; micro- and macroadenomas with acromegaly (39 operations)	8 of 39 (21%)	All 8	7 of 8	38 of 39 (97%)	8 of 39 (21%)
Theodosopoulos (Cincinnati) [47]	2010	Hitachi AIRIS II vertical-field open magnet 0.3 T	n = 27; macroadenomas	9 of 27 (33%)	4 of 9	1 of 4	18 + 1 of 27 (70%)	4 of 27 (15%)
Berkmann (Aarau) [25]	2012	Polestar N-20 0.15 T	n = 60; macroadenomas	23 of 60 (38%)	20 of 23	13 of 20	37 + 13 of 60 (83%)	20 of 60 (33%)
Tabakow (Wroclaw) [32]	2012	Polestar N-20 0.15 T	18 adenomas; Hardy I: n = 3 Hardy II: n = 7 Hardy III: n = 4 Hardy IV: n = 4	10 of 18 (56%) Hardy I: 1/3 (33%) Hardy II: 2/7 (29%) Hardy III: 3/4 (75%) Hardy IV: 4/4 (100%)	All 10	4 of 10 Hardy I: 1/1 Hardy II: 1/2 Hardy III: 2/3 Hardy IV: 0/4	12 of 18 (67%) Hardy I: 3/3 Hardy II: 6/7 Hardy III: 3/4 Hardy IV: 0/4	10 of 18 (56%)
Kim (Seoul) [31]	2013	Polestar N-20 0.15 T	n = 198; macroadenomas	46 of 198 (23%)	37 of 46	28 of 46	152 + 28 of 198 (91%)	37 of 198 (19%)
Hlavica (Zurich) [29]	2013	Polestar N-20 0.15 T	n = 104; 91 macro- and 13 giant adenomas	46 of 104 (46%)	43 of 46	37 of 43	56 + 37 of 104 (89%)	43 of 104 (41%)

and the lower margin of the chiasm. If intraoperative imaging is performed immediately after tumor resection, artifacts, such as space-occupying lesions, which are seen on imaging a few days after surgery, can be avoided. If there is a hematoma depicted, this can be evacuated during the surgical procedure, just like residual tumor. Table 1 provides an overview on the currently published results with pituitary tumors and intraoperative MRI. In all of these series, intraoperative imaging led to further resection of residual tumor in a substantial proportion of patients, and to a considerable increase in the overall complete resection rate. Several authors consider the poor depiction of parasellar structures and small tumors as the major weakness of low-field systems. There was some prolongation of the operation, but no increased complication rate. Low-field imaging in craniopharyngioma surgery, where a substantial proportion of the operations were transcranial procedures, was found to be less beneficial [39].

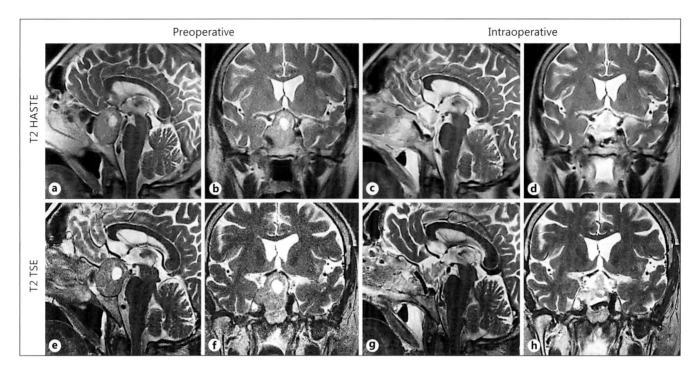

Preoperative | **Intraoperative**

T2 HASTE — a, b, c, d

T2 TSE — e, f, g, h

Fig. 3. The different image quality of intraoperative T2-weighted HASTE-sequences (upper row; acquisition time ~25 s each) in comparison to T2-weighted TSE-sequences (lower row; acquisition time ~3:50 s each) pre- (**a–d**) and intraoperatively (**e–h**) showing some residual subfrontal tumor in a 56-year-old patient with a nonfunctioning 'giant' pituitary adenoma.

Results of High-Field Studies

High-field systems are able to depict the tumor and the surrounding anatomical structures in better detail, with a higher resolution within a shorter time of data acquisition. In 2001, Dort and Sutherland [40] published a small series of 15 patients with pituitary macroadenomas and intraoperative high-field MRI. Just as in the low-field series, intraoperative MRI depicted some residual tumor in 60% of the patients and led to a further resection in 8. Consequently, the complete resection rate increased from 40 to 93%. Fahlbusch et al. [15] described 23 selected patients with acromegaly, in which the complete resection of the adenoma, as determined by intraoperative MRI, increased from 56 to 77%. Since biochemical parameters are more sensitive than imaging remission of growth hormone and IGF-1 secretion, respectively, remission was only achieved in 44% of those 18 patients in whom the tumor was completely resected. None of the patients in whom residual tumor was visible achieved remission. In a large series of 129 nonfunctioning pituitary macroadenomas, 103 were deemed completely resectable [41]. Intraoperative imaging increased the rate of complete resections from 66 to 90% in this cohort, in which the decision to operate the patient with the support of intraoperative imaging already represented a negative selection [15, 41]. Only a few of the patients were operated on in the MRI suite, namely those with tumors of reduced likelihood of total resection. Berkmann et al. [42] found that many residual tumors, as depicted by intraoperative MRI, appear smaller a few months postoperatively. Microadenomas, in which the surgical success rate is generally favorable, were excluded from most, but not all [43, 44], MR series. The quality of images clearly depends on the sequences used and, thus, also the time for image acquisition. Some information is already available after less than a minute. Higher resolution requires a longer scanning time and causes more delay with the procedure (fig. 3). The major advantage of higher field strength is also that the parasellar space can be readily assessed. Thus, residual tumor, once detected, can be attacked in a targeted fashion and mostly be reduced in its magnitude. In some patients, such an extended more radical resection has been shown to be associated with a favorable long-term outcome (fig. 4). Similarly, Meng et al. [45] increased their total resection rate in a series from Beijing. There are several reports

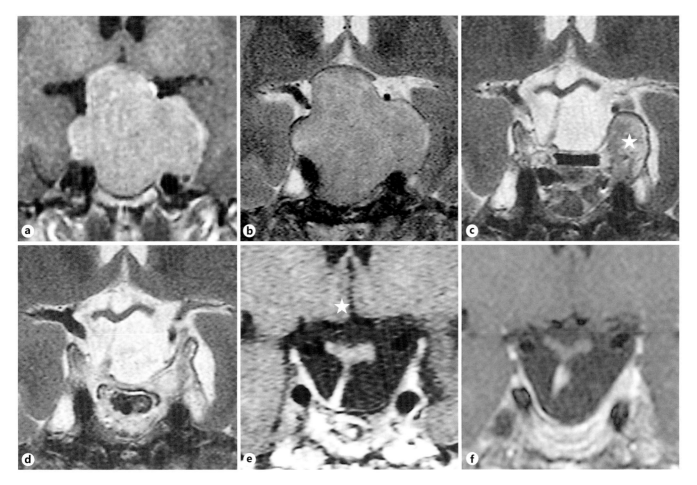

Fig. 4. A large intra- and parasellar pituitary macroadenoma in preoperative T1- (**a**) and T2-weighted (**b**) TSE MRI in a 39-year-old patient. The first intraoperative image (1.5 T, T2, TSE) with some residual tumor (☆; **c**), which was further resected (**d**). Delayed postoperative images were obtained 3 months (**e**) and 5 years (**f**) after transsphenoidal surgery. They revealed almost an identical result as the last postresection intraoperative image (**d**).

already available with 3-tesla scanners documenting an increase of total resection of pituitary adenomas, ranging from 11 [46] to 61% [43]. An overview of the currently published results of pituitary tumor surgery and intraoperative high-field MRI is given in table 2.

Use of Neuronavigation

Intraoperative imaging can also be used for navigation in that a marker is positioned and visualized when scanning is performed. If a normal anatomy is present there are anatomical landmarks like the vomer or the ostium of the sphenoid sinus which might be sufficient to guide a safe approach to the sella, even without intraoperative fluoroscopy.

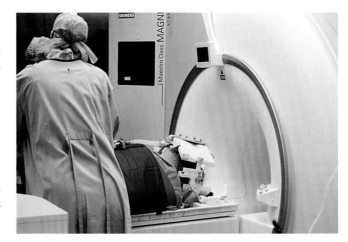

Fig. 5. Patient positioning with the head fixed in a head coil for intraoperative image acquisition and neuronavigation planning.

Table 2. Results of intraoperative high-field imaging (1.5–3.0 T) on the extent of pituitary adenoma resection: an overview of the literature

First author (city) [Ref.]	Year	Scanner used	Patients and adenomas	Suspected residual tumor on first intraoperative MRI	Eligible for further resection	Complete resection on further MRI	Complete resection at end of procedure	Intraoperative MRI leading to further tumor resection
Dort (Calgary) [40]	2001	Magnex Scientific IMRIS 1.5 T	n = 15; macroadenoma	9 of 15 (60%)	All 9	8 of 9	6 + 8 of 15 (93%)	9 of 15 (60%)
Hall (Minnesota) [51]	2005	Philips Gyroscan ACS-NT 1.5 T	n = 77; macroadenomas	–	–	–	–	–
Fahlbusch (Erlangen) [15]	2005	Siemens Magnetom Sonata Maestro 1.5 T	n = 23; macroadenomas with acromegaly; intended complete: n = 18; intended incomplete: n = 5	Intended complete: 8 of 18 (44%)	Intended complete: 5 of 8	Intended complete: 4 of 5	10 + 4 of 18 (77%); biochemical remission: 6 + 2 of 18 (44%)	5 of 23 (21%)
Nimsky (Erlangen) [10]	2005	Siemens Magnetom Sonata Maestro 1.5 T	n = 129; macroadenomas; intended complete: n = 103; intended incomplete: n = 26	Intended complete: 35 of 103 (34%)	Intended complete: all 35; intended incomplete: 12 of 26	Intended complete: 28 of 35	65 + 28 of 103 (90%)	35 + 12 of 129 (36%)
Jankovski (Brussels) [34]	2008	Philips Achieva 3 T	n = 3; macroadenomas	1 of 3 (33%)	–	–	2 of 3 (67%)	–
Pamir (Istanbul) [14]	2011	Siemens Magnetom Trio 3 T	n = 42; macroadenomas; intended complete: n = 29 intended incomplete: n = 13	Intended complete: 9 of 29 (31%)	Intended complete: 7 of 9; intended incomplete: 3 of 13	Intended complete: 4 of 7	20 + 4 of 29 (82%)	10 of 42 (24%)
Meng (Beijing) [45]	2011	1.5 T	n = 30; macroadenomas	12 of 30 (40%)	10 of 12	8 of 10	18 + 8 of 30 (87%)	12 of 30 (40%)
Lang (Calgary) [46]	2011	Siemens Magnetom Verio IMRIS 3 T	n = 9; macroadenomas	1 of 9 (11%)	1 of 1	1 of 1	8 + 1 of 9 (100%)	1 of 9 (11%)
Netuka (Prague) [43]	2011	Signa HDx General Electric 3 T	n = 86 (including 10 microadenomas); intended complete: n = 49; intended incomplete: n = 37	Intended complete: 15 of 49 (31%)	Intended complete: 13 of 15; intended incomplete: 18 of 37	Intended complete: 11 of 13	34 + 11 of 49 (92%)	21 of 86 (24%)
Szerlip (New York) [52]	2011	Siemens Magnetom Espree 1.5 T	n = 53 (49 macroadenomas); intended complete: n = 49; intended incomplete: n = 4	Intended complete: 29 of 49 (59%)	Intended complete: 28 of 29; intended incomplete: 3 of 3	Intended complete: 13 of 29	20 + 13 of 49 (67%)	29 of 53 (55%)
Qiu (Shanghai) [35]	2012	Siemens Magnetom Verio IMRIS 3 T	49 adenomas	11 of 49 (22%)	All 11	4 of 11	38 + 4 of 49 (86%)	11 of 49 (22%)
Paterno (Hannover) [53]	2014	Siemens Magnetom Espree 1.5 T	n = 72; macroadenomas; intended complete: n = 49; intended incomplete: n = 23	Intended complete: 26 of 49 (53%)	Intended complete: 23 of 23 intended incomplete: 3	Intended complete: 23 of 23	26 + 23 of 49 (100%) plus 4 of 23 of intended incomplete; 53 of 72 (74%) in total	26 of 72 (36%)
Sylvester (St. Louis) [54]	2014	Siemens Magnetom Espree IMRIS 1.5 T	n = 156; macroadenomas	112 of 156 (72%)	56 of 112	7 of 56	44 + 7 (33%)	56 of 156 (35%)
Coburger (Ulm) [55]	2014	Siemens Magnetom 1.5 T	n = 76; intended complete: n = 44		Not quoted		40 of 44 (91%) at 6-month follow-up	Not quoted
Berkmann (Erlangen) [56]	2014	Siemens Magnetom Sonata Maestro 1.5 T	n = 85; macroadenomas (with long-term follow-up)	52 of 85 (56%)	40 of 48	19 of 48	37 + 19 of 85 (65%); complete resection after follow-up (5.6 ± 1.9 years): 51 of 85 (60%)	40 of 85 (47%)

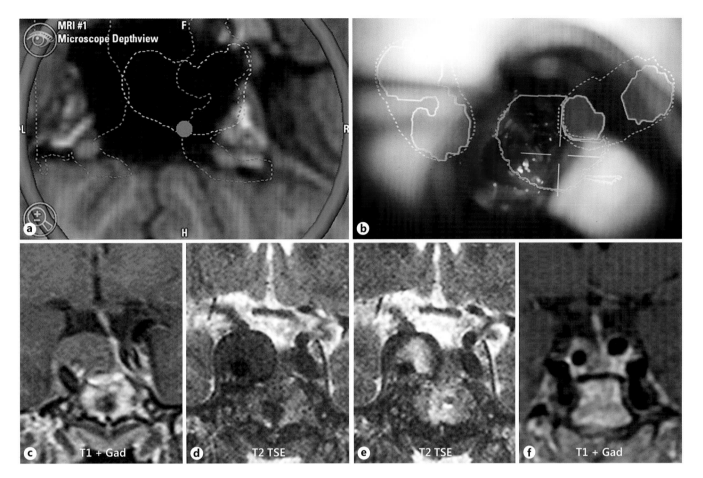

Fig. 6. Persistent and progressive parasellar pituitary adenoma in a 23-year-old male patient with difficult-to-treat acromegaly. Tumor progression occurred under combined medical therapy somatostatin analogs and the GH-receptor antagonist. The data set of intraoperative navigation planning MRI (**a**) provides crucial information to the surgeon, such as tumor volume (yellow) which can be manually segmented and visualized. **b** The view of the surgeon through the operating microscope with the superimposed structures of the carotid arteries (blue) and tumor confines (yellow). A preoperative coronal MRI section reveals the tumor (**c**) with some extension into the opticochiasmatic cistern. The task of the operation was to increase the space between the upper tumor surface and the lower margins of the optic chiasm to facilitate radiosurgery. Intraoperative images show hemorrhagic transformation and minor size reduction (**d**), while delayed postoperative standard MRI documents an even more pronounced shrinkage of the lesion (same patient as suppl. video 2).

Endoscopic surgeons usually do not use fluoroscopy for routine cases. However, in all instances of distortion of the normal anatomy due to previous operations or in patients with a poor pneumatization of the sphenoid sinus, one may appreciate using neuronavigation. Moreover, it can be used for teaching or training the transsphenoidal approach. The head of the patient usually needs to be fixed. In an intraoperative MRI unit, fiducials may be put on the patient's head or the referencing system can be integrated into the head coil (fig. 5) prior to image acquisition. It is the surgeon's choice depending on which structures he or she finds useful for navigation. Some just ask for the ideal trajectory to the tumor, whereas others prefer to also visualize tumor margins and the carotid arteries. Even when a total resection of the lesion does not seem possible, a volume reduction can be achieved (fig. 6). The contours of the structures can today be continuously or intermittently superimposed into the microscopical view of the operative field (online suppl. video 2). Neuronavigation undoubtedly increases the comfort of the surgeon. Particularly in repeat operations with distorted anatomy or dense packing of the sphenoid sinus with various materials or anatomical variants, neuronavigation helps to reach the tumor and to avoid vascular injuries [2, 4]. However, high precision is required since misleading guidance might lead to a disaster. The endoscope itself can be integrated into the neuronavigation system for orientation within the sphenoid sinus or during the approach itself.

Intraoperative Imaging and Endoscopic Surgery

It has been questioned whether the (additional) use of the endoscope or intraoperative MRI have a more important impact on the outcome of surgery. Due to the high costs of the MRI systems, only a few investigations have been conducted to address this topic. Theodosopoulos et al. [47] used a fully endoscopic operation technique and compared their visually determined impression of excision with the results of an intraoperative 0.3-tesla MRI scan. Surgery was continued in 3 out of 27 patients since residual tumor was identified by MRI that had not been previously visualized. Jane et al. [5] commented that endoscopy accurately predicted residual tumor in 55%, but erroneously assumed gross total resection in 18% of the patients. Especially intrasellar tumor residuals may appear like normal gland and are consequently not resected, although they are visualized by the surgeon. Schwartz et al. [48] assessed 15 patients operated on with a fully endoscopic transsphenoidal approach in an ultra-low-field 0.12-tesla system. In 3 patients they detected suprasellar residuals which could then be resected. Unfortunately, in 4 other patients the intraoperative MRI mimicked blood as residual tumor, which could not be confirmed on reexploration. The inconsistency was attributed to the suboptimal resolution of the low-field images. Netuka et al. [43] also used a fully endoscopic technique in 86 transsphenoidal operations of pituitary adenomas with an intraoperative 3-tesla MRI. In 24% of the patients, tumor resection was continued after MRI and an increase of the gross total resection rate from 69 to 92% resulted. Unfortunately, this investigation was not designed as a prospective study, but their data represent to date the most important expert study to compare high-field (3 T) intraoperative MRI with the endoscopic technique.

Conclusions

Today, intraoperative MRI during surgery for pituitary adenomas is an established procedure. There is a huge variety of low- and high-field systems available. High-field systems require enormous investments, since the construction of the operating theater and shielding need to be appropriate. They provide a higher resolution of images within a shorter data acquisition time. All respective publications demonstrate a higher rate of total tumor resection and a higher amount of resected tumor in adenomas which cannot be totally excised. Clearly, the technology does not make unresectable tumors resectable. Low-field systems are cheaper, can be integrated into an existing operating room more easily and also allow the estimation of the radicality of surgery better than the subjective impression of the surgeon. Almost all systems provide an opportunity to navigate procedures on the basis of an MRI data set that is acquired in the already anesthetized patient.

References

1 Bohinski RJ, Warnick RE, Gaskill-Shipley MF, Zuccarello M, van Loveren HR, Kormos DW, Tew JM Jr: Intraoperative magnetic resonance imaging to determine the extent of resection of pituitary macroadenomas during transsphenoidal microsurgery. Neurosurgery 2001;49:1133–1143; discussion 1143–1144.

2 Buchfelder M, Schlaffer S: Surgical treatment of pituitary tumours. Best Pract Res Clin Endocrinol Metab 2009;23:677–692.

3 Hardy J, Wigser SM: Trans-sphenoidal surgery of pituitary fossa tumors with televised radiofluoroscopic control. J Neurosurg 1965;23:612–619.

4 Buchfelder M, Schlaffer SM: Intraoperative magnetic resonance imaging during surgery for pituitary adenomas: pros and cons. Endocrine 2012; 42:483–495.

5 Jane JA Jr, Thapar K, Alden TD, Laws ER Jr: Fluoroscopic frameless stereotaxy for transsphenoidal surgery. Neurosurgery 2001;48:1302–1307; discussion 1307–1308.

6 Buchfelder M, Schlaffer SM: Modern imaging of pituitary adenomas. Front Horm Res 2010;38: 109–120.

7 Black PM, Moriarty T, Alexander E 3rd, Stieg P, Woodard EJ, Gleason PL, Martin CH, Kikinis R, Schwartz RB, Jolesz FA: Development and implementation of intraoperative magnetic resonance imaging and its neurosurgical applications. Neurosurgery 1997;41:831–842; discussion 842–845.

8 Pergolizzi RS Jr, Nabavi A, Schwartz RB, Hsu L, Wong TZ, Martin C, Black PM, Jolesz FA: Intraoperative MR guidance during trans-sphenoidal pituitary resection: preliminary results. J Magn Reson Imaging 2001;13:136–141.

9 Schwartz RB, Hsu L, Wong TZ, Kacher DF, Zamani AA, Black PM, Alexander E 3rd, Stieg PE, Moriarty TM, Martin CA, Kikinis R, Jolesz FA: Intraoperative MR imaging guidance for intracranial neurosurgery: experience with the first 200 cases. Radiology 1999;211:477–488.

10 Nimsky C, Ganslandt O, Fahlbusch R: Comparing 0.2 tesla with 1.5 tesla intraoperative magnetic resonance imaging analysis of setup, workflow, and efficiency. Acad Radiol 2005;12:1065–1079.

11 Nimsky C, Ganslandt O, von Keller B, Romstock J, Fahlbusch R: Intraoperative high-field-strength MR imaging: implementation and experience in 200 patients. Radiology 2004;233:67–78.

12 Steinmeier R, Fahlbusch R, Ganslandt O, Nimsky C, Buchfelder M, Kaus M, Heigl T, Lenz G, Kuth R, Huk W: Intraoperative magnetic resonance imaging with the Magnetom Open scanner: concepts, neurosurgical indications, and procedures: a preliminary report. Neurosurgery 1998;43:739–747; discussion 747–748.

13 Benes V, Netuka D, Kramar F, Ostry S, Belsan T: Multifunctional surgical suite (MFSS) with 3.0 T iMRI: 17 months of experience. Acta Neurochir Suppl 2011;109:145–149.

14 Pamir MN: 3 T ioMRI: the Istanbul experience. Acta Neurochir Suppl 2011;109:131–137.

15 Fahlbusch R, Keller B, Ganslandt O, Kreutzer J, Nimsky C: Transsphenoidal surgery in acromegaly investigated by intraoperative high-field magnetic resonance imaging. Eur J Endocrinol 2005; 153:239–248.

16 Dina TS, Feaster SH, Laws ER Jr, Davis DO: MR of the pituitary gland postsurgery: serial MR studies following transsphenoidal resection. AJNR Am J Neuroradiol 1993;14:763–769.

17 Bernstein M, Al-Anazi AR, Kucharczyk W, Manninen P, Bronskill M, Henkelman M: Brain tumor surgery with the Toronto open magnetic resonance imaging system: preliminary results for 36 patients and analysis of advantages, disadvantages, and future prospects. Neurosurgery 2000;46: 900–907; discussion 907–909.

18 Wirtz CR, Knauth M, Staubert A, Bonsanto MM, Sartor K, Kunze S, Tronnier VM: Clinical evaluation and follow-up results for intraoperative magnetic resonance imaging in neurosurgery. Neurosurgery 2000;46:1112–1120; discussion 1120–1122.

19 Lewin JS, Nour SG, Meyers ML, Metzger AK, Maciunas RJ, Wendt M, Duerk JL, Oppelt A, Selman WR: Intraoperative MRI with a rotating, tiltable surgical table: a time use study and clinical results in 122 patients. AJR Am J Roentgenol 2007;189:1096–1103.

20 Darakchiev BJ, Tew JM Jr, Bohinski RJ, Warnick RE: Adaptation of a standard low-field (0.3-T) system to the operating room: focus on pituitary adenomas. Neurosurg Clin N Am 2005;16:155–164.

21 Ahn JY, Jung JY, Kim J, Lee KS, Kim SH: How to overcome the limitations to determine the resection margin of pituitary tumours with low-field intra-operative MRI during trans-sphenoidal surgery: usefulness of Gadolinium-soaked cotton pledgets. Acta Neurochir 2008;150:763–771; discussion 771.

22 Anand VK, Schwartz TH, Hiltzik DH, Kacker A: Endoscopic transphenoidal pituitary surgery with real-time intraoperative magnetic resonance imaging. Am J Rhinol 2006;20:401–405.

23 Baumann F, Schmid C, Bernays RL: Intraoperative magnetic resonance imaging-guided transsphenoidal surgery for giant pituitary adenomas. Neurosurg Rev 2010;33:83–90.

24 Bellut D, Hlavica M, Schmid C, Bernays RL: Intraoperative magnetic resonance imaging-assisted transsphenoidal pituitary surgery in patients with acromegaly. Neurosurg Focus 2010;29:E9.

25 Berkmann S, Fandino J, Muller B, Remonda L, Landolt H: Intraoperative MRI and endocrinological outcome of transsphenoidal surgery for nonfunctioning pituitary adenoma. Acta Neurochir 2012;154:639–647.

26 Berkmann S, Fandino J, Zosso S, Killer HE, Remonda L, Landolt H: Intraoperative magnetic resonance imaging and early prognosis for vision after transsphenoidal surgery for sellar lesions. J Neurosurg 2011;115:518–527.

27 De Witte O, Makiese O, Wikler D, Levivier M, Vandensteene A, Pandin P, Baleriaux D, Brotchi J: Transsphenoidal approach with low field MRI for pituitary adenoma. Neurochirurgie 2005;51:577–583.

28 Gerlach R, du Mesnil de Rochemont R, Gasser T, Marquardt G, Reusch J, Imoehl L, Seifert V: Feasibility of Polestar N20, an ultra-low-field intraoperative magnetic resonance imaging system in resection control of pituitary macroadenomas: lessons learned from the first 40 cases. Neurosurgery 2008;63:272–284; discussion 284–285.

29 Hlavica M, Bellut D, Lemm D, Schmid C, Bernays RL: Impact of ultra-low-field intraoperative magnetic resonance imaging on extent of resection and frequency of tumor recurrence in 104 surgically treated nonfunctioning pituitary adenomas. World Neurosurg 2013;79:99–109.

30 Hlavin ML, Lewin JS, Arafah BM, Cesar A, Clampitt M, Selman WR: Intraoperative magnetic resonance imaging for assessment of chiasmatic decompression and tumor resection during transsphenoidal pituitary surgery. Tech Neurosurg 2000;6:282–288.

31 Kim EH, Oh MC, Kim SH: Application of low-field intraoperative magnetic resonance imaging in transsphenoidal surgery for pituitary adenomas: technical points to improve the visibility of the tumor resection margin. Acta Neurochir 2013; 155:485–493.

32 Tabakow P, Czyz M, Jarmundowicz W, Lechowicz-Glogowska E: Surgical treatment of pituitary adenomas using low-field intraoperative magnetic resonance imaging. Adv Clin Exp Med 2012;21: 495–503.

33 Sutherland GR, Kaibara T, Louw D, Hoult DI, Tomanek B, Saunders J: A mobile high-field magnetic resonance system for neurosurgery. J Neurosurg 1999;91:804–813.

34 Jankovski A, Francotte F, Vaz G, Fomekong E, Duprez T, van Boven M, Docquier MA, Hermoye L, Cosnard G, Raftopoulos C: Intraoperative magnetic resonance imaging at 3-T using a dual independent operating room-magnetic resonance imaging suite: development, feasibility, safety, and preliminary experience. Neurosurgery 2008;63: 412–424; discussion 424–426.

35 Qiu TM, Yao CJ, Wu JS, Pan ZG, Zhuang DX, Xu G, Zhu FP, Lu JF, Gong X, Zhang J, Yang Z, Shi JB, Huang FP, Mao Y, Zhou LF: Clinical experience of 3T intraoperative magnetic resonance imaging integrated neurosurgical suite in Shanghai Huashan Hospital. Chin Med J 2012;125:4328–4333.

36 Fahlbusch R, Ganslandt O, Buchfelder M, Schott W, Nimsky C: Intraoperative magnetic resonance imaging during transsphenoidal surgery. J Neurosurg 2001;95:381–390.

37 Wu JS, Shou XF, Yao CJ, Wang YF, Zhuang DX, Mao Y, Li SQ, Zhou LF: Transsphenoidal pituitary macroadenomas resection guided by PoleStar N20 low-field intraoperative magnetic resonance imaging: comparison with early postoperative high-field magnetic resonance imaging. Neurosurgery 2009;65:63–70; discussion 70–71.

38 Jones J, Ruge J: Intraoperative magnetic resonance imaging in pituitary macroadenoma surgery: an assessment of visual outcome. Neurosurg Focus 2007;23:E12.

39 Nimsky C, Ganslandt O, Hofmann B, Fahlbusch R: Limited benefit of intraoperative low-field magnetic resonance imaging in craniopharyngioma surgery. Neurosurgery 2003;53:72–80; discussion 80–81.

40 Dort JC, Sutherland GR: Intraoperative magnetic resonance imaging for skull base surgery. Laryngoscope 2001;111:1570–1575.

41 Nimsky C, von Keller B, Ganslandt O, Fahlbusch R: Intraoperative high-field magnetic resonance imaging in transsphenoidal surgery of hormonally inactive pituitary macroadenomas. Neurosurgery 2006;59:105–114.

42 Berkmann S, Schlaffer S, Buchfelder M: Tumor shrinkage after transsphenoidal surgery for nonfunctioning pituitary adenoma. J Neurosurg 2013; 119:1447–1452.

43 Netuka D, Masopust V, Belsan T, Kramar F, Benes V: One year experience with 3.0 T intraoperative MRI in pituitary surgery. Acta Neurochir Suppl 2011;109:157–159.

44 Tanei T, Nagatani T, Nakahara N, Watanabe T, Nishihata T, Nielsen ML, Takebayashi S, Hirano M, Wakabayashi T: Use of high-field intraoperative magnetic resonance imaging during endoscopic transsphenoidal surgery for functioning pituitary microadenomas and small adenomas located in the intrasellar region. Neurol Med Chir 2013;53:501–510.

45 Meng XH, Xu BN, Wei SB, Zhou T, Chen XL, Yu XG, Zhou DB, Tong HY, Zhang JS, Zhao Y, Hou YZ: High-field intraoperative magnetic resonance imaging suite with neuronavigation system: implementation and preliminary experience in the pituitary adenoma operation with transsphenoidal approach. Zhonghua Wai Ke Za Zhi 2011;49: 703–706.

46 Lang MJ, Kelly JJ, Sutherland GR: A moveable 3-Tesla intraoperative magnetic resonance imaging system. Neurosurgery 2011;68:168–179.

47 Theodosopoulos PV, Leach J, Kerr RG, Zimmer LA, Denny AM, Guthikonda B, Froelich S, Tew JM: Maximizing the extent of tumor resection during transsphenoidal surgery for pituitary macroadenomas: can endoscopy replace intraoperative magnetic resonance imaging? J Neurosurg 2010;112:736–743.

48 Schwartz TH, Stieg PE, Anand VK: Endoscopic transsphenoidal pituitary surgery with intraoperative magnetic resonance imaging. Neurosurgery 2006;58(suppl 1):ONS44–ONS51.

49 Martin CH, Schwartz R, Jolesz F, Black PM: Transsphenoidal resection of pituitary adenomas in an intraoperative MRI unit. Pituitary 1999;2: 155–162.

50 Walker DG, Black PM: Use of intraoperative MRI in pituitary surgery. Operative Tech Neurosurg 2002;5:231–238.

51 Hall WA, Truwit CL: Intraoperative MR imaging. Magn Reson Imaging Clin N Am 2005;13:533–543.

52 Szerlip NJ, Zhang YC, Placantonakis DG, Goldman M, Colevas KB, Rubin DG, Kobylarz EJ, Karimi S, Girotra M, Tabar V: Transsphenoidal resection of sellar tumors using high-field intraoperative magnetic resonance imaging. Skull Base 2011; 21:223–232.

53 Paterno V, Fahlbusch R: High-field iMRI in transsphenoidal pituitary adenoma surgery with special respect to typical localization of residual tumor. Acta Neurochir 2014;156:463–474.

54 Sylvester PT, Evans JA, Zipfel GJ, Chole RA, Uppaluri R, Haughey BH, Getz AE, Silverstein J, Rich KM, Kim AH, Dacey RG, Chicoine MR: Combined high-field intraoperative magnetic resonance imaging and endoscopy increase extent of resection and progression-free survival for pituitary adenomas. Pituitary 2015;18:72–85.

55 Coburger J, Konig R, Seitz K, Bazner U, Wirtz CR, Hlavac M: Determining the utility of intraoperative magnetic resonance imaging for transsphenoidal surgery: a retrospective study. J Neurosurg 2014;120:346–356.

56 Berkmann S, Schlaffer S, Nimsky C, Fahlbusch R, Buchfelder M: Follow-up and long-term outcome of nonfunctioning pituitary adenoma operated by transsphenoidal surgery with intraoperative high-field magnetic resonance imaging. Acta Neurochir 2014;156:2233–2243.

Prof. Michael Buchfelder, MD, PhD
Department of Neurosurgery
University of Erlangen-Nürnberg
Schwabachanlage 6
DE–91054 Erlangen (Germany)
E-Mail michael.buchfelder@uk-erlangen.de

Buchfelder M, Guaraldi F (eds): Imaging in Endocrine Disorders.
Front Horm Res. Basel, Karger, 2016, vol 45, pp 133–141 (DOI: 10.1159/000442329)

Molecular Imaging of Pituitary Pathology

Wouter W. de Herder

Afdeling Endocrinologie, Erasmus Medisch Centrum, Rotterdam, The Netherlands

Abstract

The presence of large numbers and/or the high affinity of dopamine D2 and/or somatostatin receptors on pituitary adenomas may enable their visualization with radionuclide-coupled receptor agonists or antagonists. However, the role of these imaging modalities in the differential diagnosis of or therapeutic purposes for pituitary lesions is very limited. Only in very specific cases might these molecular imaging techniques become helpful. These include the differential diagnosis of pituitary lesions, ectopic production of pituitary hormones, such as adrenocorticotrophic hormone, growth hormone (GH) or their releasing hormones (corticotropin-releasing hormone and GH-releasing hormone), and the localization of metastases from pituitary carcinomas.   © 2016 S. Karger AG, Basel

A variety of neoplastic and nonneoplastic lesions can occur within the sellar and parasellar regions (table 1). Among these, pituitary adenomas are the most common. Most pituitary tumors are benign adenomas and can display variable invasiveness. Generally, pituitary carcinomas can only be diagnosed in the presence of distant metastases. Historically, adenomas with a diameter less than 10 mm are classified as microadenomas, whereas those larger than 10 mm are considered macroadenomas. Pituitary adenomas are subclassified into clinically functioning – according to the hormone secreted – and clinically nonfunctioning. Among the hormone products secreted are prolactin (PRL), growth hormone (GH), adrenocorticotrophic hormone (ACTH), thyroid-stimulating hormone (TSH), gonadotropins (luteinizing hormone and follicle-stimulating hormone) and glycoprotein hormone subunits or combinations of these products. The majority of the so-called clinically nonfunctioning pituitary adenomas (NFPAs) either secrete inappropriate amounts of pituitary hormones or inactive hormonal fragments. The differential diagnosis of pituitary tumors is currently based on clinical, endocrinological and radiological characteristics. Active hormone-secreting pituitary adenomas are easily diagnosed because of signs and symptoms related to hormonal hypersecretion. NFPAs generally do not produce specific hormonal syndromes, but often hypopituitarism results from insufficient secretion of anterior pituitary hormones. The differential diagnosis of these tumors is mainly achieved using neuroradiological studies. However, even with the use of modern imaging techniques the differential diagnosis of NFPAs may still be difficult in some cases. Imaging techniques in nuclear medicine may potentially allow further characterization of these tumors. Molecular imaging can be used for the visualization and follow-up of processes at the molecular and cellular level in the intact patient without disturbing them.

Table 1. ^{111}In-pentetreotide scintigraphy in sellar and suprasellar lesions

Scan-positive
- Meningiomas
- Class III and IV gliomas
- Metastases (neuroendocrine tumors, breast and other adenocarcinomas)
- Osteosarcomas
- Hodgkin and non-Hodgkin lymphomas
- Abscesses
- Granulomatous lesions
- Angioleiomyomas
- Chordomas
- Hemangiopericytomas

Scan-negative
- Class I and II gliomas
- Neurinomas, neurofibromas
- Epidermoids
- Ependymomas
- Plasmacytomas
- Craniopharyngiomas and other cystic lesions
- Postoperative scar tissue
- Radionecrosis

Receptor Imaging of Pituitary Tumors

Dopamine D2 receptor analogs are well-accepted medical remedies for prolactinomas and a subset of GH-secreting pituitary adenomas. The currently available long-acting octapeptide somatostatin analogs (SSAs) are used as medical therapy of patients with GH- and TSH-secreting pituitary tumors. The presence of large numbers and/or the high affinity of dopamine D2 and/or somatostatin receptors (ssts) on these and other subtypes of pituitary adenomas may enable their visualization with radionuclide-coupled receptor agonists or antagonists.

Dopamine D2 Receptor Imaging of Pituitary Adenomas

Dopamine D2 receptors have been identified on the majority of prolactinomas and on subgroups of GH-secreting and gonadotropin-secreting pituitary adenomas, or NFPAs [1–3]. In prolactinomas these receptors are the pharmacological basis for first-line medical therapy with dopamine D2 receptor agonists [2, 4]. These drugs can successfully control or normalize the pathological PRL hypersecretion and can also induce a significant reduction of tumor size with long-term tumor control [2, 4].

In the past, positron emission tomography (PET) studies using ^{11}C-labeled raclopride and N-methylspiperone were used for the in vivo assessment of D2 receptors in prolactinomas, GH-secreting pituitary adenomas and NFPAs [5–7]. D2 receptor imaging in pituitary adenomas is also feasible with single-photon emission computed tomography (SPECT) using ^{123}I-S-(–)-N-[(1-ethyl-2-pyrrolidinyl) methyl]-2-hydroxy-3-iodo-6-methoxybenzamide (^{123}I-IBZM) or [123]I-(S)-N-[(1-ethyl-2-pyrrolidinyl) methyl]-5-iodo-2,3-dimethoxybenzamide (^{123}I-epidepride) [8, 9]. ^{123}I-epidepride SPECT is generally considered to be superior to ^{123}I-IBZM SPECT (fig. 1) [8, 10].

Positive ^{123}I-IBZM SPECT uptake in the pituitary region was demonstrated in the majority of dopamine agonist-sensitive PRL-secreting macroadenomas and in less than 50% of patients with NFPAs [3, 9, 11, 12]. The pituitary tumor uptake of ^{123}I-IBZM or ^{123}I-epidepride showed a relatively poor correlation with shrinkage of the NFPA with dopamine agonist treatment [3, 11–13]. Since medical therapy with dopamine agonists is generally not considered as the first- or second-line treatment of NFPA, the role of dopamine D2 receptor imaging for therapeutic decisions in NFPA patients remains limited.

With modern MRI protocols, discrimination of NFPAs from other pathologies in the sellar region is generally easy. Clinically functioning and NFPAs may present with hyperprolactinemia as a secondary phenomenon resulting from pituitary stalk compression. The specificity of D2 receptor SPECT for the differentiation of prolactinomas from these tumors will probably be low because dopamine D2 receptors have also been demonstrated on NFPAs [3, 10]. However, D2 receptor SPECT might be of additional discriminatory merit in the differential diagnosis between pituitary and nonpituitary tumors: a positive SPECT would point to the presence of a pituitary adenoma. This technique might also be applied in the postoperative period after pituitary surgery in NFPA patients to discriminate scar tissue from NFPA recurrence or residual tumor.

Dopamine D2 Receptor Imaging of Pituitary Carcinomas

In patients with metastatic pituitary carcinomas, whole-body D2 receptor SPECT can be used to localize the metastatic lesions. In a patient with a metastatic malignant prolactinoma, ^{123}I-IBZM SPECT failed to visualize the primary

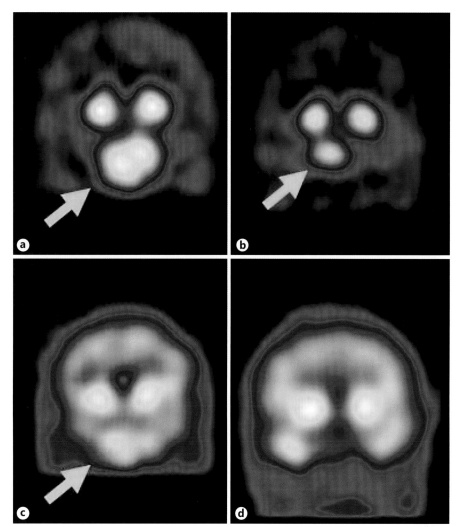

Fig. 1. Two patients with pituitary macroadenoma. ^{123}I-epidepride (**a**, **b**) and ^{123}I-IBZM (**c**, **d**) SPECT studies of the head in the coronal plane. **a**, **c** A patient with a PRL-secreting macroadenoma: uptake of ^{123}I-epidepride and of ^{123}I-IBZM in the basal ganglia and in the pituitary tumor (arrows). **b**, **d** A patient with a nonfunctioning pituitary macroadenoma: uptake of ^{123}I-epidepride and of ^{123}I-IBZM in the basal ganglia, but only uptake of ^{123}I-epidepride in the pituitary tumor (arrow).

pituitary tumor, but confirmed the presence of intracranial metastases. A partial response of this metastatic tumor to dopamine D2 receptor agonists could be demonstrated both in vivo and in vitro [14]. In patients with metastatic prolactinomas and metastatic ACTH-secreting pituitary tumors, ^{123}I-epidepride SPECT revealed previously occult bone metastases (fig. 2) [13, 15].

Somatostatin Receptor Scintigraphy of Pituitary Disorders

High numbers of specific, high-affinity ssts have been demonstrated on most neuroendocrine tumors. Five sst subtypes, named: sst_1, $sst_{2(a)}$, sst_3, sst_4 and sst_5, have been cloned.

These ssts differ with regard to their binding of natural somatostatin-14, somatostatin-28 and the currently commercially available octapeptide SSAs. Octreotide and lanreotide bind with high affinity to sst_2 and with moderate-to-low affinity to sst_3 and sst_5 [16]. The multiligand SSA pasireotide binds with high affinity to sst_1, sst_{2a}, sst_3 and sst_5. In the different pituitary tumor types, heterogeneous expression of the ssts has been found [1, 17, 18].

Until recently, sst scintigraphy (SRS) with ^{111}In-pentetreotide was almost exclusively used for the visualization of sst_2, sst_3 and sst_5. However, the nonpathologic anterior pituitary gland also takes up ^{111}In-pentetreotide [19]. Therefore, most studies have used either a visual scoring system or cut-off values were determined for an uptake index calculated from the uptake of radioactivity in the pituitary re-

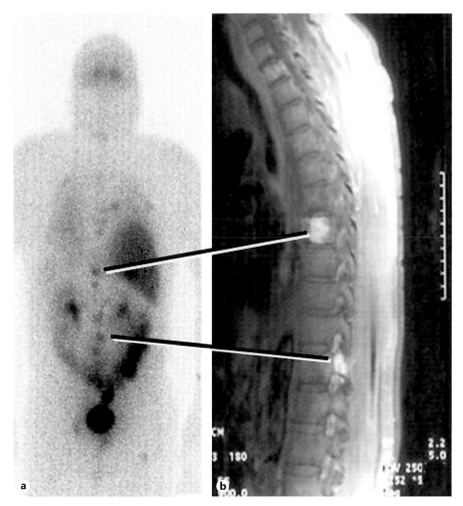

Fig. 2. A 58-year-old man with a metastatic prolactinoma. **a** Posterior planar ^{123}I-epidepride scan: normal accumulation of radioactivity in the basal ganglia, thyroid, lungs, liver, bowel and urinary bladder (but not in the pituitary area) and pathological uptake of the radiopharmaceutical in multiple thoracic (Th1, 3, 5–8, 10 and 12) and lumbar spine ($L_{1, 2, 4}$ and $_5$) sites, suggestive of metastases. **b** Sagittal T1-weighted MRI image obtained after the administration of gadolinium DTPA: hyperintensity in the body of Th6 and the left pedicle of Th10 (lines), suggestive of metastases.

gion of interest divided by the uptake in a fixed background region of interest [19].

Other radiolabeled SSAs with varying affinities for the different ssts are either still under investigation or already used in a few centers. When compared to ^{111}In-pentetreotide, ^{99m}Tc-labeled SSAs are cheaper and include ^{99m}Tc-depreotide, which preferentially binds with high affinity to $sst_{2(a)}$, sst_3, sst_5 and ^{99m}Tc-vapreotide, which preferentially binds with high affinity to $sst_{2(a)}$ and sst_5, and with lower affinity to sst_3 and sst_4. ^{111}In-DOTA-lanreotide, ^{99m}Tc-HYNIC-TOC and ^{99m}Tc-HYNIC-TATE have more or less similar sst-binding affinities as ^{111}In-pentetreotide and the comparison of imaging with these compounds has shown similar results [20, 21].

Studies in patients with GH-, PRL- and TSH-secreting pituitary tumors have shown a close association between the increased ^{111}In-pentetreotide uptake in the pituitary tu-

mor and the inhibition of the excessive tumoral hormone secretion after an acute octreotide dose [22–24] or with the effects of octreotide therapy [25]. However, other investigators could not always reproduce these findings (fig. 3) [26–28].

SRS generally does not play any role in the decision to start octapeptide SSA treatment in a patient with a GH- or TSH-secreting pituitary tumor. It might, however, play an important role in those exceptional cases where the pituitary GH hypersecretion results from stimulation by ectopically secreted GH-releasing hormone (GHRH), which is generally produced by an (occult) neuroendocrine tumor. In these patients, whole-body SRS SPECT successfully localized the source of ectopic GHRH production [29] (fig. 4). Similarly, SRS SPECT can play an important role in the detection of the source of ectopic corticotropin-releasing hormone or ACTH production [30].

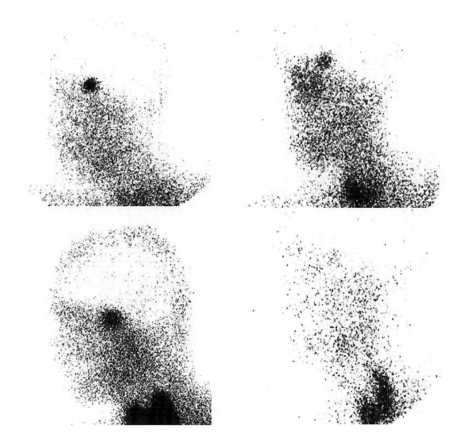

Fig. 3. Four patients with active acromegaly. ^{111}In-pentetreotide (OctreoScan®) images of the head showing variable uptake in the pituitary area that does not correlate with the size of the pituitary adenoma or with the clinical severity of the disease.

Until now, the in vivo effects of SSAs on NFPAs have also been very difficult to predict. Various studies have demonstrated positive effects of this therapy on tumor size, visual field disturbances or excessive secretion of tumor products. Like in GH-secreting adenomas, some studies in NFPAs have shown a correlation between pituitary uptake of ^{111}In-pentetreotide and: (1) the inhibition of tumor growth, (2) excessive hormonal secretion (like follicle-stimulating hormone, luteinizing hormone or glycoprotein hormone subunits in some patients) or (3) the improvement in visual field defects with SSA therapy or with peptide receptor radiotherapy using radiolabeled SSAs. Generally, negative SRS predicted the failure of SSAs to induce any kind of response in NFPAs in these studies. However, other studies also could not show any correlation between SRS positivity and tumor response in NFPAs [26, 27].

A variety of other lesions in and around the pituitary area express ssts and, therefore, can be visualized by SRS (table 1; fig. 5). Therefore, the role of SRS for the differential diagno-

sis between NFPAs and other sellar or perisellar lesions is limited.

In the last decade, PET/CT using ^{68}Ga-DOTA-labeled SSAs has been introduced for the diagnostic work-up of neuroendocrine tumors. Three different ^{68}Ga-DOTA-labeled SSAs are used in clinical practice: DOTANOC, DOTATATE and DOTATOC [31]. These compounds differ with regard to their individual affinity to the different ssts. ^{68}Ga-DOTATATE has a high affinity for $sst_{2(a)}$, ^{68}Ga-DOTATOC has a high affinity for $sst_{2(a)}$ and sst_5, and ^{68}Ga-DOTANOC is $sst_{2(a)}$, sst_3 and sst_5 specific. In neuroendocrine tumors, sst PET/CT using ^{68}Ga-DOTANOC, ^{68}Ga-DOTATATE or ^{68}Ga-DOTATOC is superior to SRS SPECT-CT, showing higher sensitivities for lesion detection (more than 90%!) particularly due to a better special resolution or better sst affinities [31]. These compounds are also more 'patient friendly' since they allow for imaging 1–3 h after intravenous injection [31]. New ^{68}Ga-DOTA-labeled SSAs for PET imaging include ^{68}Ga-DOTAVAP and ^{68}Ga-DOTALAN.

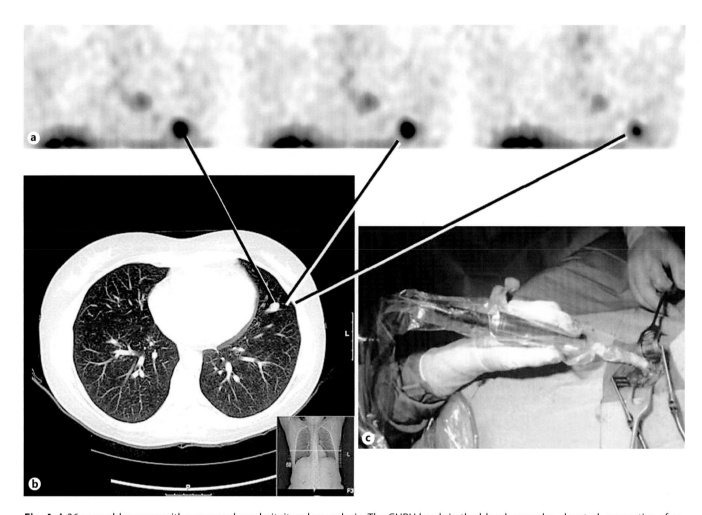

Fig. 4. A 36-year-old woman with acromegaly and pituitary hyperplasia. The GHRH levels in the blood were also elevated, suggestive of ectopic GHRH secretion and acromegaly. **a** Coronal SPECT ^{111}In-pentetreotide (OctreoScan®) images of the chest showing scan-positive pathology in the (lingula segment?) left lung and a scan-positive (mediastinal? lymph node?) lesion. **b** Transverse CT scan image showing the primary GHRH-secreting tumor in the lingula segment of the left lung. **c** Probe-guided surgery was performed after the administration of 82 MBq ^{111}In-pentetreotide. The primary lung tumor and a lymph node metastasis in the lymph node station 4L were positive. The primary tumor in the lung was localized and a segment resection was performed. A possible lymph node metastasis in the lymph node station 4L was removed together with other tumor-negative lymph nodes. Pathology showed a typical lung carcinoid (<2 mitoses per 2 mm^2) with a diameter of 0.9 cm and 1 lymph node metastasis in the lymph node station 4L. After surgery, the patient was disease free for almost 6 years.

[18]F-Fluorodeoxy-D-Glucose Positron Emission Tomography and Pituitary Pathology

[18]F-Fluorodeoxy-D-glucose (^{18}F-FDG) PET provides images based on variations in glucose metabolism between normal, nonpathologic and malignant cells and tissues. High ^{18}F-FDG uptake is usually associated with highly proliferative tumors. ^{18}F-FDG PET is rapidly becoming an integral part of routine oncology practice in most countries and this technique is generally used as an additional imaging tool next to conventional (structural) imaging, like CT and MRI.

Not surprisingly, several studies report the detection of previously occult functioning or NFPAs in patients undergoing PET for various oncological indications, like lymphoma, myeloma, non-small cell lung cancer, thyroid carcinoma and paragangliomas.

Metastases to the pituitary [32] or pituitary localizations of lymphoma [33] can also be found using ^{18}F-FDG PET, and on the other hand the technique could be used for the staging of a metastatic growth hormone-secreting pituitary carcinoma [34]. Furthermore, a case of ipilimumab-induced hypophysitis was ^{18}F-FDG PET positive [35].

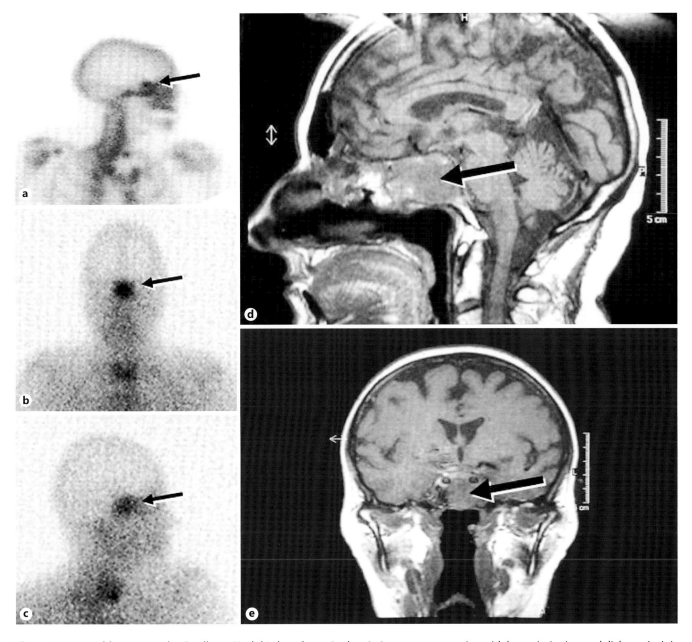

Fig. 5. A 70-year-old woman with a B cell non-Hodgkin lymphoma in the pituitary area, presenting with hypopituitarism and diabetes insipidus. **a** A ^{99m}Tc-bone scan showing uptake of the radiopharmaceutical in the bones surrounding the pituitary area. **b**, **c** ^{111}In-pentetreotide (OctreoScan®) images of the head showing uptake of the radiopharmaceutical in the pituitary area. Sagittal (**d**) and coronal (**e**) T1-weighted MRI images of the head obtained after the administration of gadolinium-DTPA showing the suprasellar lymphoma with intrasellar expansion (arrows).

In large series, ^{18}F-FDG PET positivity of the pituitary is only found in 0.007–0.2% of cases [32, 36]. The role of ^{18}F-FDG PET in patients presenting with primary pituitary tumors is limited. In a single-center study of 24 patients with pituitary lesions, ^{18}F-FDG PET was positive in the pituitary area in all patients with macroadenomas, but in only half of the patients with microadenomas and none of the patients with cystic lesions [37]. Also, in a series of 12 patients with newly diagnosed or recurrent ACTH-producing pituitary adenomas, ^{18}F-FDG PET-CT was only positive in approximately 60% and the majority of patients also had abnormal MRI readings suggestive of a pituitary adenoma. Pituitary MRI was only incidentally negative in this series [38]. It can be expected that with the improvement of modern MRI protocols for the differential diagnosis of pituitary adenomas, ^{18}F-FDG PET will continue to play a very minor role.

L-^{11}C-Methionine Positron Emission Tomography and Pituitary Pathology

L-^{11}C-methionine PET has only been used in experimental settings to study amino acid metabolism in pituitary adenomas versus other different sellar pathologies or to study the effects of drugs on these processes [39–41]. One case of a metastatic prolactinoma has also been studied [42].

Conclusions

Despite the increasing relevance of molecular imaging in oncology, its role in the differential diagnosis of pituitary lesions is limited along with its role for therapeutic purposes. Only in very specific cases might molecular imaging become helpful. These include the differential diagnosis of pituitary lesions, ectopic production of pituitary hormones or their releasing hormones, and the localization of metastases from pituitary carcinomas.

References

1 Ferone D, de Herder WW, Pivonello R, Kros JM, van Koetsveld PM, de Jong T, Minuto F, Colao A, Lamberts SW, Hofland LJ: Correlation of in vitro and in vivo somatotropic adenoma responsiveness to somatostatin analogs and dopamine agonists with immunohistochemical evaluation of somatostatin and dopamine receptors and electron microscopy. J Clin Endocrinol Metab 2008;93:1412–1417.

2 Hofland LJ, Feelders RA, de Herder WW, Lamberts SW: Pituitary tumours: The sst/D$_2$ receptors as molecular targets. Mol Cell Endocrinol 2010; 326:89–98.

3 de Herder WW, Reijs AE, Kwekkeboom DJ, Hofland LJ, Nobels FR, Oei HY Krenning EP, Lamberts SW: In vivo imaging of pituitary tumours using a radiolabelled dopamine D2 receptor radioligand. Clin Endocrinol 1996;45:755–767.

4 Colao A, Savastano S: Medical treatment of prolactinomas. Nat Rev Endocrinol 2011;7:267–278.

5 Muhr C, Bergstrom M, Lundberg PO, Bergstrom K, Hartvig P, Lundqvist H, Antoni G, Langstrom B: Dopamine receptors in pituitary adenomas: PET visualization with ^{11}C-N-methylspiperone. J Comput Assist Tomogr 1986;10:175–180.

6 Muhr C: Positron emission tomography in acromegaly and other pituitary adenoma patients. Neuroendocrinology 2006;83:205–210.

7 Lucignani G, Losa M, Moresco RM, Del Sole A, Matarrese M, Bettinardi V, Mortini P, Giovanelli M, Fazio F: Differentiation of clinically non-functioning pituitary adenomas from meningiomas and craniopharyngiomas by positron emission tomography with [^{18}F]fluoro-ethyl-spiperone. Eur J Nucl Med 1997;24:1149–1155.

8 Pirker W, Riedl M, Luger A, Czech T, Rossler K, Asenbaum S, Angelberger P, Kornhuber J, Deecke L, Podreka I, Brucke T: Dopamine D2 receptor imaging in pituitary adenomas using iodine-123-epidepride and SPECT. J Nucl Med 1996;37:1931–1937.

9 Pirker W, Brucke T, Riedl M, Clodi M, Luger A, Asenbaum S, Podreka I, Deecke L: Iodine-123-IBZM-SPECT: studies in 15 patients with pituitary tumors. J Neural Transm Gen Sect 1994; 97:235–244.

10 de Herder WW, Reijs AEM, de Swart J, Kaandorp Y, Lamberts SWJ, Krenning EP, Kwekkeboom DJ: Comparison of iodine-123 epidepride and iodine-123 IBZM for dopamine D2 receptor imaging in clinically non-functioning pituitary macroadenomas and macroprolactinomas. Eur J Nucl Med 1999;26:46–50.

11 de Herder WW, Lamberts SW: Imaging of pituitary tumours. Baillieres Clin Endocrinol Metab 1995;9:367–389.

12 Ferone D, Lastoria S, Colao A, Varrella P, Cerbone G, Acampa W, Merola B, Salvatore M, Lombardi G: Correlation of scintigraphic results using ^{123}I-methoxybenzamide with hormone levels and tumor size response to quinagolide in patients with pituitary adenomas. J Clin Endocrinol Metab 1998;83:248–252.

13 de Herder WW, Reijs AE, Feelders RA, van Aken MO, Krenning EP, Tanghe HL, van der Lely AJ, Kwekkeboom DJ: Dopamine agonist therapy of clinically non-functioning pituitary macroadenomas: is there a role for ^{123}I-epidepride dopamine D2 receptor imaging? Eur J Endocrinol 2006;155: 717–723.

14 Assies J, Verhoeff NP, Bosch DA, Hofland LJ: Intracranial dissemination of a macroprolactinoma. Clin Endocrinol 1993;38:539–546.

15 Petrossians P, de Herder W, Kwekkeboom D, Lamberigts G, Stevenaert A, Beckers A: Malignant prolactinoma discovered by D2 receptor imaging. J Clin Endocrinol Metab 2000;85:398–401.

16 Lamberts SW, van der Lely AJ, de Herder WW, Hofland LJ: Octreotide. N Engl J Med 1996;334: 246–254.

17 Gatto F, Feelders RA, van der PR, Kros JM, Waaijers M, Sprij-Mooij D, Neggers SJ, van der Lelij AJ, Minuto F, Lamberts SW, de Herder WW, Ferone D, Hofland LJ: Immunoreactivity score using an anti-sst2A receptor monoclonal antibody strongly predicts the biochemical response to adjuvant treatment with somatostatin analogs in acromegaly. J Clin Endocrinol Metab 2013;98:E66–E71.

18 Veenstra MJ, de Herder WW, Feelders RA, Hofland LJ: Targeting the somatostatin receptor in pituitary and neuroendocrine tumors. Expert Opin Ther Targets 2013;17:1329–1343.

19 Colao A, Lastoria S, Ferone D, Varrella P, Marzullo P, Pivonello R, Cerbone G, Acampa W, Salvatore M, Lombardi G: The pituitary uptake of ^{111}In-DTPA-D-Phe1-octreotide in the normal pituitary and in pituitary adenomas. J Endocrinol Invest 1999;22:176–183.

20 Cwikla JB, Mikolajczak R, Pawlak D, Buscombe JR, Nasierowska-Guttmejer A, Bator A, Maecke HR, Walecki J: Initial direct comparison of ^{99m}Tc-TOC and ^{99m}Tc-TATE in identifying sites of disease in patients with proven GEP NETs. J Nucl Med 2008;49:1060–1065.

21 Gabriel M, Muehllechner P, Decristoforo C, von Guggenberg E, Kendler D, Prommegger R, Profanter C, Moncayo R, Virgolini I: ^{99m}Tc-EDDA/HYNIC-Tyr(3)-octreotide for staging and follow-up of patients with neuroendocrine gastro-enteropancreatic tumors. Q J Nucl Med Mol Imaging 2005;49:237–244.

22 Broson-Chazot F, Houzard C, Ajzenberg C, Nocaudie M, Duet M, Mundler O, Marchandise X, Epelbaum J, Gomez De Alzaga M, Schafer J, Meyerhof W, Sassolas G, Warnet A: Somatostatin receptor imaging in somatotroph and non-functioning pituitary adenomas: correlation with hormonal and visual responses to octreotide. Clin Endocrinol 1997;47:589–598.

23 Gorges R, Cordes U, Engelbach M, Bartelt KM, Haberern G, Hey O, Beyer J, Bockisch A: Prädiktion der pharmakologischen Wirkung von Octreotid bei Akromegalie mittels ^{111}In-Pentetreotid-Szintigraphie und Berechnung eines hypophysären Uptake-Index. Nuklearmedizin 1997;36:117–124.

24 Losa M, Magnani P, Mortini P, Persani L, Acerno S, Giugni E, Songini C, Fazio F, Beck-Peccoz P, Giovanelli M: Indium-111 pentetreotide single-photon emission tomography in patients with TSH-secreting pituitary adenomas: correlation with the effect of a single administration of octreotide on serum TSH levels. Eur J Nucl Med 1997;24:728–731.

25 Boni G, Ferdeghini M, Bellina CR, Matteucci F, Castro LE, Parenti G, Canapicchi R, Bianchi R. [^{111}In-DTPA-D-Phe]-octreotide scintigraphy in functioning and non-functioning pituitary adenomas. Q J Nucl Med 1995;39:90–93.

26 Plockinger U, Reichel M, Fett U, Saeger W, Quabbe HJ: Preoperative octreotide treatment of growth hormone-secreting and clinically non-functioning pituitary macroadenomas: effect on tumor volume and lack of correlation with immunohistochemistry and somatostatin receptor scintigraphy. J Clin Endocrinol Metab 1994;79:1416–1423.

27 Plockinger U, Bader M, Hopfenmuller W, Saeger W, Quabbe HJ: Results of somatostatin receptor scintigraphy do not predict pituitary tumor volume- and hormone-response to ocreotide therapy and do not correlate with tumor histology. Eur J Endocrinol 1997;136:369–376.

28 Rieger A, Rainov NG, Elfrich C, Klaua M, Meyer H, Lautenschlager C, Burkert W, Mende T: Somatostatin receptor scintigraphy in patients with pituitary adenoma. Neurosurg Rev 1997;20:7–12.

29 van Hoek M, Hofland LJ, de Rijke YB, van Nederveen FH, de Krijger RR, van Koetsveld PM, Lamberts SW, van der Lely AJ, de Herder WW, Feelders RA: Effects of somatostatin analogs on a growth hormone-releasing hormone secreting bronchial carcinoid, in vivo and in vitro studies. J Clin Endocrinol Metab 2009;94:428–433.

30 de Herder WW, Krenning EP, Malchoff CD, Hofland LJ, Reubi JC, Kwekkeboom DJ, Oei HY, Pols HA, Bruining HA, Nobels FR, Lamberts SWJ: Somatostatin receptor scintigraphy: its value in tumor localization in patients with Cushing's syndrome caused by ectopic corticotropin or corticotropin-releasing hormone secretion. Am J Med 1994;96:305–312.

31 Sundin A: Radiological and nuclear medicine imaging of gastroenteropancreatic neuroendocrine tumours. Best Pract Res Clin Gastroenterol 2012; 26:803–818.

32 Hyun SH, Choi JY, Lee KH, Choe YS, Kim BT: Incidental focal ^{18}F-FDG uptake in the pituitary gland: clinical significance and differential diagnostic criteria. J Nucl Med 2011;52:547–550.

33 Soussan M, Wartski M, Ezra J, Glaisner S, Pecking AP, Alberini JL: Non-Hodgkin lymphoma localization in the pituitary gland: diagnosis by FDG-PET/CT. Clin Nucl Med 2008;33:111–112.

34 Ilkhchoui Y, Appelbaum DE, Pu Y: FDG-PET/CT findings of a metastatic pituitary tumor. Cancer Imaging 2010;10:114–116.

35 van der Hiel B, Blank CU, Haanen JB, Stokkel MP: Detection of early onset of hypophysitis by ^{18}F-FDG PET-CT in a patient with advanced stage melanoma treated with ipilimumab. Clin Nucl Med 2013;38:e182–e184.

36 Jeong SY, Lee SW, Lee HJ, Kang S, Seo JH, Chun KA, Cho IH, Won KS, Zeon SK, Ahn BC, Lee J: Incidental pituitary uptake on whole-body ^{18}F-FDG PET/CT: a multicentre study. Eur J Nucl Med Mol Imaging 2010;37:2334–2343.

37 Seok H, Lee EY, Choe EY, Yang WI, Kim JY, Shin DY Cho HJ, Kim TS, Yun MJ, Lee JD, Lee EJ, Lim SK, Rhee Y: Analysis of ^{18}F-fluorodeoxyglucose positron emission tomography findings in patients with pituitary lesions. Korean J Intern Med 2013;28:81–88.

38 Alzahrani AS, Farhat R, Al Arifi A, Al Kahtani N, Kanaan I, Abouzied M: The diagnostic value of fused positron emission tomography/computed tomography in the localization of adrenocorticotropin-secreting pituitary adenoma in Cushing's disease. Pituitary 2009;12:309–314.

39 Bergstrom M, Muhr C, Jossan S, Lilja A, Nyberg G, Langstrom B: Differentiation of pituitary adenoma and meningioma: visualization with positron emission tomography and [^{11}C]-L-deprenyl. Neurosurgery 1992;30:855–861.

40 Daemen BJ, Zwertbroek R, Elsinga PH, Paans AM, Doorenbos H, Vaalburg W: PET studies with L-[1-^{11}C]tyrosine, L-[methyl-^{11}C]methionine and ^{18}F-fluorodeoxyglucose in prolactinomas in relation to bromocriptine treatment. Eur J Nucl Med 1991;18:453–460.

41 Tang BN, Levivier M, Heureux M, Wikler D, Massager N, Devriendt D, David P, Dumarey N, Corvilain B, Goldman S: ^{11}C-methionine PET for the diagnosis and management of recurrent pituitary adenomas. Eur J Nucl Med Mol Imaging 2006;33: 169–178.

42 Muhr C, Bergstrom M, Lundberg PO, Hartman M, Bergstrom K, Pellettieri L, Langstrom B: Malignant prolactinoma with multiple intracranial metastases studied with positron emission tomography. Neurosurgery 1988;22:374–379.

Prof. Wouter W. de Herder, MD, PhD
Afdeling Endocrinologie, Erasmus Medisch Centrum
's Gravendijkwal 230
NL–3015 CE Rotterdam (The Netherlands)
E-Mail w.w.deherder@erasmusmc.nl

Buchfelder M, Guaraldi F (eds): Imaging in Endocrine Disorders.
Front Horm Res. Basel, Karger, 2016, vol 45, pp 142–151 (DOI: 10.1159/000442331)

Imaging of Neuroendocrine Tumors

Kjell Öberg · Anders Sundin

Department of Endocrine Oncology and Radiology, Uppsala University Hospital, Uppsala, Sweden

Abstract

Neuroendocrine tumors (NETs) comprise a heterogeneous group of malignancies with a very variable clinical expression and progression. They present unique properties that are important to consider for radiological and nuclear imaging, such as APUD-characteristics (amine precursor uptake and dearboxylation), as well as the expression of somatostatin receptors. The most common localizations are the lungs, gastrointestinal tract and pancreas. The only curative treatment is surgery, but more than 50% present metastatic disease at the time of diagnosis. The systemic treatment includes chemotherapy and targeted agents, as well as peptide receptor radiotherapy. The diagnosis and follow-up of these tumors necessitate a large number of different imaging methods, such as CT, MRI, US, SRS and PET. Ultrasonography offers the possibility to take guided biopsies from different lesions. Somatostatin receptor scintigraphy was developed in the 1990s and nowadays presents the standard of care for NETs in most countries. The procedure offers a total body examination and a better staging of the disease. However, it has been replaced in most centers by PET/CT with ^{68}Ga-DOTA-somatostatin analogues with a superior spatial resolution and faster imaging (one-stop procedure). Another tracer used for PET/CT is ^{18}FDG, particularly for high-grade tumors. Other more specific tracers are ^{18}F-L-DOPA, ^{11}C-L-DOPA and ^{11}C-5-hydroxytryptophan, which have demonstrated excellent imaging results. The new targeted agents present a challenge in the evaluation procedure of treatment and, therefore, new imaging techniques and an improvement of currently available techniques are mandatory.   © 2016 S. Karger AG, Basel

Neuroendocrine tumors (NETs) comprise a heterogenous group of tumors with a variable clinical expression and progression. They present unique properties that are important to consider for radiological and nuclear medicine imaging. NETs arise from cells of the neuroendocrine system spread out in the body with the capacity to take up precursor molecules and produce amine and peptides (amine precursor uptake and dearboxylation – APUD – characteristics). The primary tumor most frequently occurs in the lungs (bronchial carcinoids), intestine and pancreas, and less often in other parts of the diffuse neuroendocrine cell system, such as the autonomous nervous system (paraganglioma and pheochromocytoma) or the c-cells of the thyroid (medullary thyroid carcinomas) [1]. The clinical behavior, hormone production, imaging characteristics and therapeutic management of NETs largely depend on the location of the primary tumor and the degree of differentiation and dissemination, as well as the tumor's functional status and grade. The NET incidence is approximately 7.1/100,000/year, with a higher prevalence of >35/100,000/year [2].

A NET may be functioning, with symptoms related to hormonal overproduction, or nonfunctioning. The latter also produce hormones (i.e. chromogranin-A, pancreatic polypeptide, somatostatin), but usually at low quantities, or abnormal molecular forms of hormones that do not give pathognomonic symptoms, thus presenting with symptoms related only to tumor growth [1].

NETs had been previously classified, depending on the primary tumor localization, as foregut (lung, gastric, duodenal tumors), midgut (small intestinal and proximal colon tumors) and hindgut (distal colon and rectum tumors). This old classification has since been abandoned. A subsequent classification was based on the localization of the tumor plus eventual hormone production [e.g. pancreatic (p)NETs with gastrin production]. A new classification also emerged in 2010 when the WHO developed a new grading system according to which of three categories of tumor can be recognized: NET-G1 (Ki-67 <2%), NET-G2 (Ki-67 = 3–20%) and NET-G3 (Ki-67 >20%). This system, together with a TNM-staging system, has significantly improved the management of NETs [3]. Unfortunately, a new classification system has not yet been applied to lung NETs, which are still divided into typical and atypical bronchial carcinoids, and large-cell and small-cell NETs. The grading and the staging systems do not only play a role in the choice of treatment for NETs patients, but also in the decision of the most appropriate imaging techniques. This review will focus on gastrointestinal (e.g. intestinal and pancreatic) NETs.

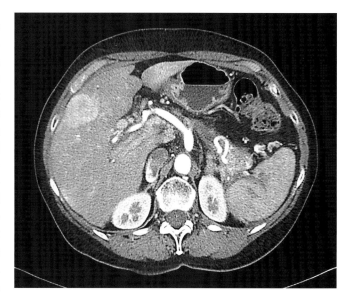

Fig. 1. Contrast-enhanced transversal CT examination in the late arterial phase (portal-venous inflow phase) showing a hypervascular contrast-enhancing (bright) liver metastasis, from a small bowel NET, in the ventral-lateral aspect of the virtually unenhanced (dark) liver.

Imaging Techniques

Computed Tomography

Computed tomography (CT) is the basic imaging modality for the initial radiological workup at presentation of the disease [4, 5], and the first choice for the monitoring of therapy outcomes in patients having undergone surgical resection with curative intent. In modern CT scanners a large number of detectors are arranged in parallel rows (multidetector CT, MDCT) and, by use of a rapidly rotating X-ray tube, hundreds of approximately 1-mm sections are produced per second. These thin-slice images are generally routinely reformatted to produce high spatial resolution 2D transversal, coronal and sagittal multiplanar reformatted volumes that are used for the actual image reading. Curved reformats may also be produced and can sometimes be helpful, for example to show the relation between a pNET and the pancreatic duct or the tumor and adjacent vessels. Since the scanning procedure is so fast, there are rarely problems with breathing artifacts and examination of the thorax and abdomen is usually completed during one breath hold. These fast MDCT scanners allow for the optimal use of intravenous contrast media, and organs of interest may be examined according to specific protocols depending on the application [4, 6, 7]. A power injector is a prerequisite to administer the contrast medium at a sufficiently high injection rate, typically 5 ml/s. An injector with two heads is preferable to inject the contrast medium followed by a saline chaser for a better use of the whole contrast medium volume. It is also advantageous to flush high-density contrast media from the brachiocephalic vein and superior vena cava that otherwise may produce image artifacts.

Early scanning after contrast medium injection start (CT angiography or early arterial phase) may occasionally be required as part of the preoperative imaging workup to display arterial anatomy. By postprocessing, 3D image volumes (maximum intensity projection) and volume-rendering images may be produced to facilitate this interpretation. Some 10–15 s later, in the late arterial phase (also called the portal-venous inflow phase), the small arterial branches are contrast enhanced and this is the best phase in which to diagnose hypervascular liver metastases (fig. 1) and pNETs (fig. 2). In the majority of patients the vascular anatomy is also sufficiently displayed in this contrast enhancement phase. As pointed out earlier, CT angiography is rarely needed and can instead be performed as a separate procedure in the few instances in which the vascular anatomy cannot be sufficiently visualized. In the venous (portal-venous) phase, approximately 60–90 s after injection start, the contrast medium has circulated through the capillary net-

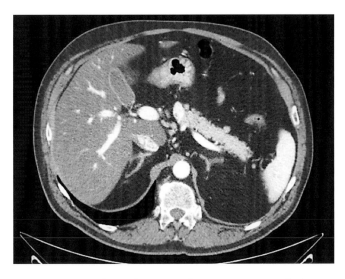 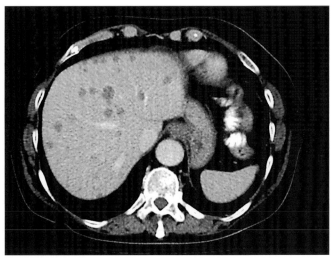

Fig. 2. Contrast-enhanced transversal CT examination in the late arterial phase (portal-venous inflow phase) showing a hypervascular contrast-enhancing (bright) pNET (insulinoma).

Fig. 3. Contrast-enhanced transversal CT examination in the venous (portal-venous) phase showing several hypovascular low-attenuating (dark) liver metastases, from a small bowel NET, in the contrast-enhanced high-attenuating (bright) liver.

work and reached the veins, including the portal vein, to enhance the normal liver parenchyma. In this phase, hypovascular liver metastases are best delineated (fig. 3). In order to achieve the correct timing of the scan start relative to the contrast medium injection, dedicated computer software in the MDCT scanner is routinely utilized, for so-called 'bolus tracking'. Repeated scanning over the liver is performed in the same bed position at a low-radiation dose, and the contrast medium arrival into the aorta may hence be monitored to initiate the scanning at the correct time point. Some prefer visual monitoring of the contrast medium arrival whereas others rely on a graphical presentation of the aortic attenuation that can be retrieved from a region of interest that is positioned in the abdominal aorta and becomes visible on the computer monitor.

Magnetic Resonance Imaging
Due to its excellent soft tissue contrast, magnetic resonance imaging (MRI) generally performs better than CT for the detection for many NET lesions, for example liver metastases and pNETs [8, 9]. MRI is also becoming more available, although it remains somewhat limited in some minor centers. The method is mainly used as a problem-solving tool when CT fails. As no radiation is used, MRI is also suitable for monitoring NET therapy in young patients in whom surveillance for many years is anticipated, in order to decrease the radiation dose. Whole-body MRI protocols cur-

rently include the neck-thorax and abdomen, and the modern high-field-strength magnets (3 T) allow for better spatial resolution and/or faster examinations as compared to MRI at 1.5 T. Nevertheless, small lung metastases may be missed and therefore CT rather than MRI should generally be used for examination of the thorax. Similarly to the iodine-based contrast media for CT, the intravenous gadolinium-based MRI contrast media are extracellular agents and the contrast-enhancement phases are the same. Repeated MRI acquisitions of the liver and pancreas, preferably in 3D, thus allows for MR angiography imaging to identify hypervascular lesions in the late arterial phase (portal-venous inflow phase), and hypovascular tumors and metastases in the venous contrast-enhancement phase [10, 11]. 'Bolus tracking' computer software is also used with MRI to achieve the correct timing of the examination start in relation to the contrast medium injection. By acquisition in 3D, the data for each respective contrast-enhancement phase may later be reconstructed in transversal, coronal and sagittal images. Today, diffusion-weighted imaging is increasingly being applied as a part of the MRI examination. By using signal sequences that reflect the water diffusion, which is restricted in tissues with high cellularity, tumors may be better depicted (fig. 4). For the locoregional assessment of pNETs, magnetic resonance cholangiopancreatography should always be included to visualize the relation of the tumor to that of the pancreatic duct and the main bile

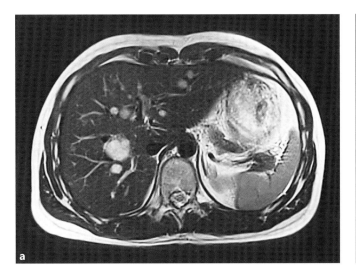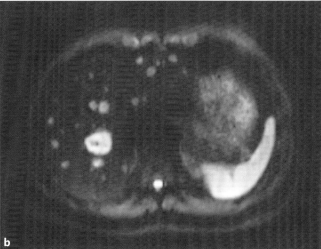

Fig. 4. a Transversal T2-weighted MRI image showing multiple high signaling (bright) liver metastases from a small bowel NET in the low signaling (dark) normal liver parenchyma. **b** Diffusion-weighted MRI at the same level showing an even better lesion to normal tissue contrast.

duct [12]. Liver-specific MRI-contrast media [13] are also available. Using gadolinium or manganese-based contrast media, the signal in the normal liver is increased and liver metastases appear hypointense (darker than the normal liver). The superparamagnetic iron oxide particles are instead taken up by the Kupffer cells of the reticuloendothelial system and decrease the MRI signal of the normal liver parenchyma, so that metastases appear hyperintense (brighter than the normal liver).

Ultrasonography

Ultrasonography (US) utilizes high-frequency (MHz) sound and, like MRI, does not expose the patient to radiation. With a high-frequency US transducer (10–12 MHz) superficial organs and tissues (i.e. thyroid and parathyroid glands) can be examined with high spatial resolution. Transducers with a lower frequency (3–7 MHz) have better penetration but lower spatial resolution and are therefore used to examine abdominal and retroperitoneal organs. In an increasing number of centers, US is performed also during intravenous contrast enhancement (CEUS) using microbubbles, making <0.5-cm liver metastases detectable [14, 15]. CEUS is also a very valuable alternative to MRI to assess previously equivocal liver lesions in the CT image. Dynamical CEUS examination over time allows for the characterization of liver lesions based on the in- and outflow pattern of the contrast medium [15]. US is also a convenient method to guide the needle for

tumor biopsies and is generally faster than biopsy with CT guidance. CT is, however, needed for biopsy of thoracic tumors since US cannot penetrate lung tissue and this drawback also restricts the possibilities of applying US for NET therapy monitoring outside of the abdomen. Moreover, for this application, examination of the whole abdomen and retroperitoneal space is time consuming and in patients with a large tumor load it may be difficult to achieve a reliable overview of the extent. For these reasons, US is not a standard technique for NET therapy monitoring. However, occasional NET patients harbor liver metastases that are difficult to depict by CT or may not be visualized at all. In these instances CEUS is very useful. The alternate use of CT and US can be considered for therapy monitoring of abdominal NETs in young patients to decrease the radiation dose when MRI is not available.

With perioperative or intraoperative US the transducer is placed directly on the organ surface. Intraoperative US facilitates the depiction of pNETs and liver metastases during surgery and should be used in connection with resection of a pNET, especially in patients with multiple endocrine neoplasia (MEN). Endoscopic US is the most sensitive technique for the diagnosis of pNETs [16–18], although its availability is still limited. Endoscopic US allows for biopsy using fine-needle aspiration for cytology or core biopsy for histopathological diagnosis [19, 20], details of which are described in the paper by Schmidt and Kuwert [this vol., pp. 37–45].

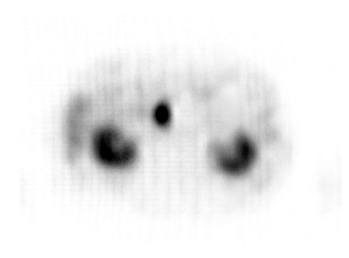

Fig. 5. SRS (Octreoscan™) SPECT transversal image showing high uptake (dark) in a retroperitoneal lymph node metastasis from a pNET.

Somatostatin Receptor Imaging

Somatostatin receptor (SSTR) imaging (SRI) can be accomplished by scintigraphy using a gamma camera or, more recently, by PET. SRI facilitates tumor staging and, compared to CT, additional lesions are generally diagnosed. It is also mandatory to perform SRI in order to obtain information on the tumor's SSTR status to assess the patient's eligibility for treatment with somatostatin analogues. SSTR scintigraphy (SRS) using ^{111}In-DTPA-octreotide (OctreoScan™) is currently the standard method for SRI [21]. According to many protocols, planar 2D whole-body images (anterior and posterior views) are acquired at 4 and 24 h, and 3D single photon computed emission tomography (SPECT) of the abdomen and/or thorax is performed 24 h after injection (fig. 5). Hybrid technology denotes that a CT scanner also incorporated is able to produce two sets of images (SPECT and CT) and, by means of computer software, a third volume image – SPECT/CT fusion – is subsequently produced whereby the anatomical CT information is superimposed onto the functional SPECT images. Previously, when only planar scintigraphic imaging was performed, examination at 48 h was sometimes employed when it was difficult to interpret the 24-hour examination because of high colonic radioactivity. Currently, when SPECT is regularly performed, and especially since the introduction of SPECT/CT, there is rarely a need for the delayed 48-hour examination, and some centers also refrain from performing the 4-hour examination. The sensitivity and specificity of SRS varies con-

siderably in different reports, which is likely explained by the variety of examination protocols being used in the different studies. A review comprising 35 centers and 1,200 patients showed a median 89% (range 67–100%) detection rate and a median 84% (range 57–93%) sensitivity [22]. Moreover, the sensitivity of SRS varies with the tumor type and its anatomical localization [23], and it is well known that the sensitivity for detecting small insulinomas is generally low.

Although SRS remains the mainstay for SRI, over the last few years the positron emitter ^{68}Ga (half-life 68 min) has been used to label somatostatin analogues for SRI by using PET/CT. The rationale for applying PET for SRI is the superior spatial resolution (approximately 0.5 cm) compared to SRS (approximately 1.5 cm). Furthermore, the tracer kinetics is much faster, allowing PET imaging 30–60 min after injection and the tissue contrast is better than that with SPECT.

Conveniently, ^{68}Ga is generator produced, similarly to ^{99m}Tc in the nuclear medicine department, and an in-house cyclotron is therefore not needed. The most commonly used preparations are ^{68}Ga-DOTATOC, ^{68}Ga-DOTATATE and ^{68}Ga-DOTANOC [24, 25] (fig. 6). Compared to octreotide, one amino acid has been exchanged in TOC and NOC, and to produce TATE (octreotate) a second amino acid has also been exchanged. This results in different affinities to the various SSTR subtypes for the three respective preparations. ^{68}Ga-DOTATOC, ^{68}Ga-DOTATATE and ^{68}Ga-DOTANOC all bind to SSTR2 and SSTR5. ^{68}Ga-DOTATATE is characterized by a very high affinity for SSTR2, whereas ^{68}Ga-DOTANOC also shows a good affinity for SSTR3. These differences between the three preparations seem, however, to be marginal in the daily clinical routine [26, 27]. PET with ^{68}Ga-labeled somatostatin analogues has been shown to be clearly superior to SRS [25] and CT/MRI [28–32] in several studies, although similar results were found in one study comparing ^{68}Ga-DOTANOC and SRS [33]. PET with ^{68}Ga-labeled somatostatin analogues has also been shown to be better than with ^{18}F-DOPA [34].

Positron Emission Tomography

Besides the ^{68}Ga-labeled somatostatin analogues, there are other PET tracers for NET imaging. ^{18}FDG accumulates only in high-grade NETs [34] and therefore ^{18}FDG-PET has not been considered useful for imaging in the majority of NET patients. In more recent studies, ^{18}FDG-PET has, however, been shown to supply additional information when used in combination with ^{68}Ga-DOTATATE [35] and SRS [36]. Also, ^{18}FDG positivity has been reported to predict

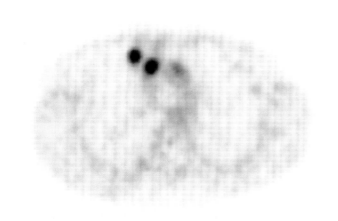

a

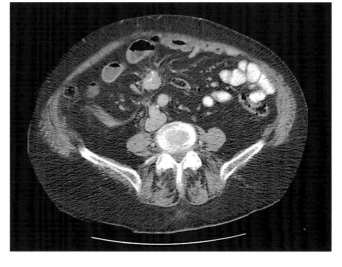

Fig. 7. Contrast-enhanced transversal CT examination in the venous (portal-venous) phase showing a centrally located mesenteric metastasis from a small bowel NET. The typical desmoplastic reaction in the surrounding fat and the multiple calcifications within the lesions can be seen.

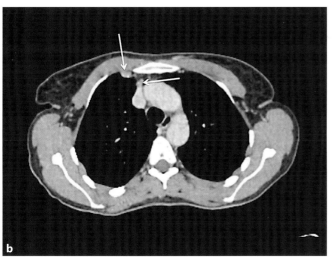

b

Fig. 6. 68Ga-DOTATOC PET/CT. **a** Transversal PET image showing high tracer uptake (dark) in two small thoracic lymph node metastases from a small bowel NET. **b** Corresponding CT showing the lymph nodes (arrows).

availability, PET with these tracers is usually applied as a problem-solving tool when other imaging techniques fail or show contradictory or equivocal results.

Neuroendocrine Tumor Characteristics, Presentation and Image Findings

Small Intestinal Neuroendocrine Tumors

Small intestinal NETs present a primary tumor that is usually located in the distal ileum, sometimes in the appendix or in the proximal colon. The primary tumors are usually small and sometimes multiple, whereas lymph nodes and liver metastases might be larger. The typical finding is the spoke-wheel formation in the abdomen around a mesenteric lymph node due to fibrotic changes in the mesentery (fig. 7). This phenomenon is usually seen in patients that present abdominal symptoms, such as pain and bowel obstruction. Initial symptoms from a small intestinal NET are usually diffuse and they are misdiagnosed for a medium of 4–5 years for diffuse conditions, such as menopause, irritable bowel syndrome and alcoholism, etc. When the tumor has metastasized to the liver the patient usually presents with a carcinoid syndrome, such as flushing or diarrhea, and sometimes right-sided heart fibrosis (carcinoid heart disease). This is seen in about 20–30% of patients at diagnosis.

early tumor progression and to be associated with a higher risk of death [27]. In a recent study on pNETs, 18FDG-PET was used to identify tumors with a higher malignant potential [37–39]. 18FDG is the recommended PET tracer in grade 3 NETs, and may also be considered in high grade 2 NETs.

NETs were formerly described as APUDomas and, based on these properties, specialized PET tracers for NET imaging have been developed. These are mainly the amine precursors 18F-L-DOPA, 11C-L-DOPA and 11C-5-hydroxytryptophan [40, 41]. These have shown excellent imaging results, surpassing those of SRS, but, because of their limited

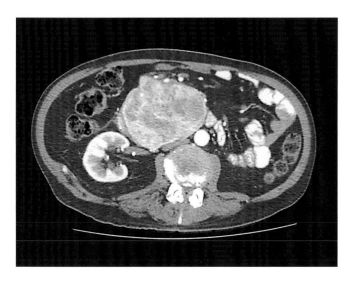

Fig. 8. Contrast-enhanced transversal CT examination in the late arterial phase (portal-venous inflow phase) showing a large hypervascular contrast-enhancing (bright) pNET (glucagonoma).

At the same time, biomarkers such as chromogranin-A and urine 5-HIAA (5-hydroxyindoleacctic acid) are elevated and are used for the diagnosis and follow-up of the patient. Carcinoids of the appendix measuring less than 2 cm are usually benign and are incidental follow-up findings in young individuals, but larger tumors (2 cm) can be metastatic and a right hemicolectomy is indicated. A particular type of tumor in this area is the so-called 'goblet cell' carcinoid which is a MANEC (mixed adenoneuroendocrine carcinoma) composed of neuroendocrine and exocrine components with mucus production. This type of tumor is usually more aggressive than the typical small intestinal and appendiceal NETs [3].

Pancreatic Neuroendocrine Tumors
The other large group of NETs are the pancreatic tumors, pNETs. They consist of functioning and nonfunctioning tumors. The functioning type are gastrin-producing tumors (Zollinger-Ellison syndrome), insulin-producing tumors (hypoglycemic syndrome), vasoactive intestinal peptide (VIP)-producing tumors (Verner-Morrison syndrome) and glucagonomas. These tumors present with symptoms related to their specific hormone production, which in a gastrinoma is usually gastrin. Two thirds of the gastrinomas are, however, not located in the pancreas but in the duodenum, and are sometimes related to MEN type 1 (MEN-1), which is an inherited disease with multiple tumors in different parts of the body. Insulin-producing tumors are the most common functioning pNETs, which usually present with low blood sugar and high insulin levels. The tumor is usually located in the pancreas. Patients with Verner-Morrison syndrome have high levels of VIP, with severe, watery diarrhea, hypokalemia, reduced glucose tolerance and flushing. These tumors can be located not only in the pancreas, but also as ganglioneuromas in the thorax and in the abdomen. Finally, glucagon-producing tumors (fig. 8) usually present with a typical skin rash (necrolytic migratory erythema) that is well recognized by dermatologists. They usually present high glucagon levels and also a propensity to develop thromboembolic complications and slight diabetes as well as anemia. This is related to the catabolic effect of glucagon. The primary tumor is located in the pancreas and is usually large because of the late detection [3].

The nonfunctioning tumors represent the largest group, constituting more than 60% of patients with pNETs. These tumors are usually larger and a correct diagnosis is made late, and sometimes misdiagnosis as adenocarcinomas of the pancreas occurs. The respective symptoms of these lesions are regular cancer symptoms such as gastrointestinal obstructions, bleeding, anemia and weight loss. In patients with MEN-1 there are typically a large number of small microtumors that might secret hormones, but nonfunctioning tumors are also seen. Other NETs in the gastroenteropancreatic area are duodenal carcinoids producing either gastrin or somatostatin.

Gastric Neuroendocrine Tumors
Gastric NETs include gastric carcinoids type 1, 2 and 3, and rare tumors such as ghrelinomas. Gastric carcinoid type 1 is often related to chronic atrophic gastritis with small multiple polyps and enterochromaffin-like cell hyperplasia. Type 2 is related to a gastrin-producing pancreatic or duodenal NET. Both of these conditions, type 1 and type 2, are driven by gastrin hypersecretion. The type 3 carcinoid is usually solitary, large and has metastatic potential. They are usually more malignant than type 1 and type 2 [3].

Colorectal Neuroendocrine Tumors
Colonic NETs (both large cell and small cell) are quite often high-grade tumors (NET-G3), whilst rectal NETs are usually small (<2 cm) and can be removed by endoscopy. The only curative treatment of NETs remains surgical resection. However, more than 50% of patients present metastatic disease at the time of diagnosis. Curative surgery is therefore rarely achieved, although nowadays debulking procedures

by resection, radiofrequency ablation and embolization are very common to reduce the tumor mass. The medical treatment includes chemotherapy, tumor-targeted agents and, in those patients with a high expression of somatostatin type 2 receptors, treatment with peptide receptor radiotherapy (PRRT; [177]lutetium, ^{90}Y-DOTATATE). The variable clinical presentation by NETs and treatment modalities necessitate a large number of imaging methods and careful follow-up of these tumors.

Imaging in Therapy Monitoring

CT is generally the imaging method employed for surveillance of the NET patient to detect recurrent disease after surgery and locally ablative procedures, and to monitor systemic therapy. US of the liver is valuable during treatment because patients occasionally develop metastases that are difficult to depict by CT and may sometimes not be seen at all. MRI is advantageous for liver and pancreatic imaging, and is preferred if available. MRI should also be considered, rather than CT, in the young patient when many years of follow-up are expected in order to decrease the radiation dose.

RECIST (Response Evaluation Criteria in Solid Tumors) is used for therapy monitoring in general oncology and relies on measurements of the longest tumor diameters at CT/MRI. RECIST 1.0 defines a maximum of 5 lesions per organ and 10 in total should be measured, the choice of which should be based on their size and on their suitability for repeated measurements. They are then considered representative for the whole tumor load [42]. The current criteria (RECIST 1.1) are easier to use and state that a maximum of 2 lesions per organ and 5 in total should be measured [42]. Disease regression or progression is evaluated by comparing the sum of the longest target lesion diameters in the follow-up examination to that of the baseline CT/MRI. In cases with a complete response all tumor lesions have disappeared, whilst in partial remission the sum of lesion diameters has decreased by 30% or more, and in progressive disease (PD) the sum of lesion diameters has increased by 20% or more and/or there are new lesions. The appearance of a new tumor is always equated with PD, irrespective of the outcome based on lesion measurements. The treatment results in stable disease when the criteria for partial remission or PD are not fulfilled (decrease less than 30%/increase less than 20%).

For several reasons, the RECIST criteria are less well suited to monitoring NET therapy. NETs are generally slow growing and the various available therapies, especially the new targeted agents, generally do not result in tumor shrinkage but rather a stabilization of the disease. In order to adapt RECIST to NETs in this respect, it has been proposed that stable disease at follow-up should be considered as a response in patients who were progressing before the start of NET therapy [43], a routine which has already been adapted in several centers.

Convincing results have not yet been reported on ^{68}Ga-DOTATOC PET/CT for the monitoring of PRRT with ^{177}Lu-DOTATATE [44], except that new tumor lesions were depicted earlier by PET/CT than with conventional radiological methods. A change in the tumor standard uptake value (SUV), from baseline to follow-up ^{68}Ga-DOTATOC PET/CT, does not reflect tumor response. One probably important factor is the amount of administered peptide that influences both the tumor and normal tissue uptake of the tracer. Another likely contributing factor is that SUV measurements do not seem to represent the tumor SSTR expression for lesions with an SUV higher than 20–25 [29]. Instead, the net uptake rate (K_i) calculated according to the Patlak method most probably provides a more accurate measure [27] of the tumor SSTR expression, but since this calculation relies on dynamic PET imaging during the 45 min after tracer injection it is difficult to apply in the daily imaging routine. Generally, a decrease in the total tumor SSTR expression represents treatment response, as seen in sequential scintigraphies during consecutive courses of PRRT with ^{177}Lu-DOTA-TATE, but this is true as long as it reflects a decrease in the total tumor volume. Thus, morphological proof of tumor regression according to RECIST is also needed because a decrease in the tumor SUV per se is not analogous to tumor regression. Although an infrequent phenomenon, de-differentiation of the NET may also occur with a loss of SSTR expression.

PET with [18]FDG, accumulating only in high- (G3) and intermediate-grade (high G2) NETs, is not suitable as a general tool for NET therapy monitoring although FDG positivity of the NET has been shown to be indicative of worse patient outcome. For PET with ^{18}F-DOPA and ^{11}C-5-HTP there are no – or only anecdotal – data on therapy monitoring and, moreover, these tracers are only available in a few centers. Thus, no nuclear medicine tracer for NET therapy monitoring is currently available for clinical application. Therefore, and in the light of the mentioned inherent problems with RECIST for NET therapy monitoring, future research in this area is urgently needed.

References

1 Gustafsson BI, Kidd M, Modlin IM: Neuroendocerine tumors of the diffuse neuroendocrine system. Curr Opin Oncol 2008;20:1–12.

2 Lawrence B, Gustafsson BI, Chan A, et al: The epidemiology of gastroenteropancreatic neuroendocrine tumors. Endocrinol Metabol Clin North Am 2011;40:1–18.

3 Salazar R, Wiedermann B, Ruszniewski P (eds): ENETS 2011 Concesus Guidlines for the Management of Patients with Digestive Neuroendocrine Tumors. Neuroendocrinology 2012;95:67–177.

4 Sundin A, Vullierme MP, Kaltsas G, Plöckinger U: ENETS Consensus Guidelines for the Standards of Care in Neuroendocrine Tumors: radiological examinations. Neuroendocrinology 2009;90:167–183.

5 Kumbasar B, Kamel IR, Tekes A, Eng J, Fishman EK, Wahl RL: Imaging of neuroendocrine tumors: accuracy of helical CT versus SRS. Abdom Imaging 2004;29:696–702.

6 Paulson EK, McDermott VG, Keogan MT, DeLong DM, Frederick MG, Nelson RC: Carcinoid metastases to the liver: role of triple-phase helical CT. Radiology 1998;206:143–150.

7 Fidler JL, Fletcher JG, Reading CC, Andrews JC, Thompson GB, Grant CS, Service FJ: Preoperative detection of pancreatic insulinomas on multiphasic helical CT. AJR Am J Roentgenol 2003;181:775–780.

8 Dromain C, de Baere T, Lumbroso J, Caillet H, Laplanche A, Boige V, Ducreux M, Duvillard P, Elias D, Schlumberger M, Sigal R, Baudin E: Detection of liver metastases from endocrine tumors: a prospective comparison of somatostatin receptor scintigraphy, computed tomography, and magnetic resonance imaging. J Clin Oncol 2005;23:70–78.

9 Seemann MD, Meisetschlaeger G, Gaa J, Rummeny EJ: Assessment of the extent of metastases of gastrointestinal carcinoid tumors using whole-body PET, CT, MRI, PET/CT and PET/MRI. Eur J Med Res 2006;11:58–65.

10 Dromain C, de Baere T, Baudin E, Galline J, Ducreux M, Boige V, Duvillard P, Laplanche A, Caillet H, Lasser P, Schlumberger M, Sigal R: MR imaging of hepatic metastases caused by neuroendocrine tumors: comparing four techniques. AJR Am J Roentgenol 2003;180:121–128.

11 Caramella C, Dromain C, De Baere T, Boulet B, Schlumberger M, Ducreux M, Baudin E: Endocrine pancreatic tumours: which are the most useful MRI sequences? Eur Radiol 2010;20:2618–2627.

12 Lopez Hänninen E, Amthauer H, Hosten N, Ricke J, Böhmig M, Langrehr J, Hintze R, Neuhaus P, Wiedenmann B, Rosewicz S, Felix R: Prospective evaluation of pancreatic tumors: accuracy of MR imaging with MR cholangiopancreatography and MR angiography. Radiology 2002;224:34–41.

13 Rockall AG, Planche K, Power N, Nowosinska E, Monson JP, Grossman AB, Reznek RH: Detection of neuroendocrine liver metastases with MnDPDP-enhanced MRI. Neuroendocrinology 2009;89:288–295.

14 Hoeffel C, Job L, Ladam-Marcus V, Vitry F, Cadiot G, Marcus C: Detection of hepatic metastases from carcinoid tumor: prospective evaluation of contrast-enhanced ultrasonography. Dig Dis Sci 2009;54:2040–2046.

15 Massironi S, Conte D, Sciola V, Pirola L, Paggi S, Fraquelli M, Ciafardini C, Spampatti MP, Peracchi M: Contrast-enhanced ultrasonography in evaluating hepatic metastases from neuroendocrine tumours. Dig Liver Dis 2010;42:635–641.

16 Ishikawa T, Itoh A, Kawashima H, Ohno E, Matsubara H, Itoh Y, Nakamura Y, Nakamura M, Miyahara R, Hayashi K, Ishigami M, Katano Y, Ohmiya N, Goto H, Hirooka Y: Usefulness of EUS combined with contrast-enhancement in the differential diagnosis of malignant versus benign and preoperative localization of pancreatic endocrine tumors. Gastrointest Endosc 2010;71:951–959.

17 Khashab MA, Yong E, Lennon AM, Shin EJ, Amateau S, Hruban RH, Olino K, Giday S, Fishman EK, Wolfgang CL, Edil BH, Makary M, Canto MI: EUS is still superior to multidetector computerized tomography for detection of pancreatic neuroendocrine tumors. Gastrointest Endosc 2011;73:691–696.

18 Versari A, Camellini L, Carlinfante G, Frasoldati A, Nicoli F, Grassi E, Gallo C, Giunta FP, Fraternali A, Salvo D, Asti M, Azzolini F, Iori V, Sassatelli R: Ga-68 DOTATOC PET, endoscopic ultrasonography, and multidetector CT in the diagnosis of duodenopancreatic neuroendocrine tumors: a single-centre retrospective study. Clin Nucl Med 2010;35:321–328.

19 Atiq M, Bhutani MS, Bektas M, Lee JE, Gong Y, Tamm EP, Shah CP, Ross WA, Yao J, Raju GS, Wang X, Lee JH: EUS-FNA for pancreatic neuroendocrine tumors: a tertiary cancer center experience. Dig Dis Sci 2012;57:791–800.

20 Pais SA, Al-Haddad M, Mohamadnejad M, Leblanc JK, Sherman S, McHenry L, DeWitt JM: EUS for pancreatic neuroendocrine tumors: a single-center, 11-year experience. Gastrointest Endosc 2010;71:1185–1193.

21 Kwekkeboom DJ, Krenning EP, Scheidhauer K, Lewington V, Lebtahi R, Grossman A, Vitek P, Sundin A, Plöckinger U: ENETS Consensus Guidelines for the Standards of Care in Neuroendocrine Tumors: somatostatin receptor imaging with ^{111}In-pentetreotide. Neuroendocrinology 2009;90:184–189.

22 Modlin IM, Kidd M, Latich I, Zikusoka MN, Shapiro MD: Current status of gastrointestinal carcinoids. Gastroenterology 2005;128:1717–1751.

23 de Herder WW, Kwekkeboom DJ, Valkema R, Feelders RA, van Aken MO, Lamberts SW, van der Lely AJ, Krenning EP: Neuroendocrine tumors and somatostatin: imaging techniques. J Endocrinol Invest 2005;28(suppl 11):132–136.

24 Ambrosini V, Campana D, Tomassetti P, Grassetto G, Rubello D, Fanti S: PET/CT with [68]Gallium-DOTA-peptides in NET: an overview. Eur J Radiol 2011;80:e116–e119.

25 Ambrosini V, Campana D, Tomassetti P, Fanti S: ^{68}Ga-labelled peptides for diagnosis of gastroenteropancreatic NET. Eur J Nucl Med Mol Imaging 2012;39(suppl 1):S52–S60.

26 Poeppel TD, Binse I, Petersenn S, Lahner H, Schott M, Antoch G, Brandau W, Bockisch A, Boy C: ^{68}Ga-DOTATOC versus ^{68}Ga-DOTATATE PET/CT in functional imaging of neuroendocrine tumors. J Nucl Med 2011;52:1864–1870.

27 Velikyan I, Sundin A, Sörensen J, Lubberink M, Sandström M, Garske-Román U, Lundqvist H, Granberg D, Eriksson B: Quantitative and qualitative intrapatient comparison of ^{68}Ga-DOTATOC and ^{68}Ga-DOTATATE: net uptake rate for accurate quantification. J Nucl Med 2014;55:204–210.

28 Gabriel M, Decristoforo C, Kendler D, Dobrozemsky G, Heute D, Uprimny C, Kovacs P, von Guggenberg E, Bale R, VirgoliniI J: ^{68}Ga-DOTA-Tyr[3]-octreotide PET in neuroendocrine tumors: comparison with somatostatin receptor scintigraphy and CT. J Nucl Med 2007;48:508–518.

29 Hofman MS, Kong G, Neels OC, Eu P, Hong E, Hicks RJ: High management impact of Ga-68 DOTATATE (GaTate) PET/CT for imaging neuroendocine and other somatostatin expressing tumours. J Med Imaging Radiat Oncol 2012;56:40–47.

30 Srirajaskanthan R, Kayani I, Quigley AM, Soh J, Caplin ME, Bomanji J: The role of ^{68}Ga-DOTATATE PET in patients with neuroendocrine tumors and negative or equivocal findings on ^{111}In-DTPA-octreotide scintigraphy. J Nucl Med 2010;51:875–882.

31 Ambrosini V, Campana D, Bodei L, Nanni C, Castellucci P, Allegri V, Montini GC, Tomassetti P, Paganelli G, Fanti S: ^{68}Ga-DOTANOC PET/CT clinical impact in patients with neuroendocrine tumors. J Nucl Med 2010;51:669–673.

32 Kumar R, Sharma P, Garg P, Karunanithi S, Naswa N, Sharma R, Thulkar S, Lata S, Malhotra A: Role of ^{68}Ga-DOTATOC PET-CT in the diagnosis and staging of pancreatic neuroendocrine tumours. Eur Radiol 2011;21:2408–2416.

33 Naswa N, Sharma P, Kumar A, Nazar AH, Kumar R, Chumber S, Bal C: Gallium-68-DOTA-NOC PET/CT of patients with gastroenteropancreatic neuroendocrine tumors: a prospective single-center study. AJR Am J Roentgenol 2011;197:1221–1228.

34 Ambrosini V, Tomassetti P, Castellucci P, Campana D, Montini G, Rubello D, Nanni C, Rizzello A, Franchi R, Fanti S: Comparison between ^{68}Ga-DOTA-NOC and ^{18}F-DOPA PET for the detection of gastro-entero-pancreatic and lung neuro-endocrine tumors. Eur J Nucl Med Mol Imaging 2008;35:1431–1438.

35 Krausz Y, Freedman N, Rubinstein R, Lavie E, Orevi M, Tshori S, Salmon A, Glaser B, Chisin R, Mishani E, J Gross D: ^{68}Ga-DOTA-NOC PET/CT imaging of neuroendocrine tumors: comparison with ^{111}In-DTPA-octreotide (OctreoScan®). Mol Imaging Biol 2011;13:583–593.

36 Haug A, Auernhammer CJ, Wängler B, Tiling R, Schmidt G, Göke B, Bartenstein P, Pöpperl G: Intraindividual comparison of ^{68}Ga-DOTA-TATE and ^{18}F-DOPA PET in patients with well-differentiated metastatic neuroendocrine tumours. Eur J Nucl Med MolImaging 2009;36:765–770.

37 Kayani I, Conry BG, Groves AM, Win T, Dickson J, Caplin M, Bomanji JB: A comparison of ^{68}Ga-DOTATATE and ^{18}F-FDG PET/CT in pulmonary neuroendocrine tumors. J Nucl Med 2009;50: 1927–1932.

38 Binderup T, Knigge U, Loft A, Mortensen J, Pfeifer A, Federspiel B, Hansen CP, Højgaard L, Kjaer A: Functional imaging of neuroendocrine tumors: a head-to-head comparison of somatostatin receptor scintigraphy, ^{123}I-MIBG scintigraphy, and ^{18}F-FDG PET. J Nucl Med 2010;51:704–712.

39 Binderup T, Knigge U, Loft A, Federspiel B, Kjaer A: ^{18}F-fluorodeoxyglucose positron emission tomography predicts survival of patients with neuroendocrine tumors. Clin Cancer Res 2010;16: 978–985.

40 Orlefors H, Sundin A, Garske U, Juhlin C, Oberg K, Skogseid B, Langstrom B, Bergstrom M, Eriksson B: Whole-body ^{11}C-5-hydroxytryptophan positron emission tomography as a universal imaging technique for neuroendocrine tumors: comparison with somatostatin receptor scintigraphy and computed tomography. J Clin Endocrinol Metab 2005;90:3392–3400.

41 Koopmans KP, Neels OC, Kema IP, Elsinga PH, Sluiter WJ, Vanghillewe K, Brouwers AH, Jager PL, de Vries EG: Improved staging of patients with carcinoid and islet cell tumors with ^{18}F-dihydroxy-phenyl-alanine and ^{11}C-5-hydroxy-tryptophan positron emission tomography. J Clin Oncol 2008;26:1489–1495.

42 Eisenhauer EA, Therasse P, Bogaerts Schwartz LH, Sargent D, Ford R, Dancey J, Arbuck S, Gwyther S, Mooney M, Rubinstein L, Shankar L, Dodd L, Kaplan R, Lacombe D, Verweij J: New response evaluation criteria in solid tumours: revised RECIST guideline (version 1.1). Eur J Cancer 2009; 45:228–247.

43 Sundin A, Rockall A: Therapeutic monitoring of gastroenteropancreatic neuroendocrine tumors: the challenges ahead. Neuroendocrinology 2012; 96:261–271.

44 Haug AR, Auernhammer CJ, Wangler B, Schmidt GP, Uebleis C, Göke B, Cumming P, Bartenstein P, Tiling R, Hacker M: ^{68}Ga-DOTATATE PET/CT for the early prediction of response to somatostatin receptor-mediated radionuclide therapy in patients with well-differentiated neuroendocrine tumours. J Nucl Biol Med 2010;51:1349–1356.

Kjell Öberg, MD
Sektionen för Endokrin Onkologi
Akademiska Sjukhuset
Ingång 40, våning 5
SE–751 85 Uppsala (Sweden)
E-Mail kjell.oberg@medsci.uu.se

Author Index

Subject Index